Entrustable Professional Activities and Entrustment Decision-Making in Health Professions Education

Edited by
Olle ten Cate, Vanessa C. Burch, H. Carrie Chen, Fremen Chihchen Chou and Marije P. Hennus

]u[

ubiquity press
London

Published by
Ubiquity Press Ltd.
6 Osborn Street, Unit 3N
London E1 6TD
www.ubiquitypress.com

First published 2024

Cover design by Britta Zwarg
Cover image credits: Joesboy / iStock / Getty Images Plus (young Herring Gull);
GlobalP / iStock / Getty Images Plus (old Herring Gull)

Print and digital versions typeset by Siliconchips Services Ltd.

ISBN (Paperback): 978-1-914481-60-4
ISBN (PDF): 978-1-914481-61-1
ISBN (EPUB): 978-1-914481-62-8
ISBN (Mobi): 978-1-914481-63-5

DOI: https://doi.org/10.5334/bdc

The full text of this book has been peer-reviewed to ensure high academic standards.
For full review policies, see https://www.ubiquitypress.com/

Suggested citation:
ten Cate O, Burch VC, Chen HC, Chou FC, Hennus MP. (Eds). 2024. *Entrustable Professional Activities and Entrustment Decision-Making in Health Professions Education.* London: Ubiquity Press. DOI: https://doi.org/10.5334/bdc. License: CC BY 4.0

To read the free, open access version of this book online, visit https://doi.org/10.5334/bdc or scan this QR code with your mobile device:

The image on the book cover metaphorically symbolizes a combination of supportive supervision, initial autonomy, safety and trust.

Contents

Foreword

When I was approached about writing the foreword for a comprehensive work about entrustable professional activities (EPAs) and entrustment decision-making, I was both honored and excited that such a resource would be available.

My introduction to the primary editor, Dr. Olle ten Cate, many years ago, did not come in the usual way, such as through a colleague or at a professional meeting. Competency-based education (CBE) ignited our ongoing collaboration and long-lasting friendship. I distinctly remember discussing his seminal 2007 article introducing the concept of EPAs with several colleagues.[a] It was during that conversation that I realized EPAs were the critical missing piece that would allow us to envision the way forward in implementing CBE for all health professions.

Dr. ten Cate has assembled a group of international authors, who have been instrumental in advancing the widespread adoption of EPAs, to tell this story. The book is a masterful work, whereby authors invite readers into their 'think tank,' deepening our understanding of familiar concepts, inviting us to connect ideas in new ways, and challenging us to imagine a future where a key barometer of CBE quality is patient outcomes. Beginning with the abstract of Chapter 2, I was hooked by the proposed alignment of the conceptual framework of canonical, contextual, and personalized competence, with the 'know, do, and be' that embody the professional identity formation of the physician.

While one of the great contributions of EPAs has been enabling more robust assessment of trainees, the authors remind us that this is but one aspect of their broader impact of defining a profession, and unifying the goals of education, training, and practice. The term 'EPAs fit for purpose,' by profession and specialty, provides the perfect description of the unique characteristic of EPAs to capture both the 'whole' of a profession through its key professional activities with a concurrent focus on the competencies and milestones or 'sum of its parts' that bring it all to life.

I 'felt' the gravitas of making entrustment decisions when reading about trust and entrustment. These complex concepts are delivered in ways that lead to a clear understanding of their

---

[a] ten Cate O, Scheele F. Competency-based postgraduate training: can we bridge the gap between theory and clinical practice? *Acad Med.* 2007;82(6):542–547. DOI: https://doi.org/10.1097/ACM.0b013e31805559c7

foundational role across the education, training, and practice continuum. Attention is also given to the pragmatic steps needed when introducing EPAs into diverse clinical learning environments, such as incorporating workplace-based assessments, and maximizing the contributions of clinical competency committees. Whether you are just beginning the journey toward incorporating EPAs into your program or well on your way to achieving this goal, this resource will expand the depth of your understanding and your ability to implement CBME in your learning environment.

Circling back to my 2007 epiphany, I initially spent time learning about EPAs and how they might align with competencies and milestones to improve assessment. In 2011, I accepted a position in our specialty that enabled me to work with pediatrics program directors and other leaders to develop both core and subspecialty EPAs for our profession. If only I had the wealth of knowledge in this book back then! I have had the good fortune to know and work with Dr. ten Cate and many of the authors who contributed to this 'must-read' book. In the diffusion of innovation, they are the early adopters, those who take on the burden of defining a way forward to reach the light they see on the horizon. Thank you all for sharing your vision and the wisdom you have gathered as you work to realize it.

Carol Carraccio, MD, MA
Former vice-president for competency-based medical education at the
American Board of Pediatrics

Preface

Entrustable professional activities (EPAs) and entrustment decision-making are concepts that have found their way into the literature and practice of health professions education in the past decades. Intimately linked to competency-based education, EPAs and entrustment decision-making are being adopted, or explored and considered, in many schools and programs around the world. The concepts continue to influence innovations in curricula and assessment in the workplace and will likely continue to do so in the foreseeable future.

While definable in a few sentences, EPAs and entrustment decision-making have implications that are potentially more profound than they might seem at first sight. Their use can be far-reaching, complex, and sometimes confusing. How EPAs are conceptualized, how they relate to competencies and competency frameworks, what role they play in curriculum development and assessment, and how clinical supervision of trainees should be modulated after decisions of entrustment with clinical tasks, are not easily or similarly understood across different programs, disciplines, professions, and settings. The rapidly growing literature, now reaching over 1,100 references in PubMed, includes many proposed EPAs but also explanations, guidelines, and studies, as well as conceptualizations and concerns about misinterpretations. As early as 2013, a colleague educator sighed that 'EPAs are now becoming a *label de jour* for almost everything,' pointing at their popularity but also at a lack of good understanding.

There has not been a standard comprehensive reference that provides an overview of the state of the art around EPAs and entrustment decision-making that can serve to inform curriculum developers and educators. Our hope with this book is to fill that gap.

To support educators in understanding and working with EPAs, there are many faculty development workshops and initiatives offered at institutional and national levels. One international initiative that began in 2018 is a multiday course, *Ins and Outs of Entrustable Professional Activities*, now delivered online several times per year and with satellite courses in different languages. Many of the contributors to the current volume have collaborated in this course as faculty members, and all have actively contributed to the literature in this area of research and development.

The purpose of the book is to provide a comprehensive overview of relevant information about EPAs and entrustment decision-making. It is meant to be a state-of-the-art reference work about conceptual and theoretical topics related to EPAs and entrustment decision-making, a field that is very dynamic and includes ongoing as-yet-to-be-settled discourses. It is also meant to serve as a practical handbook to assist educators and institutions in the development and implementation of curricula and assessment procedures built upon a foundation of EPAs. It offers a reference for faculty development courses and is available via open access for any interested reader. However, it is not a prescriptive cookbook. Many recommendations are provided but adaptation to local context and culture is key.

We are aware of the dynamic nature of health professions education. There is no doubt that the decade ahead will present new innovations that will supersede some of the insights and guidelines in this volume. That is a sign of a healthy, living domain of scholarship, continuously seeking to improve its value. We hope the book will actually stimulate such development.

We are highly indebted to a large number of authors and reviewers (internal and external) for their dedication and thoughtful contributions to this volume. Our process and design have made it possible to present every chapter as a standalone, peer-reviewed, open publication, easily accessible by a wide audience. However, this also makes it unavoidable to have some overlap among chapters on similar topics, that, while aligned in their key messages, may be framed or described using different wording. Writing this book has stimulated deep discussions among the author teams within chapters and across chapters. In sharpening constructs and definitions, occasionally new ideas have surfaced that will likely lead to additions to the literature in the near future. We added a glossary of definitions that can be used as a starting point for development, implementation, and, sometimes, debate. At times, the writing process led to slightly varying definitions and interpretations across chapters and author teams. This reflects the beauty of a domain that is continuously in development and stimulates ongoing academic debate. It resembles the scholarly atmosphere that can also be found among the International Competency-Based Health Professions Educators Collaborative (previously called ICBME), of which many authors are members.

EPAs represent first and foremost a foundation for achieving meaningful education in the health professions that stimulates the development of professional skills, professional identity, and professional responsibilities through supportive and tailored supervision. This supervision is characterized by mutual trust, which we hope will become a guiding principle among the diversity of trainees, teachers, and professionals, leading to safe and high-quality patient care.

Olle ten Cate
Vanessa C. Burch
H. Carrie Chen
Fremen Chihchen Chou
Marije P. Hennus

Author biographies

Jonathan M. Amiel, MD, is professor of psychiatry at Columbia University Irving Medical Center, New York, USA. He led the American pilot of the core EPAs for entering residency on behalf of the Association of American Medical Colleges (AAMC) and served on the working group for the foundational competencies for undergraduate medical education, also for the AAMC. ORCID: https://orcid.org/0000-0003-4027-6397

Harold G.J. Bok, DVM, PhD, is professor and associate dean of education at the Faculty of Veterinary Medicine, Utrecht University, the Netherlands. He chairs the research group 'Educational Scholarship in Veterinary Medicine.' He has been involved in numerous (inter)national projects, studies, and publications relating to assessment, competency-based education, EPAs, and workplace-based learning. ORCID: https://orcid.org/0000-0002-6435-0240

Josephine Boland, EdD, is a medical education consultant specializing in the development and implementation of competency-based medical education using EPAs. She has supported EPA development at a national level for postgraduate specialist training programs in Ireland—in general practice, anaesthesia, psychiatry, and radiology and for the new curriculum framework for the internship. ORCID: https://orcid.org/0000-0001-9580-317X

Christy K. Boscardin PhD, is professor and director of student assessment at the University of California, San Francisco, School of Medicine, California, USA. She is a medical education researcher with focus on assessment, measurement, validity and workplace assessments. ORCID: https://orcid.org/0000-0002-9070-8859

Ryan Brydges, PhD, is an associate professor in the Department of Medicine at the University of Toronto and holds the Professorship in Technology-Enabled Education at St. Michael's Hospital, Unity Health Toronto, Toronto, Ontario, Canada. He studies how clinicians learn to learn using technology, and how to develop defensible assessments in simulation-based and workplace-based settings. ORCID: https://orcid.org/0000-0001-5203-7049

Vanessa C. Burch, MD, PhD, is executive director of education and assessment, Colleges of Medicine of South Africa, and honorary professor of medicine, University of Cape Town, South Africa. She teaches and publishes on EPAs and WBA and is engaged in designing and implementing EPAs and WBA for postgraduate education in South Africa. ORCID: https://orcid.org/0000-0001-7304-4424

H. Carrie Chen, MD, PhD, is pediatrician, professor of health systems science, and associate dean for medical education research and scholarship, Kaiser Permanente Bernard J. Tyson School of Medicine, Pasadena, California, USA. She has been involved in numerous local and national EPA projects for various professions in the USA and other countries, and has published on EPAs. ORCID: https://orcid.org/0000-0003-1663-1598

Chien-Yu Jonathan Chen, MD, PhD, is the director and associate professor of education and humanities in medicine and vice academic dean at Taipei Medical University, Taipei, Taiwan. He leads the CBME Committee at the Taiwan Society of Anesthesiologists and the ACGME Taiwan Hub. ORCID: https://orcid.org/0000-0001-5895-9941

Fremen Chihchen Chou, MD, PhD, is assistant professor of medical education at China Medical University, School of Medicine and Center for Faculty Development, China Medical University Hospital, Taichung, Taiwan. He leads Taiwan's emergency medicine CBME reform, serves as ACGME regional hub leader, is an inaugural executive member of the International CBME Collaborators, and faculty member of the Ins and Outs of EPAs, an international course. ORCID: https://orcid.org/0000-0002-7932-5056

J. Damon Dagnone, MD, MSc, MMEd, is an associate professor of emergency medicine at Queen's University, Canada, and the director of standards and accreditation at the Royal College of Physicians and Surgeons of Canada. In this role, he oversees the evolution of the Competence by Design project across 68 postgraduate specialty disciplines at a national level. ORCID: https://orcid.org/0000-0001-6963-7948

Jacqueline de Graaf, MD, PhD, is professor of professional performance in PGME at Radboud University Medical Center, Nijmegen, the Netherlands, and director of PGME. As chair of the Dutch Council of Internal Medicine she introduced EPAs country-wide. She contributed and participated in several national and international projects that supported the development of EPAs in all PGME specialties. ORCID: https://orcid.org/0000-0001-7662-9284

Timo de Raad, MSc, is a physician assistant and educator at Wilhelmina Children's Hospital, University Medical Center Utrecht, the Netherlands. He is a medical education researcher, specializing in critical care, resuscitation education, simulation, and interprofessional EPA development and assessment. ORCID: https://orcid.org/0000-0002-8844-3273

Abigail T. Elmes-Patel, PharmD, MHPE, is a visiting clinical assistant professor at the University of Illinois Chicago College of Pharmacy, Chicago, Illinois, USA. She studies the quality assessment of EPAs in pharmacy education and stakeholder perspectives of the implementation of EPA-based frameworks within pharmacy experiential curricula in the United States. ORCID: https://orcid.org/0000-0002-0964-2574

Robert Englander, MD, MPH, is an adjunct professor of medical education at the University of Illinois College of Medicine, Chicago, Illinois, USA. He led the US Undergraduate Medical Education EPA development. He has also been engaged in many projects across specialties and health professions to develop, implement, and study EPAs. ORCID: https://orcid.org/0000-0001-5431-1320

Jean A. Fitzpatrick, PT, PhD, MHS, is a physical therapist and the director of the programs in PT, vice chair of rehabilitative and regenerative medicine, and assistant dean in the Vagelos College of Physicians and Surgeons at Columbia University, New York, USA. She has led EPA efforts for entrance into practice and continuing professional development. ORCID: https://orcid.org/0000-0003-1511-9170

Siobhan Fitzpatrick, BA, MA, is a technical officer for the World Health Organization, Geneva, Switzerland. She advises on policies, norms and standards to strengthen health workforce competency-based education. She led the development of the WHO Global competency and outcomes frameworks for universal health coverage (2022) and the essential public health functions (2024). ORCID: https://orcid.org/0000-0002-8414-8242

Sonia Frick, MD, is an internist and intensivist at Limmattalspital, Switzerland. She leads the workgroup for the development of EPAs for internal medicine in Switzerland and is a member of the Swiss Advisory Group for EPAs, helping numerous specialties creating EPAs. ORCID: https://orcid.org/0000-0002-8955-8451

Brian C. Gin, MD, PhD, is a pediatric hospitalist and associate professor at the University of California, San Francisco, California, USA. As a learner in the UCSF-UMCU doctoral program in health professions education, he is examining the intersection between trainee and supervisor viewpoints of entrustment, using artificial intelligence to develop methodologies for unpacking trust. ORCID: https://orcid.org/0000-0001-7655-3750

Andrew K. Hall, MD, MMEd, is vice-chair education and associate professor in the Department of Emergency Medicine, University of Ottawa, and clinician educator at the Royal College of Physicians and Surgeons of Canada, both in Ottawa, Ontario, Canada. He chairs the Competence By Design program evaluation operations team for the Royal College and is an international CBME collaborator. ORCID: https://orcid.org/0000-0003-1227-5397

Stanley J. Hamstra, PhD, is professor and vice-chair for clinical teaching, Department of Surgery, University of Toronto, and senior scientist, Holland Bone and Joint Program, Sunnybrook Research Institute, Toronto, Canada. His research focuses on learner assessment in GME, with a critical eye to how and where EPAs should be implemented in CBME. ORCID: https://orcid.org/0000-0002-0680-366X

Karen E. Hauer, MD, PhD, is vice dean for education and professor of medicine at University of California, San Francisco (UCSF), California, USA. She designed the program of assessment at UCSF School of Medicine and has published research on trust and entrustment, learner assessment, clinical competency committees, EPAs, grading, and equity in assessment. ORCID: https://orcid.org/0000-0002-8812-4045

Marije P. Hennus, MD, PhD, MClinEd, is a pediatric intensivist and associate professor of teaching at Wilhelmina Children's Hospital, University Medical Center Utrecht, the Netherlands. She was the national lead in developing and implementing EPAs for Dutch PICU fellows (2020) and has since been involved in numerous projects, studies, and publications relating to EPAs. ORCID: https://orcid.org/0000-0003-1508-0456

Eric S. Holmboe, MD, is a general internist and health services researcher who is currently working at Intealth in Philadelphia PA. He has been involved in developing competency Milestones, programs of assessment, and approaches to faculty development in work-based assessment, with a special focus on their intersection with health care outcomes. ORCID: https://orcid.org/0000-0003-0108-6021

Ylva Holzhausen, MSc, PhD, is the team lead of the 'Educational Research' division at the Dieter Scheffner Center for Medical Education and Educational Research, Charité-Universitätsmedizin Berlin, Germany. She is involved in the development and implementation of EPAs in undergraduate medical education. ORCID: https://orcid.org/0000-0001-8710-8257

Jennie B. Jarrett, PharmD, MMedEd, PhD, is a research assistant professor at the University of Illinois Chicago College of Pharmacy, Chicago, Illinois, USA. She has led development of EPA assessment tools and studied implementation of an EPA-based framework within the longitudinal, pharmacy experiential curricula in the United States. ORCID: https://orcid.org/0000-0003-0583-308X

Gersten Jonker, MD, PhD, is an anesthesiologist and director of anesthesiology residency training at University Medical Center Utrecht, the Netherlands. He is a medical education researcher and has been involved in EPA development and implementation projects in anesthesiology at local, regional, and national levels. ORCID: https://orcid.org/0000-0001-6819-9990

Natasha Khursigara-Slattery, MD, MEHP, is associate program director of the Mid-West Intern Network at University Hospital Limerick, Ireland. She is the national lead for the professionalism and professional identity pillar of the EPA-based national Irish intern curriculum and a lead of the framework for a new training body overseeing the governance of Intern training in Ireland. ORCID: https://orcid.org/0009-0000-6202-8752

Benjamin Kinnear, MD, Med, is an associate professor of internal medicine and pediatrics in the Division of Hospital Medicine at University of Cincinnati Medical Center and Cincinnati Children's Hospital Medical Center, and is associate program director for the med-peds and internal medicine residency programs. He has published work related to programmatic assessment, entrustment decision-making, competency committees, and validity arguments. ORCID: https://orcid.org/0000-0003-0052-4130

Jennifer Klasen, PD, MD, PhD, MME, is a surgical consultant at Clarunis, University Digestive Healthcare Center Basel, University Hospital Basel and St. Clara Hospital, Switzerland. She is a medical education researcher and has been involved as an adviser for EPA development and implementation projects in general and specialized surgery at local and national levels. ORCID: https://orcid.org/0000-0001-8355-1606

Roberta I. Ladenheim, MD, MHPE, is an internist with a master's in health professions education, currently directing the Postgraduate Department at Universidad Hospital Italiano de Buenos Aires. With vast experience in faculty development, she has contributed to national-level competency framework development and advocates for implementing competency-based education and EPAs in her region. ORCID: https://orcid.org/0000-0002-0088-6951

Machelle Linsenmeyer, EdD, FNAOME, is assistant vice president for institutional effectiveness and academic resources at West Virginia School of Osteopathic Medicine, Lewisburg, West Virginia, USA. She has been involved in EPA development since 2014, serving most recently (since 2018) as chair of the American Association of Colleges of Osteopathic Medicine EPA Steering Committee. ORCID: https://orcid.org/0000-0002-5796-8843

María José López, MSc, is associate professor in the Pedagogical Advising Department, School of Medical Sciences, National University of Cuyo, Argentina, director of the postgraduate program in education on health sciences and researcher in medical education. She led the designs of undergraduate and residency EPA-curricula, and the development of a national EPA framework for gynecology and obstetrics. ORCID: https://orcid.org/0000-0001-7250-9189

Adrian P. Marty, MD, MME, is a senior attending anesthesiologist and program director at the Balgrist University Hospital, Zurich, Switzerland. As a change agent, his main focus is on the meaningful implementation of EPAs and CBE for example through mobile technology. He is involved in national and international research projects on EPAs and CBE. ORCID: https://orcid.org/0000-0003-3452-9730

Eric G. Meyer, MD, PhD, is professor of psychiatry and military and emergency medicine at the Uniformed Services University of the Health Sciences, Bethesda, Maryland, USA. He has led local EPA projects related to military medicine and has published on EPAs with a focus in undergraduate medical education. ORCID: https://orcid.org/0000-0002-0538-4344

Daniel Nel, MD, MMEd, is a general surgeon and program director in the Division of General Surgery at the University of Cape Town, South Africa. He has an interest in surgical education and was involved in the national steering committee tasked with implementing WBA using EPAs across postgraduate training in South Africa. ORCID: https://orcid.org/0000-0002-3265-1049

Yoon Soo Park, PhD, is the Ilene B. Harris professor and head of the Department of Medical Education at the University of Illinois College of Medicine in Chicago, Illinois, USA. He has contributed to assessment validity and measurement studies in CBME. ORCID: https://orcid.org/0000-0001-8583-4335

Harm Peters, MD, PhD, is professor of nephrology and medical education at the Charité – Universitätsmedizin Berlin, where he directs the Scheffner Centre for Medical Education and Educational Research. He has been involved in local, national, and international EPA projects and has published on EPAs. ORCID: https://orcid.org/0000-0003-1441-7512

Severin Pinilla, MD, MEd, PhD, is a psychiatrist and medical education researcher at the University of Bern. He leads the EPA development group for psychiatry in Switzerland and is a member of the Swiss Institute for Medical Education advisory group for EPAs in graduate medical education. ORCID: https://orcid.org/0000-0002-0797-2043

Inge A. Pool, PhD, is an educationalist and manager of health professions education at the Isala Academy, Isala Hospital, Zwolle, the Netherlands. She is a health professions education researcher and was involved in implementing EPAs in postgraduate nursing education in the Netherlands. ORCID: https://orcid.org/0000-0002-3622-1273

Martin V. Pusic, MD, PhD, is an associate professor of pediatrics and emergency medicine at Harvard Medical School, Boston, Massachusetts, USA. He is also director of the Research and Education Foundation at the American Board of Medical Specialties. He is coinvestigator on an AMA-funded research project investigating the advantages and barriers to competency-based time variable training in graduate medical education. ORCID: https://orcid.org/0000-0001-5236-6598

Michael S. Ryan, MD, MEHP, is professor of pediatrics and associate dean for assessment, evaluation, and scholarship at the University of Virginia, Charlottesville, Virginia, USA. He was a steering committee and site PI for the AAMC's Core EPA pilot for its duration has published extensively on EPAs in medical school programs. ORCID: https://orcid.org/0000-0003-3266-9289

Daniel J. Schumacher, MD, PhD, MEd, is a tenured professor of pediatrics at Cincinnati Children's Hospital Medical Center, Ohio, USA. He has led the study of EPAs for general pediatrics nationally within the United States and has also studied entrustment decision-making of competency committees. ORCID: https://orcid.org/0000-0001-5507-8452

Alan Schwartz, PhD, JD, is the Michael Reese endowed professor of medical education and research professor of pediatrics at the University of Illinois Chicago, Illinois, USA. He directs the Association of Pediatric Program Directors Longitudinal Educational Assessment Research Network, which has coordinated national studies of the pediatrics EPAs in the United States. ORCID: https://orcid.org/0000-0003-3809-6637

Robert Sternszus, MDCM, MA(Ed), is associate professor in the Department of Pediatrics and the Institute of Health Sciences Education, Faculty of Medicine and Health Sciences, McGill University, Canada. He has been involved in scholarship on professional identity formation and its links to competence and CBME. ORCID: https://orcid.org/0000-0001-8115-5490

David R. Taylor, MD, MHPE, is associate professor of medicine at Queen's University, Canada. He has been involved in developing and implementing EPAs in undergraduate and postgraduate medical education as well as in other health professions. ORCID: https://orcid.org/0000-0001-9762-7878

Olle ten Cate, PhD, is an emeritus professor of medical education at Utrecht University, the Netherlands, and a professor at the University of California, San Francisco, California, USA. Since 2005 he has been involved in numerous projects, studies, and publications related to EPAs and entrustment decision-making. ORCID: https://orcid.org/0000-0002-6379-8780

Claire Touchie, MD, MHPE, is professor of medicine and associate director, educator development, for the Centre for Innovation in Medical Education (CiMED), University of Ottawa, Canada. She is a member of the International CBE Collaborators and a founding faculty of the Ins and Outs of Entrustable Professional Activities: An International Course. ORCID: https://orcid.org/0000-0001-7926-9720

David A. Turner, MD, is the vice president of competency-based medical education at the American Board of Pediatrics and an adjunct professor in pediatric critical care at Duke Children's Hospital in Durham, North Carolina, USA. He is committed to helping lead the transition to a competency-based approach to education and assessment in pediatrics in the USA and has been involved in numerous CBME and EPA projects, studies, and publications. ORCID: https://orcid.org/0000-0002-0957-1382

Eric J. Warm, MD, is professor of medicine, vice chair for graduate medical education, and internal medicine residency program director at the University of Cincinnati. He is a founding member of the RADICAL Medical Education Research Lab (Research in Assessment Designed to Improve Care and Learning). ORCID: https://orcid.org/0000-0002-6088-2434

Mabel Yap, MBBS, MSc, PhD, is director, professional training and assessment standards, Ministry of Health, Singapore. She is also an adjunct associate professor and faculty development lead, Education Office, National University Singapore Health System. She is responsible for implementing EPAs nationally in Singapore, from UME to PGME, and also for allied health professionals. ORCID: https://orcid.org/0000-0002-7589-7962

Acknowledgments

The editors wish to thank the following external reviewers for the many useful comments that have led to better chapters: Adnan Alseidi, Raphael Bonvin, Jan Breckwoldt, Monika Brodmann, William Cutrer, Arvin Damodaran, Walter Eppich, Larry Gruppen, Christina Gummesson, Rose Hatala, Louis Jenkins, Gail Jensen, Brian Kim, Kim Lomis, Sally Marotti, Patricia O'Sullivan, Anna Oswald, Rocio Quinonez, Herman Tam, Pedro Tanaka, Susan van Schalkwyk, Jennifer Weller, Timothy Wood, and John Young, as well as foreword author Carol Carraccio, who read all chapters carefully and provided additional suggestions.

Funding for the book was generously provided by Open Access Fund of Utrecht University, The Netherlands, and by faculty members of the International online course Ins and Outs of Entrustable Professional Activities, who voluntarily donated their course compensations in 2023 and 2024 to make this book possible.

SECTION A

Introduction and theoretical backgrounds

CHAPTER 1

Entrustable professional activities and entrustment decision-making for competency-based education in the health professions: an introduction

Olle ten Cate, Marije P. Hennus

Abstract

Since the turn of the millennium, competency-based education (CBE) has become a new standard for training in the health professions in many countries. Early work to operationalize CBE has included development of detailed frameworks of competencies that every physician should demonstrate. However, these models were criticized because they do not directly translate to everyday activities of practice. For that reason, entrustable professional activities (EPAs) were introduced in 2005. EPAs are units of professional practice that may be entrusted to trainees once they show the competencies needed to execute them without supervision. EPAs have become popular within competency-based programs in many countries, with numerous examples not only in medicine but in all health professions, including nursing, veterinary medicine, pharmacy, physical therapy, dentistry, and more. This chapter provides an overview of key foundational concepts related to EPAs. Beginning with a historical overview, the chapter provides a definition and rationale for EPAs. While competencies are qualities of individuals, EPAs are units of work. The two can be seen as dimensions of a matrix. Almost all activities in health care draw upon multiple, integrated competencies (communication and collaboration skill, professional behavior, content expertise, etc.). Next, entrustment decision-making as an approach to assessment is explained, as well as the associated framework of levels of supervision, ranging from 'allowed to observe' to 'ready to be a supervisor.' The chapter concludes with a summary of important considerations for building an EPA program.

How to cite this book chapter:

ten Cate O, Hennus MP. Entrustable professional activities and entrustment decision-making for competency-based education in the health professions: an introduction. In: ten Cate O, Burch VC, Chen HC, Chou FC, Hennus MP. (Eds). *Entrustable Professional Activities and Entrustment Decision-Making in Health Professions Education*, Chapter 1, pp. 3–14. [2024] London: Ubiquity Press. DOI: https://doi.org/10.5334/bdc.a

Authors

- Olle ten Cate, PhD. University Medical Center Utrecht, Utrecht, the Netherlands and University of California, San Francisco, USA. Correspondence: t.j.tencate@umcutrecht.nl
- Marije P. Hennus, MD, PhD, MSc Clin Ed. University Medical Center Utrecht, Utrecht, the Netherlands.

Introduction

Entrustable professional activities (EPAs), a concept introduced in medical education in 2005,[1] has attracted much attention among educators in the health professions. Almost 20 years and hundreds of publications later, EPAs have now been introduced in many health professional programs, in numerous countries, and across all continents. In this chapter we introduce and explain the background, nature, and use of EPAs.

Competency-based education as the soil for EPAs: a brief historical overview

Competency-based education (CBE) is rooted in a movement that started outside the health professions.[2–5] Benjamin Bloom, inspired by education scholars Tyler and Carroll, created the notion of elaborate objectives for education,[6] and launched the notion of mastery learning[7]: the idea that most learners are able to attain mastery, if given sufficient time, opportunities, and guidance. Competency-based medical education was coined in 1978[8] but only became highly popular decades later.[9]

The popularity of CBE in the health professions is unsurprising. Health care practice must be restricted, by law, to professionals who meet high standards of competence. Meeting such standards requires intensive and long periods of study, and the public must be able to put their trust in these professionals, as well as in the system that educates and assesses trainees and emerging professionals who should meet these outcome standards.

Back in the 19th century, many Western countries began to regulate the medical profession at the national level, assuming the duty to protect citizens against incompetent practitioners.[10] This led to the first conceptions of competence, and the identification of its core components for medical curricula. With the general emergence of educational objectives and the establishment of postgraduate education in the second half of the 20th century, outcome-based education, later also called CBE, then became an important guiding principle for medical educators.[11] This was followed in recent decades by undergraduate medical education and other health professions and disciplines, including nursing, veterinary medicine, pharmacy, physical therapy, and more.

Several countries have embraced CBE, using frameworks to describe the breadth of the profession in competency terms.[12–14] These frameworks (CanMEDS in Canada and the ACGME competency model in the US) have been widely adopted in various countries around the world, specifically in postgraduate medical training, which for decades was left largely unstructured. At the same time, critical voices in the literature could be heard.[15–19] The increasingly detailed competencies that had emerged in subsequent editions of national frameworks were often felt to be rather theoretical, too detailed, detached from practice, and difficult to translate into workable and reliable assessment procedures. There was a need to translate competencies better into the practice of everyday work in health care. The desire to bridge this gap between well-elaborated competency frameworks and clinical practice in patient care led to the creation of EPAs.[20]

EPAs have changed the landscape of CBE in three ways: (a) to reconceptualize the goals for training, shifting focus on competencies alone to include the tasks of health care as a focus, (b) to operationalize the individualization and time variability of training, and (c) to focus assessment on entrustment decisions for clinical tasks.

Entrustable professional activities defined, as goals of training

EPAs are the units of professional practice that constitute the tasks that clinicians (physicians, nurses, and other health professionals) do in their daily patient care work and with which trainees at some moment in their training trajectory must be entrusted.[1] These tasks can be small or big.

An attending physician on a clinical ward may be tasked to evaluate a deteriorating patient and take action to stabilize the patient's condition. This could be a typical EPA for a senior trainee in intensive care training. Similarly, a senior trainee in nursing may be asked to start providing care for an elderly patient with a complex neurological disorder and significant comorbidity. A veterinary trainee may be entrusted with suturing a dog's superficial paw laceration if nothing points toward complications. A physician assistant trainee may be asked to examine and evaluate a patient with a known chronic condition, order diagnostic tests if needed, prepare follow-up medication, and do work that only needs reviewing by a clinical staff member. These tasks can all be EPAs. Once a trainee has demonstrated they possess the required competencies for an EPA, they may be entrusted with it. A junior health profession trainee can start contributing to health care with small but significant tasks that no longer require full checks.[21] Typically, EPAs are professional activities that have a beginning and an end, are observable and measurable in their process and outcome, and are only entrusted to trained and qualified personnel, after adequate assessment. Entrustment decisions require a holistic judgment, which is more than a focus on specific knowledge or skill.

How do EPAs relate to competencies?

The distinction between EPAs and competencies is not always perceived as clear.[22] A way to think of EPAs is as the task list on a clinical ward. Administrative assistants can allocate EPAs as clinical duties to individual specialists in weekly schedules. Or EPAs could serve as duty requirements on a personnel advertisement, or they could be the to-do list in an individual health professional's calendar or notebook; EPAs are specific things that must occur in a plannable period of time. In contrast, competencies describe persons. Trainees who become competent professionals must acquire competencies that include knowledge, skills, and attitudes. These abilities allow them to perform EPAs. Professionals possess competencies but they can never 'possess' EPAs.

EPAs and competencies (or domains of competence) can be depicted as two perpendicular dimensions in a matrix model (Table 1.1). In this figure, exemplary EPAs are mapped each to the most critical domains in which the trainee should possess competence before entrustment.[23] As is clearly visible, EPAs require multiple competencies that must be applied in an integrative fashion. Even a clear task such as 'taking a patient's history' combines several domains of competence. Professionalism and communication skills are definitely necessary but medical expertise is also essential to perform a focused, efficient, and productive history.

Table 1.1: EPA and competencies as two dimensions.

Competency domains	EPA 1	EPA 2	EPA 3	EPA 4	EPA 5	EPA 6
Medical expert	xxx	xxx	xxx	xxx	x	xx
Communicator	xxx	xxx	xxx	xx	xxx	xxx
Collaborator	x	xxx	xxx	xxx	xxx	x
Scholar	x	x	xx	xxx	x	x
Leader	x	x	x	xxx	x	xxx
Health advocate	x	x	xx	xxx	xxx	xxx
Professional	xx	x	x	x	xxx	xxx

Note: EPA 1: performing a venipuncture; EPA 2: performing an appendectomy; EPA 3: hand-over at morning report after night shift; EPA 4: developing and implementation of a patient management plan; EPA 5: chairing a multidisciplinary meeting; EPA 6: requesting an organ donation. Competencies in this domain are (x) helpful, (xx) expected, or (xxx) indispensable.

As EPAs are units of *professional* practice, they are not *designed* for training, but rather *identified* and then elaborated for training purposes. To summarize: EPAs are not created for education, but education is created for EPAs.

Entrustment decisions

The decision to transfer a responsibility to a trainee is called an entrustment decision. Such decisions may be further characterized as *ad hoc* or *summative*. Ad hoc decisions happen every day in the clinical teaching environment. A supervisor must estimate whether the skills of the trainee at that moment match the complexity of the patient and the risks involved.[24] A summative entrustment decision has the nature of a formal qualification for the future responsibility of the trainee from that moment on. In workplace curricula with EPAs, summative entrustment decisions constitute the permission to carry out an EPA when there is sufficient grounding of trust among the staff that the trainee can bear this responsibility.[25] The trainee is evaluated on their ability, and bestowed with the right and duty to be engaged in clinical service to patients.[26] While this right is formally given at the end of training with a diploma, license, or certification, in EPA-based curricula it should be given for separate EPAs at various moments throughout the program, i.e., as soon there is a justified, grounded trust that the trainee has met the objectives of the program for that EPA. This way, EPA-based programs can be truly competency-based and not just time-based. Figure 1.1 shows this graphically. Rules and regulations may restrict autonomy, even if the trainee is competent, but there may be creative ways to reward trainees by minimizing supervision.

This figure, with time on the horizontal axis and proficiency on the vertical axis, includes a developmental framework of Dreyfus's five stages, from novice to expert.[27] 'Competent,' placed in the middle, can be regarded as the threshold for unsupervised professional practice. What the figure shows is that a *threshold bar of competence* is being passed at different moments for different EPAs.

A justified entrustment decision can be made when the educational team has been convinced that a trainee has met all conditions for summative entrustment, that is, readiness for more autonomous performance in future similar cases. Here is where trust becomes important, because no two patients and contexts are identical. To trust trainees with future health care tasks means more than observing adequate knowledge and skills as examined in tests. A benchmark question for an assessing supervisor might be: would you now trust your own family members with this trainee?[28] Sometimes, when formal assessments have been 'ticked off,' your gut might still tell you

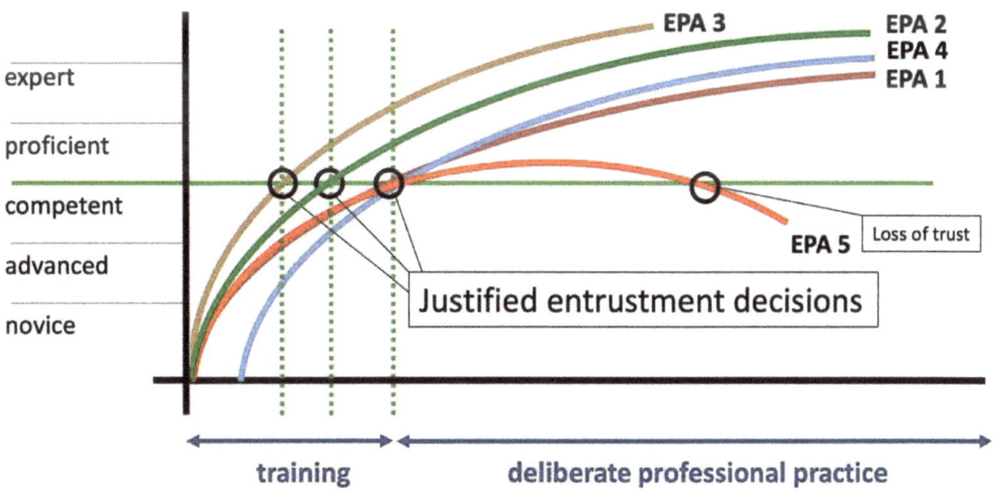

Figure 1.1: Development of clinical proficiency of one trainee for various EPAs.

differently. Gut feelings and tacit impressions might arise that can be critical[29] and should somehow be incorporated into summative entrustment decisions. Programmatic assessment,[30] elaborated in other chapters, provides the possibility to do so. Judgments from multiple individuals and various observations are combined to arrive at summative entrustment decisions, in which there is space to include both quantified and more narrative information.

The 'threshold' means there can now be sufficient trust in a trainee to work without supervision, but it does not equate to perfection. High levels of proficiency will require continued and deliberate professional practice. If that does not occur, decay may lead to substandard practice (EPA 5 in the figure), to a level that requires supervision again, even if a justified summative entrustment decision was made before.

What is needed for entrustment?

Ad hoc entrustment decisions are made for individual trainees by individual supervisors at individual moments ('Why don't you go ahead alone with this patient? I'll be at the other ward; call me if you need me, otherwise report to me an hour from now'). Even though they happen frequently, they are determined by more factors than one would initially think, including factors that are not always consciously weighed in the decision. Grouped into five, these factors include (a) the perceived trainee features, (b) a supervisor's propensity to delegate responsibility, (c) the complexity and risks of the EPA, (d) the context, such as time of the day and the need for hands, and (e) the relationship of the clinician with the trainee.[31–36] While supervisor propensity, task complexity, context factors, and relationship all affect ad hoc decisions, trainee factors are particularly relevant for workplace-based assessment to support summative decisions of entrustment, which should be context- and rater-independent. ten Cate and Chen summarize the literature and distinguish five features[23]; together, they call these the ingredients of 'A RICH' entrustment decision, after their first letters (Table 1.2).

As *summative entrustment decisions* have a certifying nature, sometimes called a *Statement of Awarded Responsibility* (STAR),[20] they should be valid and based on sufficiently grounded trust.[25] Grounded trust for a summative entrustment of an EPA must rely on sufficient occasions and observations. A valid summative entrustment decision, with important consequences not just for the trainee but also for patient safety, requires sufficient data from a variety of sources.[33] A program of assessment, using multiple sources of information, including direct observations, longitudinal monitoring, conversations with trainees, and product evaluations is needed. In addition, knowledge and skills examinations may weigh in.[37] Entrustment, as a focus of assessment, brings a different dimension to workplace-based assessment, because entrustment decisions imply an acceptance of risk for patients and, indirectly, for trainees.[26,38] Several chapters in this book (A4, D1, D2) will elaborate on this phenomenon.

Levels of supervision

So far, we have discussed entrustment decisions related to dichotomous decisions: entrust or not yet entrust, or provide supervision or not. However, it is very useful to translate entrustment decisions to decreasing levels of supervision. Five main levels have been described (Table 1.3).

Table 1.2: Trainee features as ingredients for A RICH entrustment decision.

Agency	Sufficiently self-confident, proactive toward work, team, safety, development
Reliability	Being conscientious, predictable, accountable, responsible
Integrity	Being truthful, benevolent, patient-centered
Capability	EPA-specific knowledge and skill; experience; adaptive expertise
Humility	Observing own limitations, willingness to ask help, receptive to feedback

Table 1.3: A standard framework of levels of clinical supervision.

	Supervision level	Explanation
1	Observation only	The trainee is allowed to be present and observe, not to enact an EPA
2	Direct supervision	The trainee is allowed to execute the EPA with direct or proactive supervision; a supervisor must be physically present
3	Indirect supervision	The trainee is allowed to execute the EPA with a supervisor quickly available if needed, signifying indirect, reactive supervision
4	Unsupervised practice	The trainee is allowed to work unsupervised; a supervisor may be reachable in a phone call, but not quickly present
5	Supervising a junior	The trainee may act as a supervisor for a junior trainee for this EPA

This standard framework has been recommended widely.[20,37] While the idea of using EPAs was created for postgraduate training programs, undergraduate programs have also started applying them. This has led to more detailed levels of supervision, within this framework, for undergraduate medical education.[39]

In postgraduate medical education, there may be specialty specific supervision levels. A surgery trainee will have much closer (level 2) supervision in the operating theater than an internal medicine trainee in most of their daily practice. For an anesthesiology supervisor, the question 'can I leave the operating theater, and for how long?' is most critical.[40]

Supervision levels are often used to create scales where a trainee is or should be in their development; such scales are called entrustment–supervision (ES) scales.

ES scales, in their use for assessment, can be retrospective or prospective.[34] When ES scales are used to evaluate or assess a trainee, there are two types of questions that can be posed. The first reflects the reporting of the amount of help or supervision a trainee required in a specific, observed instance. An ES scale for such use is called 'retrospective,' that is, 'looking backward,' where the preceptor answers the question 'how much help did the trainee need?' The second type of question reflects the trainee's future need for supervision, when considering entrustment. Prospective scales, looking forward, are used to recommend a supervision level in the near future: 'Based on my observation, I recommend that this trainee, for this EPA, is ready for distant supervision.'

Aligned with programmatic assessment, valid summative decisions about trainees must draw from multiple data points, preferably collected in a trainee's portfolio. Ad hoc decisions of entrustment, subsequently evaluated with the trainee and leading to recommendations for future levels of supervision, serve as input (Figure 1.2).

How EPAs serve individualized curricula

For an individual trainee, for instance in postgraduate medical training, the curriculum across postgraduate years (PGY) 1 to 4, as far as EPAs are concerned, may look like the curriculum map provided in Figure 1.3. Following principles of CBE,[41] trainees should become qualified when they are ready, not just because of a fixed period of completed time. This implies that, arguably, not every trainee progresses at the same speed as their peers.

A reasonable expectation is that most trainees meet the requirements for summative entrustment decisions at the designated level for all core EPAs of their program before graduation. But some trainees may meet them earlier, while others meet them later. Besides motivation and capacity differences, family-building and research breaks may disrupt a preset schedule. Finally, not all trainees who start have an equal background. For instance, outside North America, most countries allow entry into postgraduate medical training after varying periods of supplemental licensed clinical experience.

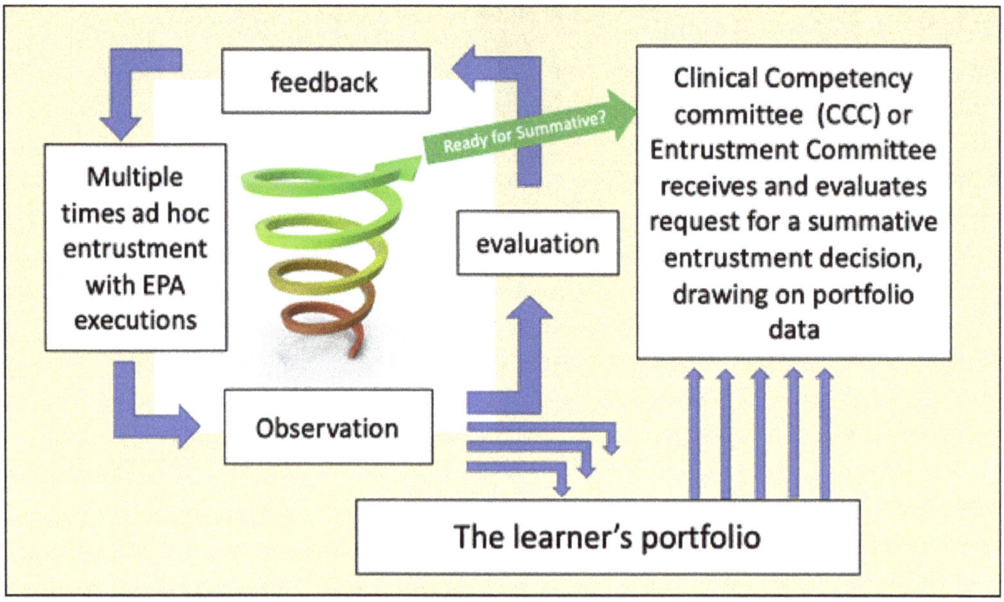

Figure 1.2: The flow of workplace-based observation data to support summative entrustment.

Depending on the sequence of the curriculum (e.g., rotations), an initial agreement may be negotiated to specify when which levels of supervision are expected, and, most importantly, when 'level 4' (ready for unsupervised practice) can be reached. Level 5 is aspirational and might apply to a limited number of senior trainees (e.g., chief residents), and not for all EPAs. Next, monitoring of the trainee will be important, as summative entrustment decisions, by a clinical competency committee (the team responsible for these decisions), must be made judiciously and based on sufficient and valid information. This can lead to deviations from the original scheme.

	PGY 1		PGY 2		PGY 3		PGY 4	
EPA a	1	2	2	2	3	4	4	5
EPA b	1	1	2	2	2	3	3	4
EPA c	2	2	3	4	5	5	5	5
EPA d	2	3	4	4	4	4	5	5

Figure 1.3: A trainee's individualized workplace curriculum in postgraduate training.

Building a program with EPAs

The introduction of EPAs and entrustment decision-making in a program is a project in itself that must be carefully planned. Several steps should be considered, even while it is good to remember that every profession, specialty, or country may have different constraints. These are some suggested steps, briefly summarized.

1. ***Identify EPAs.*** This requires a dedicated expert team and a wider group of stakeholders to arrive at consensus. The drafting of initial EPAs must be done carefully, and there are several tools to evaluate their quality. A full elaboration can be found in Hennus et al.[35]
2. ***Create full EPA descriptions.*** A fully elaborated EPA consists of eight components (title, specification & limitations, potential risks in case of failure, connection with a competency framework, sources of information to ground summative entrustment decisions, reasonable levels of supervision expected at stages of training, and optionally a period of expiration if the EPA is never practiced). ten Cate and Taylor elaborate on this description.[36]
3. ***Create tailored opportunities for learning.*** The clinical workplace cannot be recreated for learning, but trainees as well as supervisors should deliberately seek such opportunities as they present themselves in the natural course of patient care.
4. ***Design a programmatic approach to assessment.*** This should enable valid summative entrustment decisions and foster transparency. The infrastructure may differ for different programs but should include a mechanism to consolidate observational data into information that allows for advancement decisions and summative entrustment decisions.[30]
5. ***Support individual pathways with a portfolio model.*** Portfolios are increasingly considered necessary for workplace-based assessment and several commercial or home-grown EPA-based electronic tools are available.[42]
6. ***Faculty development.*** It will be necessary to inform and train faculty at different levels, such as frontline teachers, program directors, and members of clinical competency or examination committees.

Concluding remarks

EPAs represent an important step forward in translating CBE into health professions education practice. First introduced in 2005, EPAs have since become popular among programs of postgraduate and undergraduate education in medicine and other health professions. Examples of their use can also be found on the internet, including in video clips, courses, and other sources of information. This chapter provides an introduction to help readers understand the purpose and nature of EPAs and entrustment decision-making.

Acknowledgments

This chapter draws substantially from papers published by the first author.[43–45]

Competing interests

The authors declare that they have no competing interests.

Figure and table justification

Table 1.1 was modified from a figure in AMEE Guide 99 by ten Cate et al. (2015)[37]; Figure 1.3 was modified from a figure by ten Cate (2014).[46] Figure 1.1 was modified from a figure in ten Cate et al. (2010).[47] Figure 1.2 was derived from a presentation created for the international Ins and Outs of EPAs online course.

References

1. ten Cate O. Entrustability of professional activities and competency-based training. *Med Educ.* 2005;39(12):1176–1177. DOI: https://doi.org/10.1111/j.1365–2929.2005.02341.x
2. ten Cate O. Competency-based medical education. In: Cockerham WC, Dingwall R, Quah S, eds. *The Wiley-Blackwell Encyclopedia of Health, Illness, Behavior, and Society.* John Wiley & Sons; 2014:1329–1335.
3. ten Cate O. Competency-based postgraduate medical education: past, present and future. *GMS J Med Educ.* 2017;34(5):Doc69. DOI: https://doi.org/10.3205/zma001146
4. Nodine TR. How did we get here? A brief history of competency-based higher education in the United States. *Competency-Based Education.* 2016;1(1):5–11. DOI: https://doi.org/10.1002/cbe2.1004
5. Vasquez JA, Marcotte K, Gruppen LD. The parallel evolution of competency-based education in medical and higher education. *Competency-Based Education.* 2021;6(2). DOI: https://doi.org/10.1002/cbe2.1234
6. Bloom BS, Engelhart MD, Furst EJ, Hill WH, Krathwohl DR. *Taxonomy of Educational Objectives: The Classification of Educational Goals; Handbook I: Cognitive Domain.* Longmans, Green; 1956.
7. Bloom BS. Learning for mastery. Instruction and curriculum. *Evaluation Comment UCLA.* 1968;1(2):1–11.
8. McGaghie WC, Miller GE, Sajid AW, Telder TV. Competency-based curriculum development in medical education: an introduction. WHO. *Public Health Pap.* 1978;(68):11–91.
9. Carraccio C, Wolfsthal SD, Englander R, Ferentz K, Martin C. Shifting paradigms: from Flexner to competencies. *Acad Med.* 2002;77(5):361–367. DOI: https://doi.org/10.1097/00001888-200205000-00003
10. Ludmerer KM. *Learning to Heal. The Development of American Medical Education.* Basic Books; 1985.
11. Harden RM. AMEE Guide No. 14: Outcome-based education: Part 1-An introduction to outcome-based education. *Med Teach.* 1999;21(1):7–14. DOI: https://doi.org/10.1080/01421599979969
12. CanMEDS 2000: Extract from the CanMEDS 2000 Project Societal Needs Working Group Report. *Med Teach.* 2000;22(6):549–554. DOI: https://doi.org/10.1080/01421590050175505
13. Swing SR. The ACGME outcome project: retrospective and prospective. *Med Teach.* 2007;29(7):648–654. DOI: https://doi.org/10.1080/01421590701392903
14. General Medical Council. *Tomorrow's Doctors. Outcomes and Standards for Undergraduate Medical Education.* (General Medical Council, ed.). General Medical Council; 2009:1–108.
15. Brooks MA. Medical education and the tyranny of competency. *Perspect Biol Med.* 2009;52(1):90–102. DOI: https://doi.org/10.1353/pbm.0.0068
16. Glass JM. Competency based training is a framework for incompetence. *BMJ.* 2014;348:g2909. DOI: https://doi.org/10.1136/bmj.g2909
17. Grant J. The incapacitating effects of competence: A critique. *Adv Health Sci Educ Theory Pract.* 1999;4(3):271–277. DOI: https://doi.org/10.1023/A:1009845202352
18. Hodges BD. A tea-steeping or i-Doc model for medical education? *Acad Med.* 2010;85(9 Suppl):S34-S44. DOI: https://doi.org/10.1097/ACM.0b013e3181f12f32
19. Whitehead CR, Kuper A. Faith-based medical education. *Adv in Health Sci Educ.* 2017;22(1):1–3. DOI: https://doi.org/10.1007/s10459-016-9748-8
20. ten Cate O, Scheele F. Competency-based postgraduate training: can we bridge the gap between theory and clinical practice? *Acad Med.* 2007;82(6):542–547. DOI: https://doi.org/10.1097/ACM.0b013e31805559c7

21. Chen HC, Sheu L, O'Sullivan P, ten Cate O, Teherani A. Legitimate workplace roles and activities for early learners. *Med Educ.* 2014;48(2):136–145. DOI: https://doi.org/10.1111/medu.12316
22. ten Cate O, Schumacher DJ. Entrustable professional activities versus competencies and skills: Exploring why different concepts are often conflated. *Adv Health Sci Educ Theory Pract.* 2022;27(2):491–499. DOI: https://doi.org/10.1007/s10459-022-10098-7
23. ten Cate O, Chen HC. The ingredients of a rich entrustment decision. *Med Teach.* 2020;42(12): 1413–1420. DOI: https://doi.org/10.1080/0142159X.2020.1817348
24. ten Cate O. Nuts and bolts of entrustable professional activities. *J Grad Med Educ.* 2013;5(1): 157–158. DOI: https://doi.org/10.4300/JGME-D-12-00380.1
25. ten Cate O, Hart D, Ankel F, et al. Entrustment decision-making in clinical training. *Acad Med.* 2016;91(2):191–198. DOI: https://doi.org/10.1097/ACM.0000000000001044
26. ten Cate O. Entrustment as assessment: recognizing the ability, the right, and the duty to act. *J Grad Med Educ.* 2016;8(2):261–262. DOI: https://doi.org/10.4300/JGME-D-16-00097.1
27. Dreyfus HL, Dreyfus SE. *Mind over Machine.* Free Press; 1986.
28. Jonker G, Ochtman A, Marty AP, Kalkman CJ, ten Cate O, Hoff RG. Would you trust your loved ones to this trainee? Certification decisions in postgraduate anaesthesia training. *Br J Anaesth.* 2020;125(5):e408-e410. DOI: https://doi.org/10.1016/j.bja.2020.07.009
29. van Enk A, ten Cate O. 'Languaging' tacit judgment in formal postgraduate assessment: the documentation of ad hoc and summative entrustment decisions. *Perspect Med Educ.* 2020;9(6):373–378. DOI: https://doi.org/10.1007/s40037-020-00616-x
30. Hauer KE, O'Sullivan PS, Fitzhenry K, Boscardin C. Translating theory into practice: implementing a program of assessment. *Acad Med.* 2018;93(3):444–450. DOI: https://doi.org/10.1097/ACM.0000000000001995
31. Dijksterhuis MGK, Voorhuis M, Teunissen PW, et al. Assessment of competence and progressive independence in postgraduate clinical training. *Med Educ.* 2009;43(12):1156–1165. DOI: https://doi.org/10.1111/j.1365–2923.2009.03509.x
32. Hauer KE, ten Cate O, Boscardin C, Irby DM, Iobst W, O'Sullivan PS. Understanding trust as an essential element of trainee supervision and learning in the workplace. *Adv Health Sci Educ Theory Pract.* 2014;19(3):435–456. DOI: https://doi.org/10.1007/s10459-013-9474-4
33. Touchie C, Kinnear B, Schumacher D, et al. On the validity of summative entrustment decisions. *Med Teach.* 2021;43(7):780–787. DOI: https://doi.org/10.1080/0142159X.2021.1925642
34. ten Cate O, Schwartz A, Chen HC. Assessing trainees and making entrustment decisions: on the nature and use of entrustment-supervision scales. *Acad Med.* 2020;95(11):1662–1669. DOI: https://doi.org/10.1097/ACM.0000000000003427
35. Hennus MP, Jarrett JB, Taylor DR, ten Cate O. Twelve tips to develop entrustable professional activities. *Med Teach.* 2023;45(7):701–707. DOI: https://doi.org/10.1080/0142159X.2023.2197137
36. ten Cate O, Taylor DR. The recommended description of an entrustable professional activity: AMEE Guide No. 140. *Med Teach.* 2021;43(10):1106–1114. DOI: https://doi.org/10.1080/0142159X.2020.1838465
37. ten Cate O, Chen HC, Hoff RG, Peters H, Bok H, van der Schaaf M. Curriculum development for the workplace using entrustable professional activities (EPAs): AMEE Guide No. 99. *Med Teach.* 2015;37(11):983–1002. DOI: https://doi.org/10.3109/0142159X.2015.1060308
38. ten Cate O. Entrustment decisions: bringing the patient into the assessment equation. *Acad Med.* 2017;92(6):736–738. DOI: https://doi.org/10.1097/ACM.0000000000001623
39. Chen HC, van den Broek WES, ten Cate O. The case for use of entrustable professional activities in undergraduate medical education. *Acad Med.* 2015;90(4):431–436. DOI: https://doi.org/10.1097/ACM.0000000000000586
40. Weller JM, Misur M, Nicolson S, et al. Can I leave the theatre? A key to more reliable workplace-based assessment. *Br J Anaesth.* 2014;112(6):1083–1091. DOI: https://doi.org/10.1093/bja/aeu052

41. Carraccio C, Lentz A, Schumacher DJ. Dismantling fixed time, variable outcome education: abandoning 'ready or not, here they come' is overdue. *Perspect Med Educ.* 2023;12(1):68–75. DOI: https://doi.org/10.5334/pme.10
42. Marty AP, Linsenmeyer M, George B, Young JQ, Breckwoldt J, ten Cate O. Mobile technologies to support workplace-based assessment for entrustment decisions: Guidelines for programs and educators: AMEE Guide No. 154. *Med Teach.* 2023;45(11):1203–1213. DOI: https://doi.org/10.1080/0142159X.2023.2168527
43. ten Cate O. A primer on entrustable professional activities. *Fundation Education Medica.* 2017;20(3):95–101.
44. ten Cate O. A primer on entrustable professional activities. *Korean J Med Educ.* 2018;30(1):1–10. DOI: https://doi.org/10.3946/kjme.2018.76
45. ten Cate O. An updated primer on entrustable professional activities (EPAs). *Rev Bras Educ Med.* 2019;43(1 suppl 1):712–720. DOI: https://doi.org/10.1590/1981-5271v43suplemento1-20190238.ing
46. ten Cate O. AM last page: what entrustable professional activities add to a competency-based curriculum. *Acad Med.* 2014;89(4):691. DOI: https://doi.org/10.1097/ACM.0000000000000161
47. ten Cate O, Snell L, Carraccio C. Medical competence: the interplay between individual ability and the health care environment. *Med Teach.* 2010;32(8):669–675. DOI: https://doi.org/10.3109/0142159X.2010.500897

CHAPTER 2

Entrustable professional activities, entrustment, and the conceptualization of competence in the health professions

Olle ten Cate, Marije P. Hennus, Natasha Khursigara-Slattery, María José López, Robert Sternszus

Abstract

The use of entrustable professional activities (EPAs) and entrustment decision-making in health professional education was proposed to operationalize competency-based education. To ground its use, a common conceptualization of 'competence' is needed. Based on theoretical notions of epistemology (distinguishing propositional, procedural, and experiential knowledge) and inspired by the theoretical insights of Vygotsky, Maslow, Billett, and others, the authors elaborate a three-layered model that includes canonical competence (what every professional should have mastered, independent of context), contextual competence (the ability to work in relevant contexts and apply canonical competence), and personalized competence (the individual approach to high-level practice). The model aligns well with curricula that stress knowing, doing, and being, combining competency-based standards with professional identity formation.

EPAs and entrustment decision-making typically regard the contextual layer of competence. This is because entrustment decisions, to support trainees in their progressive, professional autonomy, happen in clinical contexts where canonical, context-independent knowledge and skill are necessary but insufficient. Passing the threshold of entrustment with clinical responsibilities draws on both canonical competence and the ability to work in clinical contexts, responding to the needs of patients, of collaborators, and working within the rules and habits of the local environment. Once a trainee is entrusted with clinical

How to cite this book chapter:

ten Cate O, Hennus MP, Khursigara-Slattery N, López MJ, Sternszus R. Entrustable professional activities, entrustment, and the conceptualization of competence in the health professions. In: ten Cate O, Burch VC, Chen HC, Chou FC, Hennus MP. (Eds). *Entrustable Professional Activities and Entrustment Decision-Making in Health Professions Education*, Chapter 2, pp. 15–24. [2024] London: Ubiquity Press. DOI: https://doi.org/10.5334/bdc.b

responsibilities, and feels confident about the first two layers of competence, personalized competence can emerge more prominently, leading to integrated professional and personal identity formation.

The three layers of competence together establish the conditions to think, act, and feel like a health professional: the knowing, the acting, and the being.

Authors

- Olle ten Cate, PhD. University Medical Center Utrecht, Utrecht, the Netherlands and University of California, San Francisco, USA. Correspondence: t.j.tencate@umcutrecht.nl
- Marije P. Hennus, MD, PhD, MSc Clin Ed. University Medical Center Utrecht, the Netherlands.
- Natasha Khursigara-Slattery MD, MEHP. Mid-West Intern Network, University of Limerick, Limerick, Ireland.
- María José López MSc. Facultad de Ciencias Médicas, Universidad Nacional de Cuyo, Mendoza, Argentina.
- Robert Sternszus MDCM, MA(Ed). Department of Pediatrics & Institute of Health Sciences Education, McGill University, Montreal, Canada.

Introduction

Entrustable professional activities (EPAs) represent core components of a profession that their members are privileged to perform, often exclusively. Although there is more to professional formation than professional activities, EPAs are crucial in directing the education and assessment of trainees to become professionals. Professionals must become competent to carry out these tasks and this competence must largely be acquired during a period of education, professional training, and practice experience. Health professionals who have completed training must be declared competent by their schools, by their programs, and in many countries by medical and specialty boards, and thus deemed qualified to perform all of the EPAs of their profession in an unsupervised manner. Because the practice of health care is restricted to trained, qualified professionals, assessment of their readiness can be viewed as an entrustment decision. In other words, society, represented by educational institutions and licensing bodies, decides that professionals who have completed appropriate education are sufficiently competent to practice and can be entrusted exclusively with the care of population health.

EPAs must thus be embedded within a conceptualization of medical[a] competence. To enable schools, programs, and licensing bodies to create assessments that can attest to readiness to practice—an entrustment decision—competence must be defined. This, however, is not easy. One of the many attempts to define medical competence is 'the habitual and judicious use of communication, knowledge, technical skills, clinical reasoning, emotions, values, and reflection in daily practice for the benefit of the individual and community being served.'[1] Although this is a well-known and attractive, holistic definition, it does not provide practical anchors for assessment. More detailed descriptions are found in competency frameworks,[2–4] which break down medical competence into detailed competencies (such as the 'ability to share health care goals and plans with patients and their families'), categorized within larger competency domains (such as medical expertise, communication, collaboration, professionalism).[5,6]

These frameworks, however, have also been criticized because of their reductionist nature.[7,8] As such, competence has been defined either too broadly (not practical) or too narrowly and in too much detail (and missing some of the essence); both directions have disadvantages. And, yet, a deep understanding of what competence is appears essential in health professions education, because, unlike many other educational institutions, where the retrospective achievement of requirements is sufficient, the prospective permission to practice (in fact, entrustment) conferred by educational institutions and certifying bodies cannot be validly determined without it.

This chapter aims to provide a theoretical foundation[9] for the practical use of EPAs and entrustment decision-making in health professions education that is rooted in a deep understanding of medical competence.

A note on the epistemology of medical competence

Epistemology is the philosophy of knowledge, which studies its nature, origin, sources, justifications, and the sense of truth. In different domains, different epistemic frameworks are used. In mathematics, logical deduction can yield truths that are undisputed. In social sciences, 'truths' are less obvious and often determined by convictions that are not always shared. In health care, a domain somewhere in between, a body of knowledge exists that can be considered undisputed ('the organ between the esophagus and the duodenum is the stomach') but other instances of knowledge ('patient X in room Y is very sick') may be debatable or influenced by a personal

[a] In this chapter, when we say 'medical' we expressly mean to include all professions in the healthcare domain.

frame of reference. Epistemology distinguishes propositional knowledge (knowing that) from procedural knowledge (knowing how) and knowledge by acquaintance (knowing from personal experience[b]). 'Truths' can vary from totally undisputed, shared beliefs to probabilistic and highly contextual propositions. In medicine, shared convictions based on published evidence grow into 'truths,' because these convictions justify the actions and decisions that 'must' be made (for 'best' treatment, for referral, for next investigations, etc.). They are based on research findings, usually with confidence intervals to make them plausible rather than absolute.

When we say that trainees must acquire competence to be assessed for license, it is useful to distinguish between propositional and procedural knowledge. Without procedural knowledge (*how to* knowledge), propositional knowledge alone would not suffice for clinical practice. Knowing what to do may require propositional knowledge but also requires procedural knowledge and often experiential knowledge ('I know what to do because I have seen or done this before'). More than with propositional knowledge, procedural knowledge is not absolute and is affected by contextual, ethical, biographical, and sometimes even political considerations. What to do, for instance, when a critically ill patient arrives for intensive care when all IC beds are filled with critical Covid-19 patients? *Knowing what to do* belongs to the physician's assumed knowledge base but does not imply absolute truths, because contextual variations can make circumstances unpredictable. Similarly, on a meta level, educators must know when to begin entrusting a trainee with critical responsibilities, 'knowing' that the trainee will know what to do, depending on the circumstances. Entrustment decisions involve trust, that is, an estimation of a trainee's capacity to adapt and manage unfamiliar situations.

Medical competence as a multilayered construct

The origin of competency-based medical education lies strongly in behaviorist thinking. In the 1950s and 1960s, the dominant movement toward behavioral objectives for education stemmed from the reasoning that education must lead to measurable results of predefined objectives.[11,12] Bloom created a model of knowledge, skills, and attitudes that has influenced most of the education in the world[13,14] and certainly health professions education. In addition, his mastery learning concept[15] strongly influenced the idea that deliberate effort can bring all trainees to predefined standards of competence, with sufficient motivation, time, and practice opportunities, as Ericsson and McGaghie and his colleagues have shown.[16–18] However, if sufficient medical competence is regarded as a condition to entrust trainees and professionals with privileged health care tasks, competence may be defined more broadly than skills that grow through deliberate practice. Entrustment decisions are not easily made solely upon passing standardized tests. Observing trainees in clinical workplaces reveals components of competence that would go unnoticed in written examinations,[19] such as how a trainee connects with a patient and explores and interprets their medical history, and for which expert judgment is needed.[20] This more holistic approach to workplace-based assessment of competence is relatively new.[21] Indeed, the process of professional identity formation, whereby trainees come to think, act, and feel like physicians[22] (or other health professionals), is not easily captured in a competency framework.[23]

---

[b] Knowledge by acquaintance as one of the components of epistemology was defined by Bertrand Russell as 'knowledge of which we are directly aware, without the intermediary of any process of inference or any knowledge of truths.' It is strictly not identical to experiential knowledge (which may include inferences) but close enough to distinguish from propositional and procedural knowledge. In medical education, experiential knowledge (even sometimes without full awareness) is a more commonly used construct that we will use in this chapter. See Dings (2023) for a deeper discussion.[10]

In 2024, ten Cate et al. proposed medical competence as a construct with three layers, each with different implications for standards and assessment: a canonical layer, a contextual layer, and a personalized layer.[9] In the summary below we explain how EPAs and entrustment decision-making are situated within the contextual layer of competence.

Canonical layer of competence. Medicine and other health professions cannot be practiced without a thorough knowledge of at least anatomy, physiology, and pathology—that is, within the current body of knowledge, undisputed and generalized across the contexts, cultures, and countries in which patient care is practiced. This is knowledge that can be acquired through reading, listening, discussion, and other educational methods, and that can be tested with written or online methods. This is largely propositional knowledge, but some procedural knowledge belongs to the canon, such as the application of knowledge in clinical reasoning. Basic physical skills, including the examination of patients, and even foundational principles of ethics and professional behavior may be assumed to be canonical, that is, 'what everyone of the profession should know or be able to do,' independent of the context. Standards of expected competence at this layer can be defined, and the assessment can meet established criteria of psychometric quality to enable confidence that candidates who pass indeed possess the required canonical competence. In other words, this speaks to the 'knows,' 'knows how,' and 'shows how' levels of Miller's pyramid.[24]

Contextual layer of competence. Possessing canonical competence is insufficient to practice health care. While the classroom is not the only place to acquire canonical competence, the step to the application of knowledge in practice has always been considered a significant and difficult transition for medical students.[25] It requires a different way of thinking (problem- and action-oriented, rather than systematic and reproductive) and because clinical contexts have unique and thus different intricacies. It also requires adaptive competence,[26] further complicated by continuous changes within the ecology of the clinical environment itself in response to outside pressures or changed needs of health care.[27] Working in clinical contexts thus requires a different type of competence, including an ability to apply canonical competence in a variety of circumstances. This important layer of competence is more difficult than canonical competence to capture through standards and assessment processes. No one would entrust a graduate from a medical program, solely based on passing all exams, if they have never attended to a patient. A phase of clinical experience is indispensable, and requires more experienced colleagues (attendings, consultants, supervisors, and others) to confirm their readiness for unsupervised practice. Central in the assessment of contextual competence is the notion of entrustment. If a credible group of health professionals, familiar with the context, confirms that essential patient care activities can be *entrusted* to a trainee to perform with minimal supervision, standards can be considered to have been met. This notion requires quite a different approach to standard setting and assessment, as fair and valid decisions of entrustment require grounding in data from observation. Yet entrustment implies acceptance of risk, caused by a level of unpredictability of future situations. This in turn implies that absolute standards of competence do not hold in this layer of competence. Standards must comply with local rules, protocols, culture, and patient populations, and trainees must be evaluated with local sources of information, including experts who form judgments.

Personalized layer of competence. Following Billett,[28] we recognize that the competence of an individual professional reflects not just the possession of canonical knowledge and skills and the ability to practice health care according to standards but also includes style, insights, specific skills, interests, habits, and convictions that make a professional unique. While standards of canonical and contextual competence must be met to permit unsupervised practice, professionals can differ in their competence in a personal manner, above and beyond these standards. The constructivist view on education and development posits that humans actively construct new insights on a foundation of existing knowledge. They have ontogenetically (i.e., through their histories) shaped knowledge from learning and personal experiences, mediated by sensory, neural, and cognitive systems, in interaction with a social environment.[28] Vygotsky, the Russian developmental psychologist (1896–1934) who coined the term 'zone of proximal development' and contributed to cultural-historical activity theory, also elaborated on the concept of *perezhivanie*, which explains this idea of personal development well. *Perezhivanie*, in this context, can be best translated as the subjectivity which makes individuals unique in their creative performance, being the resultant of the combined cognitive and emotional experiences, built across one's lifetime, integrated in the long-term memory, and informing one's frame of reference in viewing the world.[9,29,30]

This sounds highly theoretical, but examples may help to understand it. It is essential that clinicians communicate compassionately with patients. While there are 'key features' to compassionate communication (i.e., listening, sitting, eye contact), the way in which clinicians interact with patients will vary between individuals and is shaped by their personal voice, style, experience, and identity. The ability of the physician to communicate their compassion effectively and authentically will affect patient satisfaction, and in some cases the outcomes of care. Or a clinician with a sound fund of knowledge may encounter adverse events in clinical practice,[31] leading to strong emotions that shape their individual style and convictions in subsequent clinical judgment and practice. This is why the *perezhivanie* of one person can never be fully understood by others, as Vygotsky contended when studying artistic excellence.[30] The personalized layer of clinical competence adds a component that can be conceived of as the art of clinical practice, by the personal touch of the individual professional. It also brings us back to epistemology. The 'epistemic framework' of the individual is a personal system of knowledge and thought, rarely made explicit. Barreiro and Castorina distinguish 'excisional' and 'relational' views of epistemic frameworks,[32] and argue that the excisional view (i.e., viewing individual knowledge as disconnected from the social environment) disregards the strong social and development psychologists' arguments (including from Vygotsky and Piaget) that nature, society, and culture affect one's epistemic framework in continuous interaction.

Setting standards for the assessment of the personalized layer of competence does not make sense, because legitimate diversity and differences between individual professionals characterizes this layer. However, the individual's *pursuit* of expansion of this layer may be valued and rewarded. This is, to some extent, captured in the Accreditation Council for Graduation Medical Education's competency domain of 'Practice-Based Learning and Improvement,' which has been defined as 'the ability to investigate and evaluate one's care of patients, to appraise and assimilate scientific evidence, and to continuously improve patient care based on constant self-evaluation and life-long learning.'[6] The effort may be valued but the desired result cannot be standardized.

A hierarchical model, but not fully sequential

The model, as depicted in Figure 2.1, is hierarchical in nature but not fully sequential. That is, contextual competence requires a canonical foundation because, when the application in a context

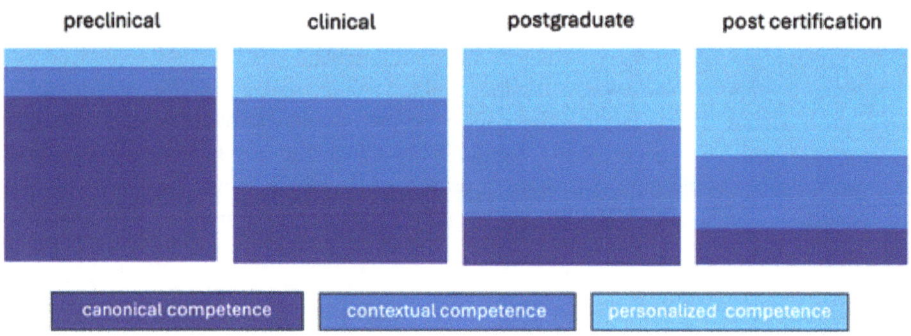

Figure 2.1: Visualization of the multilayered competence model across the continuum.

occurs, there must be something present to apply. Similarly, a personal style of practice, developed across a period of experience, requires a level of confidence that is often acquired in the first years after formal training. These years are known to be very demanding, when junior attendings or consultants are occupied by the desire and urge to meet all professional expectations and still encounter new challenging situations[33] A more relaxed phase of 'self-actualization' or the fulfillment of personal potential follows later, a state that, as proposed by Maslow, is reached after other needs have been satisfied (physiological, safety, love and belonging, esteem, competence, and aesthetic needs).[34] This happens when one feels mastery of one's domain of practice. An analogy with jazz music can help. Before being sufficiently skilled to improvise on a melody, the musician must first master the instrument, then know the basic melody at stake and understand its associated chords and harmonies, and also acquaint themselves with fellow musicians and other components of context. However, the hierarchical nature of the model is not meant to suggest that all canonical competence must first be mastered before contextual competence is acquired, with personalized competence finally emerging only at the end. On the contrary, vertical integration in medical curricula, which includes early acquaintance with clinical contexts while the teaching of the canon of basic sciences remains ongoing, has shown benefits for cognition and motivation.[35] Likewise, the seeds of personalized competence can be sowed early, when students explore and discover personal strengths and interests that guide career choices and that may eventually merge personal identity with professional identity.

The model thus addresses the tensions between the need for standardized assessment of competence to allow for access to the practice of health care, and the acknowledgment that processionals are unique, and that diversity must not only be tolerated but genuinely valued and supported. It provides a place for identity formation in competency-based education[23] and aligns with medical curricula that stress the knowing, doing, and being of health professionals.[36]

Implications for EPAs and entrustment

Within this model, entrustment decision-making typically aligns with assessment of the contextual layer of competence. Summative entrustment decisions, with critical impact for both patient safety and trainee progress, typically focus on thresholds, such as readiness for unsupervised practice (in postgraduate contexts) or for indirect supervision (undergraduate). While the stakes in assessment of canonical competence typically regard trainee progress, in the assessment of contextual competence the protection of patients is also a critical component. 'High-stakes decisions' therefore have a wider connotation in contextual competence. They must include an estimation of risks for patient safety, which is a prospective judgment.[37] Entrustment decisions must be based on more than technical skills (including interpersonal techniques). ten Cate and Chen[19] have argued that, besides capability (activity-specific knowledge, skill and experience, and adaptive expertise), four general features are relevant: integrity (truthful, good intentions, patient-centered), reliability (conscientious, predictable, accountable, responsible), humility (observing limits, willing to ask help, receptive to feedback), and agency (self-confident, proactive toward work, team, safety, and self-regulation). This array of features requires thoughtful consideration by observers, dialogues with trainees, and negotiations within clinical educator teams to arrive at intersubjective judgment and decisions. Here is where epistemology theory also becomes relevant. Epistemic humility refers to the limitations of knowledge, and acknowledges that decisions, such as in patient care, can not always be justified as being completely right or wrong.[38] Decisions of entrustment regarding trainees similarly involve a leap of faith (small or big) that supervisors and teams need to consider with some epistemic humility. Entrustment with patient care tasks requires a more holistic picture than rating scales can offer. The binary entrustment decision (yes or no) is a holistic decision that combines the evaluation of competence, the gauging of risks, and the granting of autonomy, and can only be made by examiners who know the trainee and who have the authority for patient care in the context of interest. The information determining the decision thus combines contextual features with trainee features. All features can weigh in but there is no formula to predict the outcome of the decision.

While the training and assessment of competence at the canonical layer is basically not individualized, the training and assessment of contextual competence is individualized. Competency-based curricula for the acquisition of contextual competence require sufficient flexibility and time-variability for all trainees to meet contextual standards, i.e., entrustment with all relevant EPAs, regardless of the time needed (albeit within limits).[39]

Finally, how does personalized competence relate to entrustment decision-making? While we have contended that decisions of readiness to practice require standards of canonical and contextual competence, not standards of personalized competence, there are two relationships with personalized competence. The first relates to the assessor or supervisor. Their own art and style of professional practice, fueled by their *perezhivanie*, includes not only the art of patient care but also the observation and assessment of trainees, and includes convictions about assessing quality of practice. Superb assessors, however, employ some epistemic humility in their judgment, by realizing their own limitations of knowing what is 'best.' The second relates to the trainee. Allowing the trainee to deviate within the margins of acceptable care, and assessing them with this view in mind, can contribute to the trainee's development of a personalized competence.

These three layers of competence together establish the conditions to think, act, and feel like a health professional[40]: the knowing, the acting, and the being.[36]

Acknowledgments

This chapter draws substantially from an article published in *Medical Education* and a public lecture by the first author on August 31, 2023.[9,41]

Competing interests

The authors declare that they have no competing interests.

Figure reprint

Figure 2.1 was reprinted from ten Cate et al. (2024), an open access publication with copyright residing with the authors.

References

1. Epstein RM, Hundert EM. Defining and assessing professional competence. *JAMA*. 2002;287(2):226–235. DOI: https://doi.org/10.1001/jama.287.2.226
2. Frank JR, Jabbour M. *Skills for the new millennium: report of the Societal Needs Working Group CanMEDS 2000 Project*. Royal College of Physicians and Surgeons of Canada.; 1996:1–21.
3. Frank JR, Snell L, Sherbino J. *CanMEDS 2015 Physician Competency Framework*. The Royal College of Physicians and Surgeons of Canada; 2015:36.
4. Swing SR, International CBME collaborators. Perspectives on competency-based medical education from the learning sciences. *Med Teach*. 2010;32(8):663–668. DOI: https://doi.org/10.3109/0142159X.2010.500705

5. Pangaro L, ten Cate O. Frameworks for learner assessment in medicine: AMEE Guide No. 78. *Med Teach.* 2013;35(6):e1197–1210. DOI: https://doi.org/10.3109/0142159X.2013.788789
6. Englander R, Cameron T, Ballard AJ, Dodge J, Bull J, Aschenbrener CA. Toward a common taxonomy of competency domains for the health professions and competencies for physicians. *Acad Med.* 2013;88(8):1088–1094. DOI: https://doi.org/10.1097/ACM.0b013e31829a3b2b
7. Grant J. The incapacitating effects of competence: A critique. *Adv Health Sci Educ Theory Pract.* 1999;4(3):271–277. DOI: https://doi.org/10.1023/A:1009845202352
8. Brooks MA. Medical education and the tyranny of competency. *Perspect Biol Med.* 2009;52(1):90–102. DOI: https://doi.org/10.1353/pbm.0.0068
9. ten Cate O, Khursigara-Slattery N, Cruess RL, Hamstra SJ, Steinert Y, Sternszus R. Medical competence as a multilayered construct. *Med Educ.* 2024;58(1):93–104. DOI: https://doi.org/10.1111/medu.15162
10. Dings R. Experiential knowledge: from philosophical debate to health care practice? *J Eval Clin Pract.* 2023;29(7):1119–1126. DOI: https://doi.org/10.1111/jep.13845
11. Tyler RW. *Basic Principles of Curriculum and Instruction.* University of Chicago Press; 1949.
12. Mager RF. *Preparing Educational Objectives.* 3rd ed. David S. Lake Publishers; 1984:1–136.
13. Bloom BS, Engelhart MD, Furst EJ, Hill WH, Krathwohl DR. *Taxonomy of Educational Objectives: The Classification of Educational Goals; Handbook I: Cognitive Domain.* Longmans, Green; 1956.
14. Krathwohl DR, Bloom BS, Masia BB. *Taxonomy of Educational Objectives: The Classification of Educational Goals; Handbook II: Affective Domain.* David McKay Co, Inc; 1973.
15. Bloom BS. *Learning for Mastery. Instruction and Curriculum.* Evaluation Comment UCLA. 1968.
16. McGaghie WC, Miller GE, Sajid AW, Telder TV. *Competency-based curriculum development in medical education: an introduction.* WHO. Public Health Pap. 1978;(68):11–91.
17. McGaghie WC. Mastery learning: it is time for medical education to join the 21st century. *Acad Med.* 2015;90(11):1438–1441. DOI: https://doi.org/10.1097/ACM.0000000000000911
18. Ericsson KA. Acquisition and maintenance of medical expertise: a perspective from the expert-performance approach with deliberate practice. *Acad Med.* 2015;90(11):1471–1486. DOI: https://doi.org/10.1097/ACM.0000000000000939
19. ten Cate O, Chen HC. The ingredients of a rich entrustment decision. *Med Teach.* 2020;42(12):1413–1420. DOI: https://doi.org/10.1080/0142159X.2020.1817348
20. ten Cate O, Regehr G. The power of subjectivity in the assessment of medical trainees. *Acad Med.* 2019;94(3):333–337. DOI: https://doi.org/10.1097/ACM.0000000000002495
21. Schuwirth LWT, van der Vleuten CPM. A history of assessment in medical education. *Adv Health Sci Educ Theory Pract.* 2020;25(5):1045–1056. DOI: https://doi.org/10.1007/s10459-020-10003-0
22. Cruess SR, Cruess RL, Steinert Y. Supporting the development of a professional identity: general principles. *Med Teach.* 2019;41(6):641–649. DOI: https://doi.org/10.1080/0142159X.2018.1536260
23. Sternszus R, Slattery NK, Cruess RL, ten Cate O, Hamstra SJ, Steinert Y. Contradictions and opportunities: reconciling professional identity formation and competency-based medical education. *Perspect Med Educ.* 2023;12(1):507–516. DOI: https://doi.org/10.5334/pme.1027
24. Miller GE. The assessment of clinical skills/competence/performance. *Acad Med.* 1990;65 (9 Suppl):S63-S67. DOI: https://doi.org/10.1097/00001888-199009000-00045
25. O'Brien BC, Poncelet AN. Transition to clerkship courses: preparing students to enter the workplace. *Acad Med.* 2010;85(12):1862–1869. DOI: https://doi.org/10.1097/ACM.0b013e3181fa2353
26. Teunissen PW, Watling CJ, Schrewe B, et al. Contextual competence: how residents develop competent performance in new settings. *Med Educ.* 2021;55(9):1100–1109. DOI: https://doi.org/10.1111/medu.14517

27. Ellaway RH, Bates J, Teunissen PW. Ecological theories of systems and contextual change in medical education. *Med Educ.* 2017;51(12):1250–1259. DOI: https://doi.org/10.1111/medu.13406
28. Billett S. Developing domains of occupational competence: workplaces and learner agency. In: Mulder M, ed. *Competence-Based Vocational and Professional Education. Vol 23. Technical and Vocational Education and Training: Issues, Concerns and Prospects.* Springer International Publishing Switzerland; 2017:47–66.
29. Fleer M, González Rey F, Veresov N, eds. *Perezhivanie, Emotions and Subjectivity*; vol 1. Springer Singapore; 2017. DOI: https://doi.org/10.1007/978-981-10-4534-9
30. González Rey F. Vygotsky's concept of *Perezhivanie* in *The Psychology of Art* and at the final moment of his work: advancing his legacy. *Mind, Culture, and Activity.* 2016;23(4):305–314. DOI: https://doi.org/10.1080/10749039.2016.1186196
31. Helo S, Moulton C-AE. Complications: acknowledging, managing, and coping with human error. *Transl Androl Urol.* 2017;6(4):773–782. DOI: https://doi.org/10.21037/tau.2017.06.28
32. Barreiro A, Castorina JA. Dialectical inferences in the ontogenesis of social representations. *Theory Psychol.* 2017;27(1):34–49. DOI: https://doi.org/10.1177/0959354316681863
33. Teunissen PW, Westerman M. Junior doctors caught in the clash: the transition from learning to working explored. *Med Educ.* 2011;45(10):968–970. DOI: https://doi.org/10.1111/j.1365–2923.2011.04052.x
34. Maslow AH. A theory of human motivation. *Psychol Rev.* 1943;50(4):370–396. DOI: https://doi.org/10.1037/h0054346
35. Wijnen-Meijer M, van den Broek S, Koens F, ten Cate O. Vertical integration in medical education: the broader perspective. *BMC Med Educ.* 2020;20(1):509. DOI: https://doi.org/10.1186/s12909-020-02433-6
36. Boland J, Offiah G. *Curriculum Framework for the Internship Programme in Ireland.* Health Service Executive; 2023.
37. ten Cate O. Entrustment as assessment: recognizing the ability, the right, and the duty to act. *J Grad Med Educ.* 2016;8(2):261–262. DOI: https://doi.org/10.4300/JGME-D-16-00097.1
38. Schwab A. Epistemic humility and medical practice: translating epistemic categories into ethical obligations. *J Med Philos.* 2012;37(1):28–48. DOI: https://doi.org/10.1093/jmp/jhr054
39. Schumacher DJ, Caretta-Weyer H, Busari J, et al. Competency-based time-variable training internationally: ensuring practical next steps in the wake of the COVID-19 pandemic. *Med Teach.* 2021;43(7):810–816. DOI: https://doi.org/10.1080/0142159X.2021.1925098
40. Merton RK, Reader RG, Kendall P. *The Student-Physician: Introductory Studies in the Sociology of Medical Education.* Harvard University Press; 1957:1–371.
41. ten Cate O. Health professions education: retrospective and prospective. Lecture at the Occasion of Completion of the Professoriate in Medical Education at Utrecht University, August 31, 2023; Utrecht University/UMC Utrecht, the Netherlands.

CHAPTER 3

Graded autonomy and grounded self-determination in health professions education

H. Carrie Chen, Roberta I. Ladenheim, Daniel J. Schumacher, Fremen Chihchen Chou, Olle ten Cate

Abstract

A key goal in health professions education is to support trainee development toward readiness for unsupervised clinical practice. Curricula can use entrustable professional activities (EPAs) and entrustment decision-making to structure and optimize this development. Trainees begin at the periphery of the health care community and gradually learn to think, feel, and act as a professional as they increasingly engage with the work of the community, step by step and EPA by EPA. Learning in the classroom and in the clinical workplace should be approached as integrated rather than separate phases. Classroom learning aims to prepare trainees for clinical practice, and learning through clinical practice can start early, with full supervision that decreases over time. Clinical supervisors must balance supervision for patient safety and trainee support with trainee autonomy and practice of clinical responsibilities. Under- or over-supervision has negative implications not just for patient safety but also for learning and development. Various theories and models support the importance of graded autonomy, including self-determination theory, cognitive apprenticeship theory, and learning-oriented teaching. Curricula designed to support graded autonomy need to adequately prepare trainees to contribute to the workplace via classroom education and exposure to the workplace followed by clinical experiences that allow for increasing trainee contributions to patient care. Entrustment is a forward-facing decision. As trainees achieve levels of entrustment for patient care activities, this achievement is not just a completion of a learning stage but a start of the acquisition of more responsibilities as health care team members.

How to cite this book chapter:

Chen HC, Ladenheim RI, Schumacher DJ, Chou FC, ten Cate O. Graded autonomy and grounded self-determination in health professions education. In: ten Cate O, Burch VC, Chen HC, Chou FC, Hennus MP. (Eds). *Entrustable Professional Activities and Entrustment Decision-Making in Health Professions Education*, Chapter 3, pp. 25–33. [2024] London: Ubiquity Press. DOI: https://doi.org/10.5334/bdc.c

Authors

- H. Carrie Chen, MD, PhD. Kaiser Permanente Bernard J. Tyson School of Medicine, Pasadena, CA, USA. Correspondence: H.Carrie.Chen@kp.org
- Roberta I. Ladenheim, MD. Instituto Universitario Hospital Italiano de Buenos Aires, Argentina.
- Daniel J. Schumacher, MD, PhD. Cincinnati Children's Hospital Medical Center/University of Cincinnati College of Medicine, Cincinnati, Ohio.
- Fremen Chihchen Chou, MD, PhD. School of Medicine, China Medical University/director of Center for Faculty Development, China Medical University Hospital, Taichung, Taiwan.
- Olle ten Cate, PhD. University Medical Center Utrecht, Utrecht, the Netherlands and University of California, San Francisco, USA.

Introduction

The purpose of health professions education is to prepare future health care providers who can respond to the health needs of society by providing safe, effective, quality care. Not only is this social responsibility an expected outcome but it also requires embedding in the process of health professional education. Learning to provide patient care and the development of competence requires practice. However, this practice must occur within a training environment that also meets the standards of safe, effective, high-quality patient care.

In all aspects of education, trainees develop over time. Rather than merely focusing on trainee acquisition of knowledge and skills, health professions curricula can deliberately focus on the development of trainees as emerging professionals and their preparation to bear increasing clinical responsibilities.[1] Upon commencement of their health professions education, trainees begin a journey of becoming (that is, thinking, acting, and feeling like) health professionals as they are enculturated into the practice of health care.[2,3] This is particularly relevant for learning in the health care workplace environment, where learning happens through participation in patient care.

Various developmental frameworks describe the progressive development of trainee competence. Dreyfus and Dreyfus describe a general model of skill acquisition with novices progressing through five stages to achieve expert status.[4] In undergraduate medical education, RIME—an acronym for 'reporter–interpreter–manager–educator'—provides a framework for the progressive roles and activities of junior trainees in patient care.[5] Within both frameworks, trainees engage in deliberate practice to develop and eventually achieve the necessary competence. In health professions, trainees practice by participating and taking on ever greater responsibilities in actual care of patients. This contribution to patient care by individuals who are still learning and working toward readiness for unsupervised practice inherently carries risks for patient safety. However, trainees do not practice in the workplace on their own. They join a community of practice within the workplace, whereupon they are given limited roles and responsibilities that are commensurate with their level of development and supervised by members of the community who are granted supervisory responsibility. As trainees progress in gaining competence and further identifying with the community of practice, they are gradually awarded additional roles and responsibilities with increasing autonomy and decreasing supervision, moving from the periphery to the center of a professional community of practice (Figure 3.1). This process is not linear in nature; it can involve different developmental trajectories among different trainees and for various tasks.

Balancing autonomy and supervision

Adequate supervision is the solution to ensuring optimal patient care while also needing to train the next generation of clinicians.[6] The role of the clinical supervisor is, therefore, to make decisions about which activities and responsibilities to entrust to a trainee and with what degree of graded autonomy and supervision. Autonomy and supervision are not simply the opposite ends of the same scale. Providing autonomy is allowing an individual to act of their own volition and with their own behavioral choices. Thus, even a trainee who is being supervised can be allowed to let their own clinical decisions and plans prevail. This happens within an institutional context in which trainees are assigned tasks and where records exist to establish what activities each person can do and with what level of supervision.

Graded autonomy is ideally negotiated over time between clinical supervisors and trainees, balancing trainee competence and readiness, trainee learning needs, workplace needs, and patient safety. Trainees are encouraged to take responsibility for not just their own learning but for con-

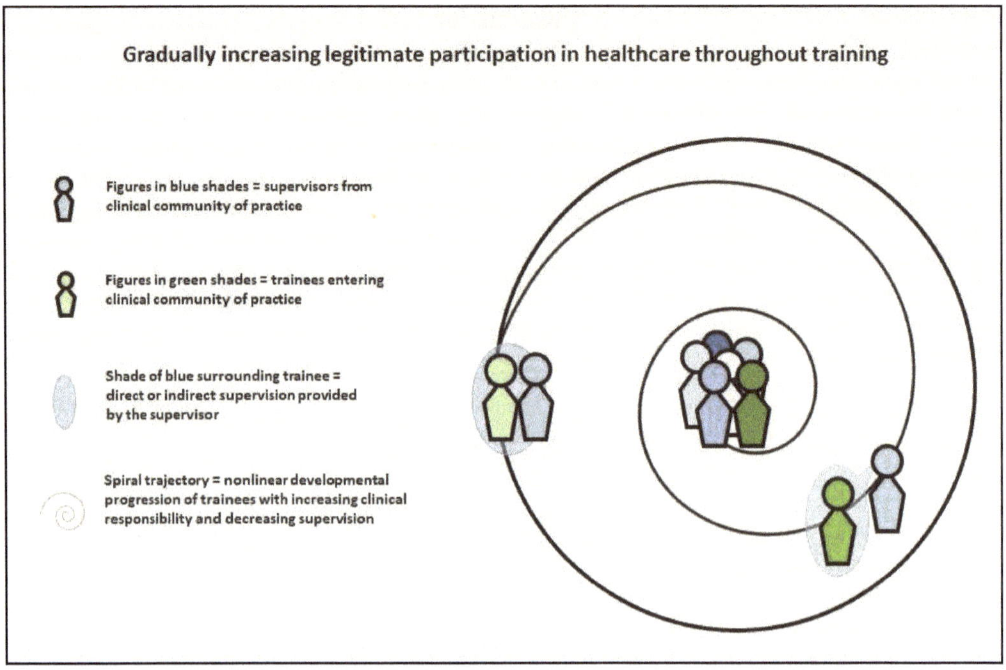

Figure 3.1: Trainee development in a professional community of practice.

tributing to the work of caring for patients and ensuring safe, effective patient care. Even as trainees achieve licensure and regulatory permission for unsupervised practice, they will face a need for continuing professional development as health care evolves. They must be able to recognize the need for ongoing learning and when to seek outside expertise. The determination of how much autonomy is granted and supervision is needed is ideally based on individual trainee's readiness and what the trainee is able to do with appropriate support. Providing an inappropriate level of supervision has implications not only for patient care but also for learning. Underestimating the level of a trainee's readiness for additional responsibility threatens their sense of competence, autonomy, and intrinsic motivation to learn. Overestimating a trainee's level of readiness places the trainee in situations where they feel they are not competent or do not have adequate supervision or support in place to act, resulting in suboptimal learning and patient care. Thus, matching levels of supervision and autonomy with levels of competence is critical for patient safety and driving trainees' desire to learn. Within competency-based education, entrustable professional activities (EPAs) seek to achieve this balance by linking entrustment decisions to a trainee's readiness to perform a given professional activity under a specified level of supervision.

In practice, decisions around autonomy and supervision are also influenced by factors beyond trainee readiness. The characteristics and experience of the clinical supervisor, their relationship with the trainee, the complexity or risk of the patient care activity, and the clinical and workplace context all impact a clinical supervisor's decision.[7] Furthermore, the desired levels of autonomy and supervision for trainee development and safe patient care may not always fully align with local regulations. Local rules and regulations often determine the limits of autonomy based on certifications or fixed stages of training (student, intern, senior resident, etc.) and are not tailored to specific trainees or for specific activities. Many regulations often demand continued high levels of supervision throughout training, limiting trainee autonomy even after trainees have demonstrated readiness for more autonomy. In addition to the negative impacts on learning noted above, this can result in trainees lacking responsibility experience and graduating less than ready for unsupervised practice. Recent graduates must then practice unsupervised in systems that cannot always ensure appropriate levels of supervision, resulting in stress for the graduates and threats to patient safety. Therefore, the sweet spot in health professions education should ensure adequate supervision for safe, effective patient care and adequate autonomy for trainee development and eventual readiness for practice.

Theoretical support for graded autonomy

A variety of existing theoretical lenses support and provide context for understanding the importance of graded autonomy over time. Three important lenses to address include self-determination theory, situated learning theory, and the learning-oriented teaching model.[8] Self-determination theory (SDT), created by Deci and Ryan, posits that an individual's natural propensity for learning is driven by simultaneously fulfilling three innate psychological needs: sense of relatedness, sense of autonomy, and sense of competence.[9,10] Relatedness focuses on feeling part of a community and of a profession. Thus, allowing trainees to meaningfully contribute to patient care as a member of a health care team is important to their becoming a professional. Lave and Wenger, using situated learning theory, advocate 'legitimate peripheral participation,' where even the newest or most junior team members are given tasks and roles that are important to the team rather than merely serving as observers (Figure 3.1).[11] This fosters relatedness but also gives trainees meaningful work to advance their development in a relevant manner, promoting the second SDT psychological need to be satisfied, a sense of competence, defined as feeling that one knows and is able to do something. While a sense of competence naturally arises from experience and the development of one's abilities, it is important to note that even trainees early in their development can feel a sense of competence when their work is aligned with their abilities and when appropriate scaffolding is provided to push their continued development. In addition, a sense of competence and self-efficacy is also derived from feedback, i.e., from an environment that reinforces one's competence.[8] An entrustment decision is a powerful implicit confirmation of efficacy and competence. Finally, autonomy speaks to the importance of feeling that one is an individual acting of one's own volition. Autonomy, as it is defined within SDT, should not be confused with performing in the absence of a team or supervision as trainees can be allowed to act of their own volition and take responsibility for their clinical actions even while acting as a member of a team or being supervised.[12] Rather, it advocates for clinical supervisors allowing for trainees' plans or ideas to prevail when accompanied by a clear, reasonable, and well-supported rationale.

Situated learning theory, developed in the 1980s to 1990s, contends that learning is constructed from, and inextricably linked to, the environment, the situations, and culture surrounding an individual.[13] Trainees, as apprentices to health care professionals, acquire necessary skills and are socialized into a profession by participating in legitimate work activities and interacting with members of the profession. *Cognitive apprenticeships*, a concept within situated learning theory, structure apprenticeship experiences with a deliberate focus on learning the thought processes of the profession from someone who is part of the culture and context of the profession. The training of health professions trainees in the clinical workplace typically aligns with this model as trainees learn to think, act, and feel like health professionals. Here, trainees seek, and workplace supervisors choose for them, experiences and tasks based on both workplace needs and the learning needs and readiness of the trainee. Supervisors developmentally sequence tasks and provide coaching and guidance to support trainee contributions to the workplace and promote ongoing development. This tailoring of workplace learning experiences and tasks has been identified as a core principle in competency-based education.[14]

In 2004, ten Cate et al. proposed a learning-oriented model of teaching with a focus on the gradual transition from full guidance by the educational program (including teachers) to fully internalized guidance by the trainee; a model rooted in situated learning theory. Here, learning is defined at three levels: cognitive (the what of leaning), affective (the why of learning), and meta-cognitive (the how of learning). The teacher's role is to support learning at all three levels and provide *constructive friction*.[15,16] Constructive friction occurs when trainees are placed into their zone of proximal development. The zone of proximal development is the space of development where a trainee cannot yet perform on their own but can perform with adequate guidance and assistance.[17] Constructive friction is where trainees experience slight discomfort, provoking deliberate learning efforts that lead to optimal learning.[3] Too little friction or too much support does not lead to effort to learn and develop; too little support creates too much friction and can be destructive when trainees experience learning and development challenges beyond their reach.

Entrustment as both a conclusion and a start

In conventional curricular philosophy, teachers set learning objectives for each course, clinical rotation, or training phase. Trainees, guided by teachers and clinical supervisors, strive to meet these objectives by completing assignments or tasks. Teachers and clinical supervisors, in turn, assess how trainees demonstrate their knowledge and skills and whether these tasks have been successfully completed. This focus in trainee assessment is exemplified by Miller's pyramid, which outlines the progression from knowledge acquisition to the application of that knowledge in practical scenarios. The preset learning objectives and assessment focused on a trainee's demonstrations of proficiency to date reflect a retrospective approach to both teaching and determination of competence where competence is the conclusion.[18]

The EPA framework introduces an alternate curricular and assessment model that is forward-facing. In this model, the curriculum is designed with a focus on the future professional responsibilities of trainees. Trainees are granted incremental autonomy, where they are increasingly entrusted with patient care responsibilities as they move closer to becoming unsupervised health professionals. Assessments are prospective and anchored upon entrustment decision-making. Rather than determining the competence of trainees based on retrospective assessments of proficiency demonstrated to date, assessors engage with trainees in a process of *determining readiness* for the next phase of learning and patient care responsibility—competence as a start. Trainees who are deemed ready are awarded increased responsibility and empowered to explore the next stage of learning with graded autonomy. This awarding or entrustment of responsibility is based on the estimation that the trainee can manage the associated risks with decreased supervision and whether their supervisors can bear the risks associated with the trainees' decreased supervision.

Accustomed to old paradigms of assignment completion and retrospective assessments, trainees and supervisors may reflexively view the attainment of an entrustment level as the 'end' or the completion of an assignment. However, entrustment with the need for less supervision indicates a move from the periphery to a more central position within the patient care community (Figure 3.1). This represents the opening, rather than the closing, of a door. A higher level of responsibility with more autonomy and less supervision for the same EPA corresponds to increasing levels of mastery. Entrustment by a clinical supervisor is therefore an acknowledgment of readiness to assume more patient care responsibility on their trajectory to becoming an unsupervised health professional.

Beyond supervisor and trainee—curriculum to support graded autonomy

Considerations of graded autonomy go beyond the discussion around individual supervisors and trainees. It is also key to curricular designs that support trainees on their developmental journey to becoming professionals—both preparing trainees for their graded responsibilities in patient care and actually providing increased responsibilities once trainees demonstrate their readiness. Health professions curricula do not always operationalize entrustment as a start of increased contributions to care or award increased autonomy with the awarding of entrustment.[19] This risks the adoption of an EPA framework becoming more of an administrative burden than a true change in the paradigm of health professions education. Emphasizing achievement of entrustment levels as a start of rather than end of learning can help focus institutional, curricular, teacher, and trainee attention on the importance of advancing responsibilities along the continuum of learning.

There are three main types of educational activities that help prepare trainees and represent this continuum of learning and increased responsibility: classroom education, clinical education without contributions to patient care, and clinical education with contributions to patient care. Classroom or non-workplace-based/nonclinical curricula prepare trainees with the core knowledge and skills (or the canonical competence) required to participate in patient care activities.[20] This includes primarily foundational science and clinical knowledge, clinical reasoning skills, and professionalism habits. Clinical education without contributions to patient care include two things: (a) attention to communications and physical examination skills via role plays, peer practice, and simulation and (b) a focus on building understanding of the clinical workplace, health system, and the variety of professional roles and specialties. The latter is often accomplished by brief observerships or clinical exposure placements in clinics and hospitals. Both classroom education and clinical education without contributions to patient care should be designed to equip students with the knowledge and skills and contextual awareness to enter the clinical workplace as participants in patient care. Clinical education with contributions to health care is the final step, in which trainees engage in longer clinical placements and are ideally embedded within a health care team and given responsibilities for patient care. Here trainees practice applying their canonical competence and develop contextual competence.[20] The clinical placements are designed such that, as trainees develop and progress, they are provided with gradually increasing responsibilities, with greater autonomy and contributions to patient care.

An ideal design for curricula supporting graded autonomy is that of the 'vertically integrated' or 'Z-shaped' curriculum. This is in contrast with the more traditional 'H-shaped' curriculum (Figure 3.2). Vertical integration does not just mean early scheduling of clinical experiences.

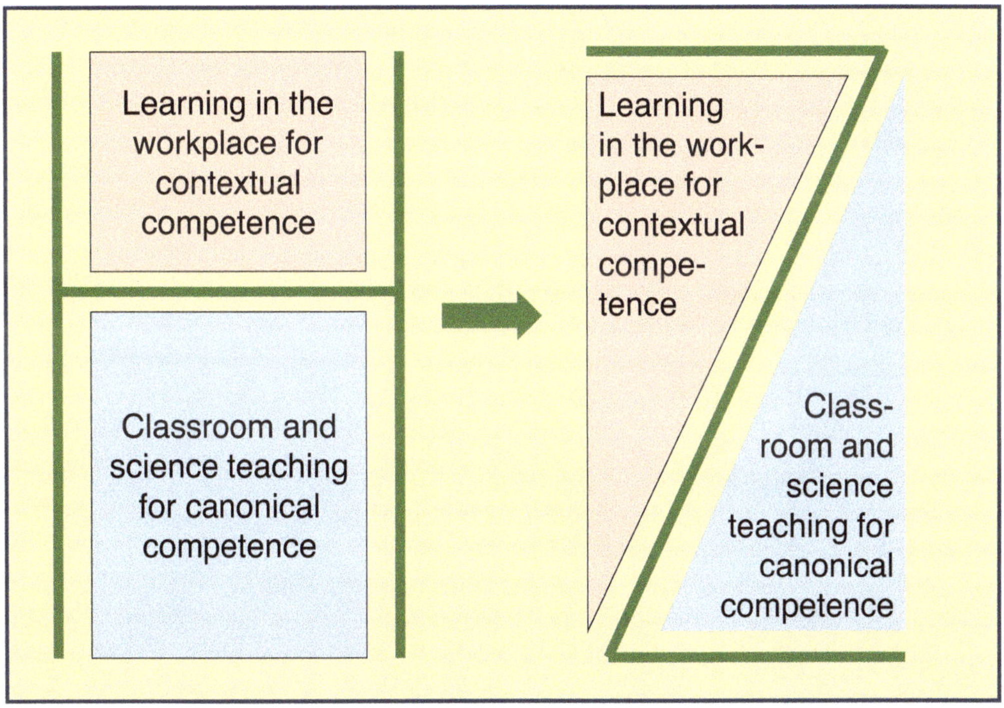

Figure 3.2: Modernization of health professions education toward vertically integrated or Z-shaped curricula with a focus on becoming a professional.

Rather, it involves a deliberate focus on the development of the knowledge, skills, and attitudes required for trainees to assume increasing clinical responsibilities.[1] It addresses the needs of trainees as emerging health professionals with a growing capability, responsibility, and right to care for patients.[2,3] This 'Z-shaped' design aligns with the multilayer model of canonical and contextual competence described above and with the application of entrustment principles.[20]

Conclusion

Health professions education aims to support trainee development toward readiness for unsupervised clinical practice within a professional community of practice. Ideally, an integrated curriculum would prepare trainees early for clinical practice and support that practice with supervision that decreases over time. Clinical supervision should balance supervision for patient safety and trainee learning with increasing clinical responsibilities and contributions to the clinical workplace. This graded increase of autonomy, responsibility, and identification with a profession is not simply an educational method or a different approach to clinical teaching. It is a philosophical frameshift that is supported by various education theories and models, and central to the mission of health professions training. EPAs and entrustment decision-making align with this philosophy and offer a framework that can structure and optimize the development of trainees, by explicitly advancing trainee autonomy, patient care responsibilities, and identification with and entry into the professional community.

Figure justification

Figure 3.2 was adapted with permission from Wijnen-Meijer M, ten Cate OThJ, Rademakers JJDJM, Van der Schaaf MF, Borleffs JCC. The influence of vertical integration in medical school on the transition to postgraduate training. *Med Teach.* 2009;31:11:e528-e532.

Competing interests

The authors declare that they have no competing interests.

References

1. Wijnen-Meijer M, van den Broek S, Koens F, ten Cate O. Vertical integration in medical education: the broader perspective. *BMC Med Educ.* 2020;20(1):509.
2. Cruess RL, Cruess SR, Boudreau JD, Snell L, Steinert Y. Reframing medical education to support professional identity formation. *Acad Med.* 2014;89(11):1446–1451.
3. Merton RK, Reader RG, Kendall P. *The Student-Physician: Introductory Studies in the Sociology of Medical Education.* Harvard University Press; 1957.
4. Dreyfus HL, Dreyfus SE. *Mind over Machine.* Free Press; 1986.
5. Pangaro L. A new vocabulary and other innovations for improving descriptive in-training evaluations. *Acad Med.* 1999;74(11):1203–1207.
6. ten Cate O. *Supervision and Entrustment in Clinical Training: Protecting Patients, Protecting Trainees.* WebM&M Case Studies; 2018;1. https://psnet.ahrq.gov/webmm/case/461
7. Hauer KE, ten Cate O, Boscardin C, Irby DM, Iobst W, O'Sullivan PS. Understanding trust as an essential element of trainee supervision and learning in the workplace. *Adv Health Sci Educ Theory Pract.* 2014;19(3):435–456.

8. Bandura A. Self efficacy: toward a unifying theory of behavioral change. *Psychol Rev.* 1977;84(2):191–215.
9. Ryan RM, Deci EL. Self-determination theory and the facilitation of intrinsic motivation, social development, and well-being. *Am Psychol.* 2000;55(1):68–78.
10. ten Cate TJ, Kusurkar RA, Williams GC. How self-determination theory can assist our understanding of the teaching and learning processes in medical education. AMEE guide No. 59. *Med Teach.* 2011;33(12):961–973.
11. Lave J, Wenger E. *Situated Learning: Legitimate Peripheral Participation (Learning in Doing: Social, Cognitive and Computational Perspectives).* 1st ed. Cambridge University Press; 1991.
12. Schumacher DJ, Bria C, Frohna JG. The quest toward unsupervised practice: promoting autonomy, not independence. *JAMA.* 2013;310(24):2613–2614.
13. Brown JS, Collins A, Duguid P. Situated cognition and the culture of learning. *Educational Researcher.* 1989;18(1):32–42.
14. Van Melle E, Frank JR, Holmboe ES, et al. A core components framework for evaluating implementation of competency-based medical education programs. *Acad Med.* 2019;94(7):1002–1009.
15. ten Cate O, Snell L, Mann K, Vermunt J. Orienting teaching toward the learning process. *Acad Med.* 2004;79(3):219–228.
16. Vermunt JD, Verloop N. Congruence and friction between learning and teaching. *Learning and Instruction.* 1999;9(3):257–280.
17. Chaiklin S. The zone of proximal development in Vygotsky's analysis of learning and instruction. In: Kozulin A, Gindis B, Ageyev VS, Miller SM, eds. *Vygotsky's Educational Theory in Cultural Context.* Cambridge University Press; 2003:39–64.
18. Schumacher DJ, Cate OT, Damodaran A, et al. Clarifying essential terminology in entrustment. *Med Teach.* 2021;43(7):737–744.
19. ten Cate O, Jarrett JB. *Would* I trust or *will* I trust? The gap between entrustment determinations and entrustment decisions for trainees in pharmacy and other health professions. *Pharmacy (Basel).* 2023;11(3).
20. ten Cate O, Khursigara-Slattery N, Cruess RL, Hamstra SJ, Steinert Y, Sternszus R. Medical competence as a multilayered construct. *Med Educ.* 2024;58(1):93–104.

CHAPTER 4

Theoretical foundations of trust and entrustment in health professions education

Brian C. Gin, Ylva Holzhausen, Natasha Khursigara-Slattery, H. Carrie Chen, Daniel J. Schumacher, Olle ten Cate

Abstract

The purpose of this chapter is to conceptualize trust within the context of entrustment in clinical education—to clarify what its purpose is, what its components are, how decisions about it are made, and what other forms of trust it relates to. In a general context, trust is a ubiquitous and intuitive construct that emerges within relationships, enabling individuals to cooperate and collaborate to perform tasks that they might not otherwise be able to perform alone. The trust specific to entrustment emerges from the interdependent goals of patient care and trainee learning, creating reciprocity between supervisor and trainee. Starting from a definition of trust in which risk assessment is central, proposed by Mayer et al. in 1995, additional details are added to conceptualize entrustment's unique form of trust. Considerations include contrasting the trustworthiness of clinical trainees with that of general trustworthiness, and consolidating the factors that influence entrustment decision-making. The connections between entrustment and other forms of trust within the patient–supervisor–trainee triad are also considered: trainee trust in their supervisors, and patient trust in trainees—including entrustment's role in ensuring patients' presumptive trust in trainees is justified. A unified model of entrustment is presented that incorporates these dimensions of trust and their theoretical conceptualizations.

How to cite this book chapter:

Brian CG, Holzhausen Y, Khursigara-Slattery N, Chen CH, Schumacher DJ, ten Cate O. Theoretical foundations of trust and entrustment in health professions education. In: ten Cate O, Burch VC, Chen HC, Chou FC, Hennus MP. (Eds). *Entrustable Professional Activities and Entrustment Decision-Making in Health Professions Education*, Chapter 4, pp. 35–50. [2024] London: Ubiquity Press. DOI: https://doi.org/10.5334/bdc.d

This chapter uses cross-references to other chapters of the same book. For those who read this chapter as a standalone publication: all cross-references can be found at: https://doi.org/10.5334/bdc

Authors

- Brian C. Gin, MD, PhD. University of California San Francisco, San Francisco, California, USA. Correspondence: brian.gin@ucsf.edu
- Ylva Holzhausen, PhD. Charité-Universitätsmedizin Berlin, Berlin, Germany.
- Natasha Khursigara-Slattery, MD, MEHP. Mid-West Intern Network, University of Limerick, Limerick, Ireland.
- H. Carrie Chen, MD, PhD. Kaiser Permanente Bernard J. Tyson School of Medicine, Pasadena, California, USA.
- Daniel J. Schumacher, MD, PhD, MEd. Cincinnati Children's Hospital Medical Center/ University of Cincinnati College of Medicine, Cincinnati, Ohio, USA.
- Olle ten Cate, PhD. University Medical Center Utrecht, Utrecht, the Netherlands and University of California, San Francisco, USA.

The purpose of trust within the concept of entrustment

Trust is intuitive—everyone knows what trust is—yet a unifying definition of trust evades description. Definitions of trust[1] appear to take various forms dependent on context and application. As such, considering trust's purpose is a prerequisite to conceptualizing it in the context of entrustment.[a]

Broadly considered, trust emerges in response to needs for social cooperation in specific settings and relationships. Trust emerges in relationships of all kinds—from a child dependent on their caregiver, to coworkers bound toward a common goal, or even to strangers walking and driving past each other at a stoplight. Trust is not uniquely human; it appears to emerge in animal relationships and societies as well, and perhaps between all sentient[b] beings that are interdependent, or at least expect something of one another. Trust appears to enable individuals to cooperate or collaborate to achieve more complex goals than they may be able to reach on their own.[2,3] It also appears to reduce the complexity individuals face when operating within a complex environment, and to contend with the myriad of outcomes that they cannot directly control.[4] Trust, whether instinctual or learned, appears to be a foundational part of development that allows an individual to function within relationships, social groups, and larger systems.[5] In the clinical learning environment, trust is necessary for patients, supervisors, and trainees to navigate the sometimes contradictory goals of delivering safe and consistent patient care versus educating trainees who arrive with a wide range of experience.[6]

The purpose of trust in clinical learning is to support safe and standards-based patient care in conjunction with trainee learning. A supervisor's entrustment of a trainee with a task is a multifaceted decision that enables them to delegate a specific level of responsibility for patient care to the trainee. The entrustment concept operationalizes this trust to deliver a framework applicable to both formative and summative assessment. Lower-stakes entrustment includes supervisors' so-called ad hoc entrustment decisions—day-to-day decisions about how much supervision to provide trainees in actual practice scenarios. Summative entrustment captures higher-stakes decisions training programs make about trainees' readiness for advancement in clinical responsibility. Indeed, trust and entrustment have recently become a major component of the discourse in health professions education and assessment.[6] While entrustment decisions vary in scale and scope, they share a common requirement: for assessments based on supervisor trust to be valid, there must be transparency around how trust is defined and how trainee trustworthiness is determined.

Trust and risk

Differences in definitions of trust include whether trustworthiness is distinct from trust, what trustworthiness is, and whether trust implies reciprocity.[7] Despite these differences, most definitions of trust appear to involve the assumption of risk or vulnerability by the trustor to be subject to or dependent upon future action of the trustee. Consistent with this common thread, the entrustment literature (and other literature on trust in clinical settings) appears to most frequently cite the definition of Mayer et al.: 'willingness of a party to be vulnerable to the actions of another based on the expectation that the other will perform a particular action important to the trustor, irrespective of the ability to monitor or control that other party,'[1] or, in short, 'willingness to be vulnerable to another party who cannot be monitored or controlled.'[8]

---

[a] Validity frameworks also advocate for articulating the purpose, intended interpretations, and consequences of an assessment as a prerequisite to its design[68]—including one operationalizing trust as a form of assessment (i.e. entrustment).

[b] Sentient, since they must be able to make a decision (or not) to trust. Note that the decision need not be conscious.

If entrustment derives from the trust a supervisor has in a trainee to perform a clinical task for a patient, then the vulnerability or risk that the supervisor assumes depends inversely upon the trainee's ability to perform the task well. Yet trust cannot be about risk and vulnerability only. After all, placing a bet also entails determining and assuming risk—but betting on someone is not the same as trusting them.[c] For a supervisor's assumed risk to amount to trust, it must also include specific beliefs about the trainee's trustworthiness, and occur in the setting of a trusting relationship with the trainee.

Trustworthiness

Specific requirements for a trustee's trustworthiness distinguish trust from merely being an exercise in risk management. A trustor must not only assess the risk posed by delegating a task to a trustee but also be motivated to accept that risk based on belief in the trustee's *trustworthiness* to perform that task. Per Mayer et al. the characteristics of trustworthiness fall into three factors: *ability, benevolence*, and *integrity*.[1,8] A trustee's *ability* and *integrity* may also be assessed by a bettor, investor,[d] or actuary, but *benevolence* is a characteristic that appears to set trust apart from these other forms of risk management. Belief in the benevolence of a trustee means that the trustor believes the trustee will approach a task with their best intentions—in the case of entrustment, this is the shared (and primary) goal of patient care, and the secondary goal of learning and self-improvement.

When considering the trustworthiness of trainees in the clinical learning environment, additional features beyond Mayer's three factors must be considered. ten Cate and Chen developed a framework specific to trainee trustworthiness by examining how supervisors evaluate trainee characteristics to make entrustment decisions. Synthesizing findings from empirical studies, they described five themes: *agency, reliability, integrity, capability*, and *humility*—called the A RICH model (Table 4.1).[9] Considering how Mayer's general trustworthiness overlaps with A RICH, *ability* and *integrity* tie directly to *capability* and *integrity*. *Benevolence*, on the other hand, manifests in multiple A RICH themes—in *reliability*, 'conscientious behavior driven by a sense of accountability and responsibility' to patients; in *integrity*, 'decisions ... motivated by concern for and made in the best interest of patients'; and, in *humility*, 'receptivity to insights of patients and co-workers.'

Despite their overlap, a defining feature that distinguishes trainee trustworthiness from general trustworthiness is the key role that trainee *humility* plays in entrustment. In entrustment, the supervisor has the option to intervene in the performance of the clinical task (see Figure 4.4 and the final discussion below), which is not generally the case with all forms of trust. This places a degree of responsibility on the trainee to seek help when necessary, based on understanding their own limitations. A trainee's humility reflects both their willingness and effectiveness to utilize their supervisor's support in a way that balances patient safety with their own growth, reflecting an (implicit or explicit) agreement inherent to clinical entrustment. Indeed, empirical studies by

---

[c] While risk and vulnerability may be necessary for trust, they are not sufficient. Trust cannot be solely about vulnerability and risk, even if related to the accomplishment of tasks that are critically important to the trustor. For example, an investor may assume risk by acquiring equity in an entity which they do not trust, with the hope of nevertheless achieving a positive return. In this scenario, the investor may fulfill Mayer's definition of trust by becoming vulnerable to another party to 'perform a particular action important to the trustor,' yet the investor has made a bet, rather than putting trust in the entity. Similarly, in the context of clinical training, betting on someone would not be the same as trusting them.

[d] While financial/investment advisers and portfolio managers may have the 'fiduciary responsibility' to act in the best interest of their clients, the same cannot be said of investors in general. For instance, when investors participate in 'short selling,' they are betting on the failure of a company's stock.

Table 4.1: Dimensions of trainee trustworthiness: the A RICH model.[9]

A Agency	R Reliability	I Integrity	C Capability	H Humility
Proactive attitude toward work, team, safety and personal development that includes awareness of and acting upon the need for action even when outside of the strict definition of one's responsibilities and practice of adaptive expertise. Agency can manifest within the context of one or more of the other four factors	Consistent, predictable, and conscientious behavior driven by a sense of accountability and responsibility	Truthfulness, benevolence, and patient-centeredness, where expertise is employed to benefit patients and decisions are motivated by concern for and made in the best interest of patients	The ability to perform a specific task in a variety of contexts and within an appropriate time frame, requiring a reasonable understanding and overall view of the clinical situation and ability to communicate and work effectively with others within a system	Discernment of one's limitations; willingness and ability to ask for help and feedback; receptivity to insights of patients and coworkers; and ability to learn and develop from mistakes, feedback, and the expertise of others

Schumacher et al. and others have demonstrated trainee humility to be a foundational feature of clinical entrustment.[10,11]

Trusting relationships

In the context of entrustment, a trusting relationship and mutual trust arise from the paired goals of patient care and learning—which are important not only to the trustor (supervisor) but also to the trustee (trainee). The optimal level of trust balances risks to patient care (which might drive more supervision) and opportunities for trainee growth (which might impel less supervision). Even if learning were not included, the shared goal of patient care would be sufficient to necessitate reciprocity: the trainee also assumes risk when being entrusted—risk that they will receive the appropriate amount of support from the supervisor to perform the task, and that the supervisor will provide supervision appropriate for their experience and ability. As such, the trainee must also trust their supervisor, and thus reciprocity appears to derive from the interdependence of supervisor and trainee for patient care and learning.[12,13] Indeed, several empirical studies support this finding, suggesting that trusting relationships are also a key feature of supervisor–trainee trust.[14,15] Within the context of clinical entrustment, it appears that the formation of a trusting relationship reflects the reciprocity inherent in depending on each other to achieve these common goals.

Entrustment decision-making

In addition to the trainee's trustworthiness and the relationship between supervisor and trainee, additional factors that contribute to entrustment decisions include a supervisor's propensity to trust, the context of entrustment, and characteristics of the task under consideration.[16–20] The supervisor's propensity to trust relates to their personal risk tolerance and individual

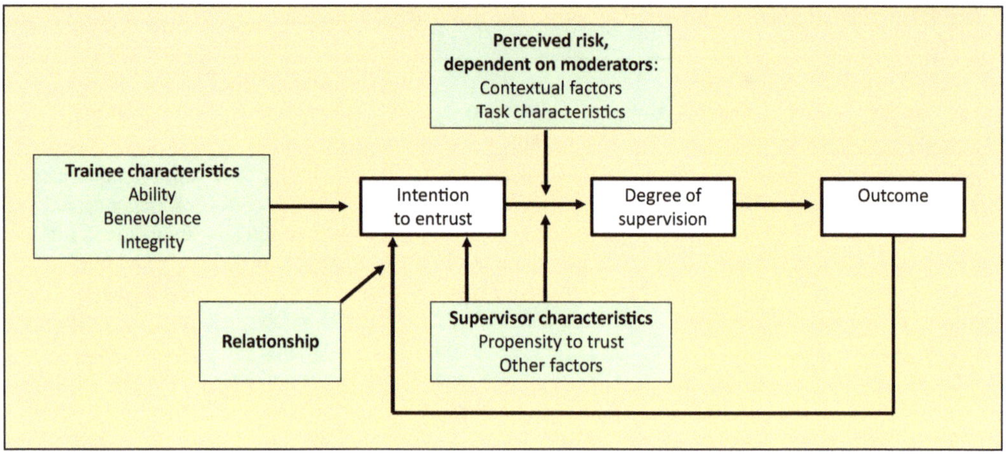

Figure 4.1: Adapted from the expanded Holzhausen model of trust.[16]

estimation of risk. This tolerance may be shaped by emotion[21] and by the supervisor's subjective assessment of the overall situation shaped by their personal experiences and emotions, or *perezhivanie*[22] (also see Chapter 2). The relationship between supervisor and trainee may further modulate this tolerance, via shared risk and responsibility toward achieving common goals. The relationship factor also depends on longitudinality[23] and the accumulation of shared experiences.[24] Indeed, cumulative interactions can move entrustment decisions toward grounded trust (based on accumulated evidence of trustworthiness) as compared to initial (swift) trust (based on initial impressions or scant data), or presumptive trust (based on credentials alone).[25]

Contextual and task factors modulate risk via considerations external to the supervisor and trainee, such as the logistical availability of support, patient load/census, and the complexity and/or acuity of the patient's presentation. Even so, these external factors are shaped by subjective experiences of them. For example, perceptions of complexity may differ between an experienced supervisor and a novice trainee.[26] As such, all factors may interact toward determining entrustment. Adapting Mayer et al.'s model of trust to entrustment, and combining this model with insights from Hauer et al.[17] and Cianciolo et al.,[2] Holzhausen et al. and Conroy et al. described how these factors are interrelated and can lead to a positive feedback cycle of trust development between supervisor and trainee (Figure 4.1).[16,27] Ultimately, entrustment need not only be a decision that occurs in the mind of a supervisor but can also be considered a negotiation between a supervisor and trainee, and their environment.

Trust and entrustment decisions by supervisors inherently include personal perceptions and thus a subjective component. While subjectivity cannot be avoided in expert judgment and decision-making, a distinction can be made between legitimate subjectivity and unwanted bias.[28] Prejudice and irrelevant influences should be avoided through awareness training and shared decision-making for both high and low-stakes entrustment (see Chapters 17 and 21).[29]

Beyond supervision—a triad of trust in the clinical learning environment

Entrustment does not occur in a vacuum but rather within a web of interrelated relationships, motivations, and vulnerabilities in the clinical learning environment. While entrustment within the supervisor–trainee dyad represents only a small piece of this puzzle (i.e., a supervisor's trust in a trainee), it is related to, and is dependent on, other manifestations of trust as well.

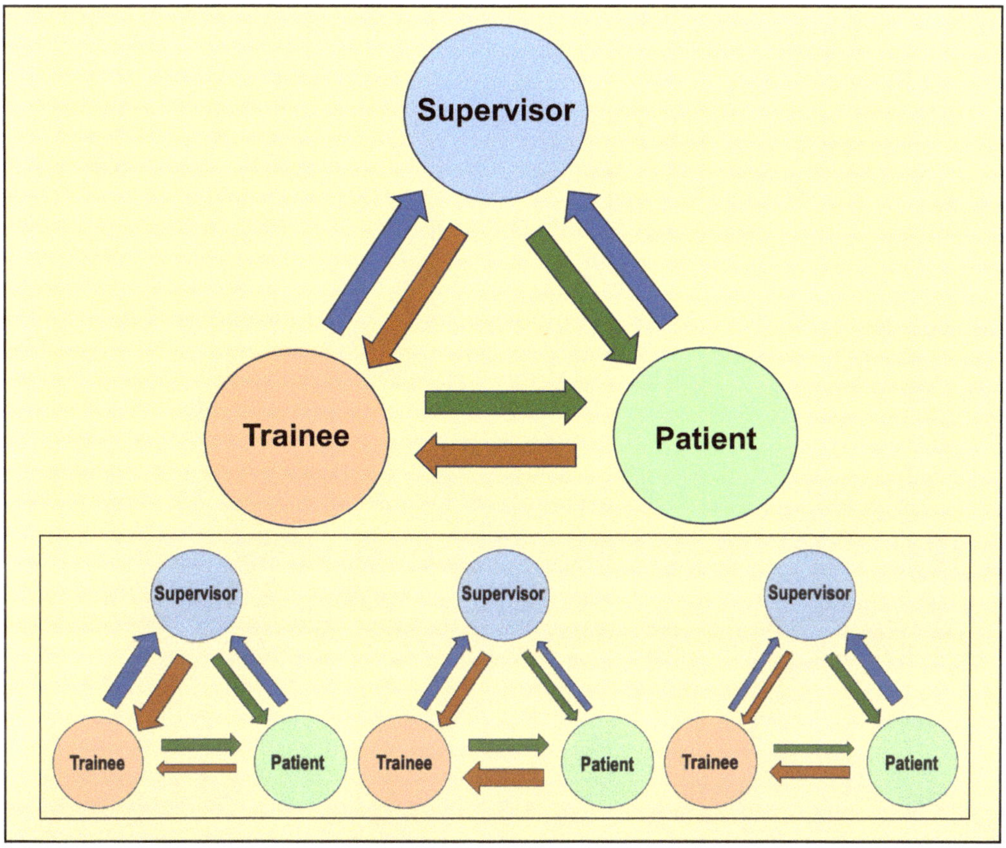

Figure 4.2: Variations of trust relationships in the triad of clinical supervision.

Including the patient in the supervisor–trainee dyad creates a triadic relationship held together by distinct forms of trust needed to facilitate patient care and trainee learning. Patients need to be able to trust those upon whom they are dependent, which includes trainees, to be able to provide the care they need in a safe, effective, caring, and honest manner.[30–32] Trainees need to be able to trust their supervisors (and overall training program) to provide the support they need when caring for patients safely.[33–35] Finally, reflecting entrustment, supervisors need to be able to trust trainees to perform clinical tasks without supervision when appropriate, and to inform the supervisor when they need assistance.[10]

Figure 4.2 shows the interdependent triad of trainee, patient, and supervisor trust. The wideness of the arrows represents the strength of trust, which can vary in six directions. Occasionally patients may have more trust in the trainee than in their supervisor, but it could be the other way around. Likewise, a trainee might trust their supervisor more, or less, to support them if needed and to provide psychological safety.[36] A supervisor might know and trust a patient to be willing to work with a trainee or not, and, finally, the supervisor might trust a particular trainee more, or less, with this patient and this activity. All dynamics together affect the supervisor's ad hoc decision to entrust the trainee with the activity.

Two components of this triadic relationship closely related to entrustment include trainee trust in supervisors and patient trust in trainees—explored further below. Other aspects of the triad are also considered in Table 4.2. The triadic relationship itself lies within a broader landscape of interprofessional and institutional trust.[37–40]

Table 4.2: Various directions of trust in the clinical learning environment in the trainee–supervisor–patient triad.

Trustor	Trustee	Aim of trust	Hypothetical quotes from a trustor reflecting trustee trustworthiness	Hypothetical quotes from a trustor reflecting their decision to trust	References
supervisor	**trainee**	entrustment with a clinical task	'this trainee seems ready for this responsibility'	'I can leave the room,' 'I'll recommend a summative entrustment decision for Level 4'	17,20,25,55 56,57 15,24,48,58
trainee	**patient**	receiving feedback	'this is a thoughtful patient with a valuable perspective'	'I'll ask for feedback from the patient,' 'I'll use that feedback and share it with a preceptor'	53
patient	**supervisor**	receiving good care	'this doctor knows what they're doing,' 'previous decisions were right'	'I'll do whatever they recommend,' 'I can reveal honesty and confidential information'	59,60
supervisor	**patient**	expecting honesty and cooperation	'this patient is highly cooperative,' 'understands my questions,' 'gives sensible and honest answers,' and 'will do what they promise to do'	'I will propose and discuss all reasonable diagnostic and therapeutic options,' 'I will make an agreement on therapeutic adherence and will ask the patient to report any problems to me'	61
patient	**trainee**	receiving good care	'this trainee seems to know what they're doing,' 'is honest about what they cannot yet do,' and 'knows when and how to ask for help if needed'	'I will consider them to be my doctor'	31,32,40,62
trainee	**supervisor**	receiving good guidance/instruction, receiving unbiased and fair ratings/assessment, receiving adequate autonomy, supervisor is available or accessible if needed	'this preceptor has impressive content expertise and experience,' 'is benevolent toward patients and toward me,' 'will not deceive me,' and 'keeps their word'	'I'll do what the preceptor asks me, even if I'm not fully convinced,' 'I'll ask for honest feedback,' 'I'll report that careless mistake I just made'	33,34,41,44,47
trainee	**trainee**	maintaining patient safety while learning via self-regulation and balance between independence and help-seeking	'I don't need to convince myself that I'm a legitimate provider, yet at the same time I know I also don't need to know everything'	'I know that I am able to perform this task without supervisor assistance, but if I ever get outside of my comfort zone, I'll ask for help'	63,64 26,65,66 67

Trainee trust in their supervisor

While decisions to assign clinical responsibility may fall on a supervisor, the trainee's trust in their supervisor may affect their motivation to fully engage in those responsibilities, and their ability to learn from them. Trainees need to be able to trust that their supervisor will support them to care for patients safely, and to evaluate their deficiencies in a manner that leads to learning rather than rejection or rebuke.[33,34,41] While trainees' acknowledgment of their own limitations is a key component of their trustworthiness,[10] this candidness must be met with the expectation that supervisors will respond positively to trainees' display of vulnerability. This is not the case by default, as trainees may struggle with the tension between a desire to perform well but also to receive feedback on their true level of ability.[42] Trust between trainees and supervisors, along with a shared understanding of the purpose of assessment, may help to alleviate this tension. Indeed, trainee trust in their supervisor, and their belief in the supervisor's benevolence—a ubiquitous factor in trustworthiness—supports their acceptance of feedback.[43–46] Such a reciprocal relationship has been described by Telio et al. as an 'educational alliance' akin to the 'therapeutic alliance' supporting openness between patients and providers.[47]

With respect to entrustment, trainees must also trust their supervisors to make appropriate entrustment decisions that enable them to both learn and take care of patients. Empiric studies suggest that trainees who perceived their supervisors' trust to be appropriately matched to their self-perceived trustworthiness experienced subjectively better learning and engagement with patients and medical teams.[48] When trainees believed they were trusted less than they deserved, they often felt detached from their patients, less motivated to learn, and micromanaged.[15] At the other extreme, Klasen et al. have recently explored the concept of allowing trainees to fail. While trainees could view these scenarios as representing a lack of support, they also perceived them to be potentially valuable learning opportunities, colored by their perception of their supervisor's intentions—intentions that may be shaped by the trainee's trust in their supervisor.[35]

Patient trust in trainees as care providers

While supervisors can make decisions to trust trainees (or not) based on grounded trust (i.e., well-documented past performances and interactions), patients are not privy to the same information[e] or choice. Since patients cannot directly oversee trainee providers, training institutions have the obligation to ensure that patients' presumptive, and indeed obligatory, trust in trainees is justified. Despite this obligation to patients, program directors occasionally decide to graduate trainees who they would not necessarily trust with their own family members.[49] In informal polls across various audiences at workshops and conferences in 2022 and 2023, ten Cate asked the question: 'Have you ever *personally* signed off for completion of a program or rotation, while not fully confident that the trainee had met critical objectives?' Many of the 329 respondents said they remembered such cases (Figure 4.3). The entrustment concept is intended to address this issue by providing transparency in trainee trust—in 'educating trainees to be worthy' of their patients' trust.

Patient trust in providers has been a well-studied area in the literature, with multiple instruments designed to measure this construct. In these studies, patient trust in providers is most often interpreted as the patient's perception of their provider's trustworthiness. Mayer et al.'s model has been used in this context as well, as many models include the three factors of ability, benevolence, and integrity in some form.[11] For example, Greene et al. describe dimensions of

---

[e] Also, trainees do not have online reviews that licensed professionals usually may have (and whether such reviews are reliable is also a matter of contention).

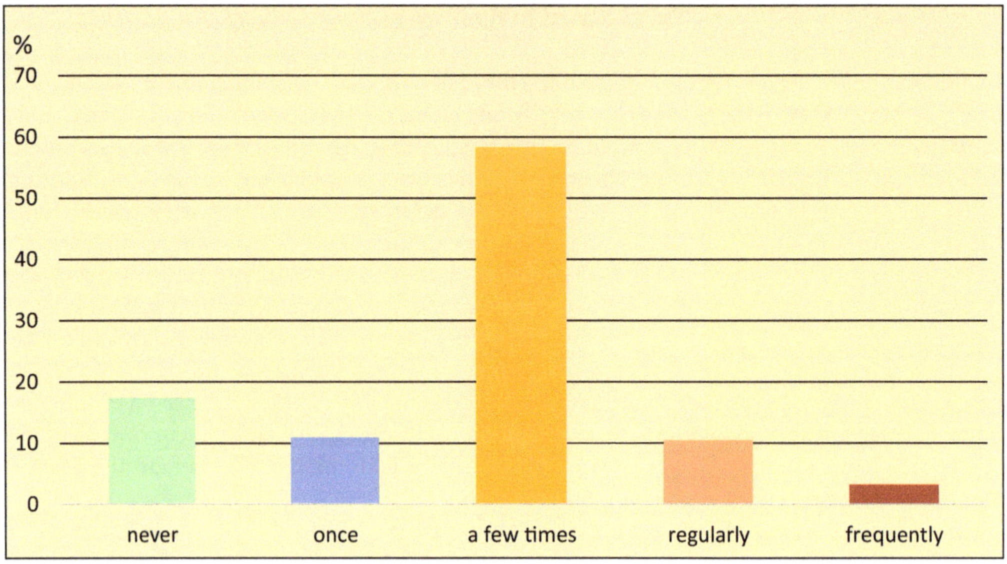

Figure 4.3: Percentage of clinical educators answering the question: 'Have you ever *personally* signed off for completion of a program or rotation, while not fully confident that the trainee had met critical objectives?' (N=329, across 10 occasions).

competence, caring, and communication.[30] Despite the qualitative distinctness of these factors, quantitative studies indicate patient trust is a unidimensional construct, suggesting inextricable overlap between these factors.[39,50]

The subset of literature on patient trust in providers who are specifically trainees appears to be less well developed. Bonds et al. explored factors associated with trust in resident physicians in a primary care setting, finding that patients' trust in trainees was also strongly dependent on the patients' trust in the hospital system with which the trainees were affiliated.[40] The role of institutional trust was also seen in a study of trainees' reflections on their interactions with patients, which also hinted at reciprocal trust between patient and trainee that facilitated patients' willingness to be vulnerable.[51] Tiyyagura et al. explored how ongoing parental concerns over trainee inexperience may limit supervisors' intentions to allow trainees to perform procedures in the pediatric emergency department, despite reassurances about adequate procedural supervision.[52] El-Haddad et al. have explored the approach of involving patients in entrustment decision-making and considering patient expectations of trainees in the performance of patient care tasks.[31,32]

A unified model of entrustment

We conclude by presenting a unified model of entrustment that summarizes the key features of our discussion in this chapter (Figure 4.4). Trust is defined by Mayer et al. as the acceptance of risk within a relationship,[1] which when applied to entrustment refers to a supervisor's trust in a trainee. The dual goals[7] of patient care and learning create reciprocity in the trust between supervisor and trainee. Not only does a supervisor assess the trustworthiness of the trainee (by assessing the trainee's agency, reliability, integrity, capacity, and humility)[9] but also the trainee accepts (or rejects) the trust that they receive from their supervisor (by assessing their supervisor's credibility, ability to provide support, and benevolence).[33,34,53] This initial step represents an 'intention to entrust,'[7,16] which is determined in relation to the perceived risk and benefit to stakeholders in the

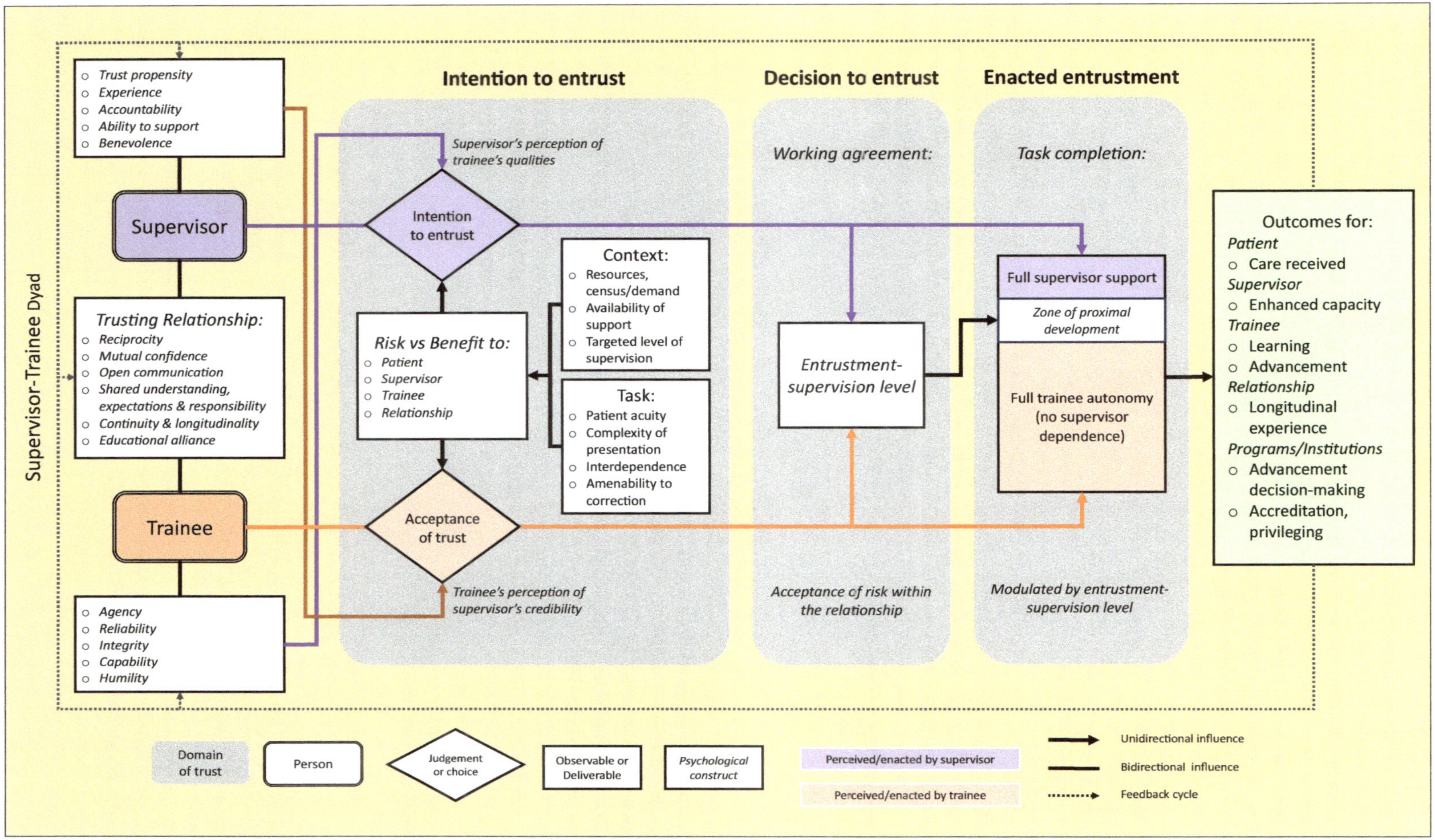

Figure 4.4: A unified model of entrustment, based on several models including Mayer et al.,[1] Castelfranchi et al.,[7] Holzhausen et al.,[16] and ten Cate and Chen.[9]

triadic relationship between patient, supervisor, and trainee. These risks and benefits themselves are influenced by context and task, related to the availability of resources and complexity of the patient presentation.[17]

The 'intention to entrust' is followed by a 'decision to entrust,'[7] which manifests as the entrustment–supervision level.[54] This decision is carried to patient care tasks as 'enacted entrustment,'[7] where it modulates the amount of support the supervisor provides and the degree of autonomy the trainee experiences. The ability of the supervisor to intervene with task completion and to decide when to support the trainee is a characteristic that distinguishes entrustment from generalized trust (the latter in which a trustor is willing 'to be vulnerable to another party who cannot be monitored or controlled'[8]). When supervisors interpose a gap between their level of support and the trainees' prior experiences (or expectations) of autonomy, trainees may experience growth as they push themselves toward practice in this so-called 'zone of proximal development.'[25,54] The outcome of 'enacted entrustment' feeds back on the triadic relationship (affecting each member as shown), while also influencing future entrustment decisions.

It is hoped that this formulation of entrustment and the discussions in this chapter provide clarity on the unique perceptions, circumstances, and forms of trust upon which entrustment depends—while suggesting a research agenda to further elucidate entrustment's many facets.[f] By exploring these dependencies, entrustment can be considered not only as supervisor trust in a trainee but also as a complex social interaction set in the context of a reciprocal relationship—a patient-centered triad.

References

1. Mayer RC, Davis JH, Schoorman FD. An integrative model of organizational trust. *Acad of Manage R.* 1995;20(3):709. DOI: https://doi.org/10.2307/258792
2. Cianciolo AT, Kegg JA. Behavioral specification of the entrustment process. *J Grad Med Educ.* 2013;5(1):10–12. DOI: https://doi.org/10.4300/jgme-d-12-00158.1
3. Cianciolo AT, Evans KM, DeCostanza AH, Pierce LG. Trust in distributed operations. In: *Trust in Military Teams.* CRC Press; 2011:89–106. DOI: https://doi.org/10.1201/9781315549637-6
4. Luhmann N. *Trust and Power.* Wiley; 1979.
5. Munley PH. Erik Erikson's theory of psychosocial development and vocational behavior. *J Couns Psychol.* 1975;22(4):314–319. DOI: https://doi.org/10.1037/h0076749
6. Damodaran A, Shulruf B. Trust in healthcare professions' education: an interdisciplinary research agenda. In: Mayer RC, Mayer BM, eds. *A Research Agenda for Trust.* Edward Elgar Publishing; 2024:185–197.
7. Castelfranchi C, Falcone R. *Trust Theory: A Socio-Cognitive and Computational Model.* Wiley; 2010.
8. Mayer RC, Mayer BM, eds. *A Research Agenda for Trust.* Edward Elgar Publishing; 2024.
9. ten Cate O, Chen HC. The ingredients of a rich entrustment decision. *Med Teach.* 2020;42(12):1413–1420. DOI: https://doi.org/10.1080/0142159X.2020.1817348
10. Schumacher DJ, Michelson C, Winn AS, Turner DA, Elshoff E, Kinnear B. Making prospective entrustment decisions: knowing limits, seeking help and defaulting. *Med Educ.* Published online 2022. DOI: https://doi.org/10.1111/medu.14797
11. Pingree EW, Huth K, Harper BD, et al. Encouraging entrustment: a qualitative study of resident behaviors that promote entrustment. *Acad Med.* 2020;95(11):1718–1725. DOI: https://doi.org/10.1097/ACM.0000000000003487

---

[f] The bulk of empiric support for entrustment decision-making centers on trainee and task characteristics. As such, additional studies on other aspects of this model (including supervisor, relationship, context, and factors affecting trainee trust in supervisor) would be most welcome.

12. Sebok-Syer SS, Chahine S, Watling CJ, Goldszmidt M, Cristancho S, Lingard L. Considering the interdependence of clinical performance: implications for assessment and entrustment. *Med Educ.* Published online 2018. DOI: https://doi.org/10.1111/medu.13588
13. Sebok-Syer SS, Shaw JM, Asghar F, Panza M, Syer MD, Lingard L. A scoping review of approaches for measuring 'interdependent' collaborative performances. *Med Educ.* Published online 2021. DOI: https://doi.org/10.1111/medu.14531
14. Bonnie LHA, Visser MRM, Kramer AWM, van Dijk N. Insight in the development of the mutual trust relationship between trainers and trainees in a workplace-based postgraduate medical training programme: a focus group study among trainers and trainees of the Dutch general practice training programme. *BMJ Open.* 2020;10(4):e036593. DOI: https://doi.org/10.1136/bmjopen-2019-036593
15. Gin BC, Tsoi S, Sheu L, Hauer KE. How supervisor trust affects early residents' learning and patient care: a qualitative study. *Perspect Med Educ.* 2021;10(6):327–333. DOI: https://doi.org/10.1007/S40037-021-00674-9
16. Holzhausen Y, Maaz A, Cianciolo AT, ten Cate O, Peters H. Applying occupational and organizational psychology theory to entrustment decision-making about trainees in health care: a conceptual model. *Perspect Med Educ.* 2017;6(2):119–126. DOI: https://doi.org/10.1007/s40037-017-0336-2
17. Hauer KE, ten Cate O, Boscardin C, Irby DM, Iobst W, O'Sullivan PS. Understanding trust as an essential element of trainee supervision and learning in the workplace. *Advances in Health Sciences Education.* 2013;19(3):435–456. DOI: https://doi.org/10.1007/s10459-013-9474-4
18. Dijksterhuis MGK, Voorhuis M, Teunissen PW, et al. Assessment of competence and progressive independence in postgraduate clinical training. *Med Educ.* 2009;43(12):1156–1165. DOI: https://doi.org/10.1111/j.1365-2923.2009.03509.x
19. Kennedy TJT, Regehr G, Baker GR, Lingard L. Point-of-care assessment of medical trainee competence for independent clinical work. *Acad Med.* 2008;83(Supplement):S89-S92. DOI: https://doi.org/10.1097/ACM.0b013e318183c8b7
20. Sterkenburg A, Barach P, Kalkman C, Gielen M, ten Cate O. When do supervising physicians decide to entrust residents with unsupervised tasks? *Acad Med.* 2010;85:1408–1417. DOI: https://doi.org/10.1097/ACM.0b013e3181eab0ec
21. Gomez-Garibello C, Young M. Emotions and assessment: considerations for rater-based judgements of entrustment. *Med Educ.* 2018;52(3):254–262. DOI: https://doi.org/10.1111/medu.13476
22. ten Cate O, Khursigara-Slattery N, Cruess RL, Hamstra SJ, Steinert Y, Sternszus R. Medical competence as a multilayered construct. *Med Educ.* 2023;(June):1–12. DOI: https://doi.org/10.1111/medu.15162
23. Hirsh DA, Holmboe ES, ten Cate O. Time to trust: longitudinal integrated clerkships and entrustable professional activities. *Acad Med.* Published online 2014. DOI: https://doi.org/10.1097/ACM.0000000000000111
24. Caro Monroig AM, Chen HC, Carraccio C, Richards BF, ten Cate O, Balmer DF. Medical students' perspectives on entrustment decision making in an entrustable professional activity assessment framework: a secondary data analysis. *Acad Med.* 2021;96(8):1175–1181. DOI: https://doi.org/10.1097/ACM.0000000000003858
25. ten Cate O, Hart D, Ankel F, et al. Entrustment decision making in clinical training. *Acad Med.* 2016;91(2):191–198. DOI: https://doi.org/10.1097/ACM.0000000000001044
26. Marty A, Frick S, Bruderer Enzler H, Zundel S. An analysis of core EPAs reveals a gap between curricular expectations and medical school graduates' self-perceived level of competence. *BMC Med Educ.* 2021;21(1):105. DOI: https://doi.org/10.1186/s12909-021-02534-w
27. Conroy M, McCallister J, Gustin J. Entrustment decision making in the intensive care unit: it's about more than the learner. *ATS Sch.* Published online 2023:1–18. DOI: https://doi.org/10.34197/ats-scholar.2023-0060oc

28. Kleijer EFW, Schuurmans MJ, ten Cate O, Pool IA. Preceptors' considerations when entrusting professional activities to postgraduate nursing students: a qualitative study. *Nurse Educ Today*. Published online 2023. DOI: https://doi.org/10.1016/j.nedt.2023.105799
29. ten Cate O, Regehr G. The power of subjectivity in the assessment of medical trainees. *Acad Med*. Published online 2019. DOI: https://doi.org/10.1097/ACM.0000000000002495
30. Greene J, Ramos C. A mixed methods examination of health care provider behaviors that build patients' trust. *Patient Educ Couns*. 2021;104(5):1222–1228. DOI: https://doi.org/10.1016/j.pec.2020.09.003
31. El-Haddad C, Hegazi I, Hu W. A patient expectations questionnaire for determining criteria for entrustment decisions. *Med Teach*. 2021;43(9):1031–1038. DOI: https://doi.org/10.1080/0142159X.2021.1907324
32. El-Haddad C, Damodaran A, McNeil HP, Hu W. A patient-centered approach to developing entrustable professional activities. *Acad Med*. 2017;92(6):800–808. DOI: https://doi.org/10.1097/ACM.0000000000001616
33. Castanelli DJ, Weller JM, Molloy E, Bearman M. How trainees come to trust supervisors in workplace-based assessment: a grounded theory study. *Acad Med*. 2022;97(5):704–710. DOI: https://doi.org/10.1097/ACM.0000000000004501
34. Castanelli DJ, Weller JM, Molloy E, Bearman M. Trust, power and learning in workplace-based assessment: the trainee perspective. *Med Educ*. 2021;(August):1–12. DOI: https://doi.org/10.1111/medu.14631
35. Klasen JM, Teunissen PW, Driessen E, Lingard LA. Trainees' perceptions of being allowed to fail in clinical training: A sense-making model. *Med Educ*. 2023;57(5):430–439. DOI: https://doi.org/10.1111/medu.14966
36. McClintock AH, Fainstad T, Blau K, Jauregui J. Psychological safety in medical education: A scoping review and synthesis of the literature. *Med Teach*. Published online 2023. DOI: https://doi.org/10.1080/0142159X.2023.2216863
37. Muller-Juge V, Cullati S, Blondon KS, et al. Interprofessional collaboration between residents and nurses in general internal medicine: A qualitative study on behaviours enhancing teamwork quality. *PLoS One*. 2014;9(4):1–8. DOI: https://doi.org/10.1371/journal.pone.0096160
38. Thannhauser J, Russell-Mayhew S, Scott C. Measures of interprofessional education and collaboration. *J Interprof Care*. 2010;24(4):336–349. DOI: https://doi.org/10.3109/13561820903442903
39. Hall MA, Dugan E, Zheng B, Mishra AK. Trust in physicians and medical institutions: what is it, can it be measured, and does it matter? *Milbank Quarterly*. 2001;79(4):613–639. DOI: https://doi.org/10.1111/1468-0009.00223
40. Bonds DE, Foley KL, Dugan E, Hall MA, Extrom P. An exploration of patients' trust in physicians in training. *J Health Care Poor Underserved*. 2004;15(2):294–306. DOI: https://doi.org/10.1353/hpu.2004.0018
41. Molloy E, Bearman M. Embracing the tension between vulnerability and credibility: 'intellectual candour' in health professions education. *Med Educ*. 2019;53(1):32–41. DOI: https://doi.org/10.1111/medu.13649
42. Brand PLP, Jaarsma ADC, van der Vleuten CPM. Driving lesson or driving test? a metaphor to help faculty separate feedback from assessment. *Perspect Med Educ*. 2021;10(1):50–56. DOI: https://doi.org/10.1007/s40037-020-00617-w
43. Eva KW, Armson H, Holmboe E, et al. Factors influencing responsiveness to feedback: on the interplay between fear, confidence, and reasoning processes. *Advances in Health Sciences Education*. 2012;17(1):15–26. DOI: https://doi.org/10.1007/s10459-011-9290-7
44. van de Ridder JMM, Berk FCJ, Stokking KM, ten Cate OTJ. Feedback providers' credibility impacts students' satisfaction with feedback and delayed performance. *Med Teach*. 2015;37(8):767–774. DOI: https://doi.org/10.3109/0142159X.2014.970617

45. van de Ridder JMM, Peters CMM, Stokking KM, de Ru JA, ten Cate OTJ. Framing of feedback impacts student's satisfaction, self-efficacy and performance. *Advances in Health Sciences Education*. 2015;20(3):803–816. DOI: https://doi.org/10.1007/s10459-014-9567-8
46. Cordovani L, Tran C, Wong A, Jack SM, Monteiro S. Undergraduate learners' receptiveness to feedback in medical schools: a scoping review. *Med Sci Educ*. 2023;33(5):1253–1269. DOI: https://doi.org/10.1007/s40670-023-01858-0
47. Telio S, Ajjawi R, Regehr G. The 'educational alliance' as a framework for reconceptualizing feedback in medical education. *Acad Med*. 2015;90(5):609–614. DOI: https://doi.org/10.1097/ACM.0000000000000560
48. Karp NC, Hauer KE, Sheu L. Trusted to learn: a qualitative study of clerkship students' perspectives on trust in the clinical learning environment. *J Gen Intern Med*. 2019;34(5):662–668. DOI: https://doi.org/10.1007/s11606-019-04883-1
49. Jonker G, Ochtman A, Marty AP, Kalkman CJ, ten Cate O, Hoff RG. Would you trust your loved ones to this trainee? Certification decisions in postgraduate anaesthesia training. *Br J Anaesth*. Published online 2020. DOI: https://doi.org/10.1016/j.bja.2020.07.009
50. Hall MA, Zheng B, Dugan E, et al. Measuring patients' trust in their primary care providers. *Medical Care Research and Review*. 2002;59(3):293–318. DOI: https://doi.org/10.1177/1077558702059003004
51. Shaughnessy AF, Vicini, SJ A, Zgurzynski M, O'Reilly-Jacob M, Duggan AP. Indicators of the dimensions of trust (and mistrust) in early primary care practice: a qualitative study. *BMC Primary Care*. 2023;24(1):150. DOI: https://doi.org/10.1186/s12875-023-02098-2
52. Tiyyagura G, Balmer D, Chaudoin L, et al. The greater good: how supervising physicians make entrustment decisions in the pediatric emergency department. *Acad Pediatr*. 2014;14(6):597–602. DOI: https://doi.org/10.1016/j.acap.2014.06.001
53. Eijkelboom MCL, De Kleijn RAM, Van diemen WJM, Maljaars CDN, Van Der Schaaf MF, Frenkel J. Patients as feedback providers: exploring medical students' credibility judgments. *Perspect Med Educ*. 2023;12(1):129–140. DOI: https://doi.org/10.5334/pme.842
54. ten Cate O, Schwartz A, Chen HC. Assessing trainees and making entrustment decisions: on the nature and use of entrustment-supervision scales. *Acad Med*. Published online 2020: 1662–1669. DOI: https://doi.org/10.1097/ACM.0000000000003427
55. Gingerich A, Daniels V, Farrell L, Olsen SR, Kennedy T, Hatala R. Beyond hands-on and hands-off: supervisory approaches and entrustment on the inpatient ward. *Med Educ*. 2018;52(10):1028–1040. DOI: https://doi.org/10.1111/medu.13621
56. Sheu L, Kogan JR, Hauer KE. How supervisor experience influences trust, supervision, and trainee learning: a qualitative study. *Acad Med*. 2017;92(9):1320–1327. DOI: https://doi.org/10.1097/ACM.0000000000001560
57. Hatala R, Ginsburg S, Gauthier S, Melvin L, Taylor D, Gingerich A. Supervising the senior medical resident: entrusting the role, supporting the tasks. *Med Educ*. 2022;56(12):1194–1202. DOI: https://doi.org/10.1111/medu.14883
58. Duijn CCMA, Welink LS, Mandoki M, ten Cate OTJ, Kremer WDJ, Bok HGJ. Am I ready for it? Students' perceptions of meaningful feedback on entrustable professional activities. *Perspect Med Educ*. 2017;6(4):256–264. DOI: https://doi.org/10.1007/s40037-017-0361-1
59. Taylor LA, Nong P, Platt J. Fifty years of trust research in health care: a synthetic review. *Milbank Quarterly*. 2023;101(1):126–178. DOI: https://doi.org/10.1111/1468-0009.12598
60. Pokhilenko I, van Esch TEM, Brabers AEM, de Jong JD. Relationship between trust and patient involvement in medical decision-making: a cross-sectional study. *PLoS One*. 2021;16(8 August). DOI: https://doi.org/10.1371/journal.pone.0256698
61. Grob R, Darien G, Meyers D. Why physicians should trust in patients. *JAMA*. Published online 2019. DOI: https://doi.org/10.1001/jama.2019.1500

62. Crossley J, Eiser C, Davies HA. Children and their parents assessing the doctor-patient interaction: a rating system for doctors' communication skills. *Med Educ.* 2005;39(8):820–828. DOI: https://doi.org/10.1111/j.1365-2929.2005.02230.x
63. Sagasser MH, Kramer AWM, Fluit CRMG, van Weel C, van der Vleuten CPM. Self-entrustment: how trainees' self-regulated learning supports participation in the workplace. *Advances in Health Sciences Education.* 2017;22(4):931–949. DOI: https://doi.org/10.1007/s10459-016-9723-4
64. Sturman N, Parker M, Jorm C. Clinical supervision in general practice training: the interweaving of supervisor, trainee and patient entrustment with clinical oversight, patient safety and trainee learning. *Advances in Health Sciences Education.* 2021;26(1):297–311. DOI: https://doi.org/10.1007/s10459-020-09986-7
65. Padilla EP, Stahl CC, Jung SA, et al. Gender differences in entrustable professional activity evaluations of general surgery residents. *Ann Surg.* 2022;275(2):222–229. DOI: https://doi.org/10.1097/SLA.0000000000004905
66. Marty AP, Schmelzer S, Thomasin RA, et al. Agreement between trainees and supervisors on first-year entrustable professional activities for anaesthesia training. *Br J Anaesth.* 2020;125(1):98–103. DOI: https://doi.org/10.1016/j.bja.2020.04.009
67. Klassen RM, Klassen JRL. Self-efficacy beliefs of medical students: a critical review. *Perspect Med Educ.* 2018;7(2):76–82. DOI: https://doi.org/10.1007/s40037-018-0411-3
68. Yaneva V, von Davier M. *Advancing Natural Language Processing in Educational Assessment.* Routledge; 2023. DOI: https://doi.org/10.4324/9781003278658

CHAPTER 5

Validity theory applied to entrustment as an approach to assessment

Claire Touchie, Olle ten Cate, Yoon Soo Park, Benjamin Kinnear, David R. Taylor

Abstract

In adopting entrustment-based assessments, the construct has shifted from assessing learners' capability to provide competent care to their readiness for the responsibility for the welfare of patients and permission to perform clinical care with appropriate autonomy. Competence committees charged with making entrustment-based decisions must make decisions that are valid, fit for purpose, and interpreted appropriately. However, entrustment as a construct is complex and warrants a discussion regarding its relation to validity.

While many different validity questions may be asked in the context of entrustable professional activities (EPAs), this chapter focuses on what we believe is the most salient and novel feature of EPA-based programs, which is the introduction of entrustment decision-making as an approach to assessment of health professionals in training. Validity theory, with reference to the models of Messick and Kane, is discussed in the context of entrustment. This leads to reflections on how some assumptions regarding validity may need to be reconceptualized, how sources of evidence and validity arguments can support defensible decisions, and how threats to validity must be considered and minimized.

How to cite this book chapter:

Touchie C, ten Cate O, Park YS, Kinnear B, Taylor D. Validity theory applied to entrustment as an approach to assessment. In: ten Cate O, Burch VC, Chen HC, Chou FC, Hennus MP. (Eds). *Entrustable Professional Activities and Entrustment Decision-Making in Health Professions Education*, Chapter 5, pp. 51–63. [2024] London: Ubiquity Press. DOI: https://doi.org/10.5334/bdc.e

This chapter uses cross-references to other chapters of the same book. For those who read this chapter as a standalone publication: all cross-references can be found at: https://doi.org/10.5334/bdc

Authors

- Claire Touchie, MD, MHPE. University of Ottawa, Ottawa, Canada. Correspondence: ctouchie@toh.ca.
- Olle ten Cate, PhD. University Medical Center Utrecht, the Netherlands.
- Yoon Soo Park, PhD. University of Illinois College of Medicine, Chicago, Illinois, USA.
- Benjamin Kinnear, MD, MEd. Cincinnati Children's Hospital Medical Center/University of Cincinnati College of Medicine, Cincinnati, Ohio, USA.
- David R. Taylor, MD, MHPE. Queen's University, Kingston, Canada.

Introduction

The emergence of EPAs and entrustment-based decisions in the context of competency-based education has led to questions of validity.[1,2] Many schools and programs have legitimate questions: Is the effort to change a program or improve assessment of trainees worth the investment? Will the change lead to better programs, better doctors, or safer patient care? As with other major shifts in educational approaches (e.g., problem-based learning), it is imperative that we provide validity evidence that these new approaches are fit for purpose. By this we mean the extent to which an educational and/or assessment approach fulfills its purpose or its function.[3]

Box 5.1 addresses some 'fit for purpose' validity questions relevant to EPAs. This chapter will focus on what we believe is the most salient and novel feature of EPA-based programs: the introduction of *entrustment decision-making* as an approach to assessment of health professionals in training. We will address how we think validity theory can be applied to this approach.[4]

Entrustment

Entrustment in health professions education involves confiding to a trainee the care of an individual or the execution of a task.[4] Entrustment happens when trainees are asked to look after a patient or perform tasks without direct supervision. Entrustment decisions can be made *in the moment*, when

Box 5.1: Examples of 'fit for purpose' validity questions around EPAs and entrustment.

Examples of 'fit for purpose' validity questions	Possible translations to operational questions	Examples of studies
How valid is this EPA?	Does this particular EPA reflect a relevant task? Can trainee readiness be measured?	Undergraduate medical education (UME) core EPA 5[5]
How valid is this EPA framework?	Does the framework of EPAs cover the breadth of activities in this profession? Is the framework workable in practice? Do these EPAs meet the expectations of employers or follow training?	EPAs in general surgery in the US,[6] pharmacy,[7] family medicine,[8] medical radiation technologists[9]
How valid is the entrustment-based discussion (EBD)?	Does the EBD increase a supervisor's insight into the readiness of the trainee for increased risks, compared to an alternative workplace-based assessment?	The procedure has been argued[10] but the validity question not investigated
How valid is the implementation of entrustment decision-making?	Do trainees qualified to be ready for distant supervision for an EPA actually receive the ensuing responsibility?	A survey-based study in dermatology addressed this[11]
How valid are entrustment-supervision (ES) scales to measure growth?	Do trainees with more experience require less supervision (or score better) on entrustment/supervision scales?	ES scales in anesthesia,[12,13] surgery,[14,15] pediatrics,[16,17,18] nursing,[19] internal medicine,[20,21] emergency medicine,[22] and UME[23] programs
How valid are ES scales compared to other measures?	Do scores on different scales to measure growth correlate with other scales?	ES scales in UME compared[24,25] ES scales versus milestone scales[26]
How do valid entrustment decisions come about?	Which trainee attributes account for the validity of entrustment decisions?	Supervisors'[27] or program directors'[28] opinions[29]

a trainee is asked to take over the care for a patient (which is ad hoc entrustment). The implicit assessment (i.e., observation + judgment ± feedback) of a trainee's readiness at the point of care (POC) is intended to direct learning and progression and to provide feedback to enhance growth as an emerging professional. These POC assessments are meant to be low in stakes, to be formative in purpose, and, on their own, not to be used to make promotion or credentialling decisions. However, such frontline assessments can be documented and integrated with other data points from different approaches to make a holistic, higher-stakes, summative decision about a trainee's capacity and permission to engage in patient care under less supervision. These summative entrustment decisions bring inherent consequences for both trainees and patients. Ensuring the validity of these entrustment decisions is a key step in incorporating them into an assessment strategy.[30]

Validity and entrustment

Validity in education refers to 'the degree to which evidence and theory support the interpretations and uses of scores of an assessment or test.'[31] The proposed interpretation of an assessment includes specifying the construct that is intended to be measured. In adopting entrustment, the construct has shifted from assessing trainees' *capability* to provide competent care to their readiness to be entrusted with the *responsibility* for the welfare of patients when performing an EPA with less or no supervision. Entrustment is a much more complex construct than capability; it requires additional consideration of other trainee qualities (e.g., conscientiousness, integrity, humility) as well as trainee-independent factors (e.g., patient acuity and complexity, and supervisor propensity to trust trainees); see also Chapter 4.[29,32] While entrustment is more meaningful for the purpose of making decisions to award clinical responsibility and autonomy, its complexity poses challenges from a construct validity perspective.

In addition, in gathering validity evidence, there is often reference to the objectivity of assessments. The search for objectivity (or measurement precision) in workplace-based assessment (WBA) has been pervasive; the lack of objectivity has often been framed as a lack of validity evidence for the use of competency-based frameworks in assessment, including that of EPAs.[2,33,34] However, the perceived necessity of objectivity in WBA has been challenged.[35,36,37] ten Cate and Regehr propose the concept of 'shared subjectivity,' where there is convergence of socially constructed perspectives rather than a focus on objectivity.[38] Constructing assessment approaches in health care often relies on consensus in the choice of test items, in standard setting, in the use of assessment tools, and similarly in judgments about trainee proficiency. Acknowledging that (a) expert judgment is indispensable and (b) experts differ in their unique and subjective judgments, subjectivity and its contribution to the variability of measurement should not be qualified as unwanted error.

On the contrary, using various perspectives to arrive at a coherent 'rich picture' through consensus rather than assuming a 'single truth' implies accepting, or even embracing, subjectivity or what could be called 'relevant variance.'[35,39,40,41] Nonetheless, in order to support the purpose of assessment, validity evidence must be gathered to support or refute the interpretation of whether an educator considers a trainee trustworthy for a clinical task and caring for patients. Readiness of trainees for unsupervised practice after training is a concern voiced in the literature and the importance of the validity of decisions to grant permission to act without supervision cannot be stressed enough.[42,43]

Understanding validity in the context of entrustment decision-making: Messick's and Kane's frameworks

Two dominant validity frameworks have been applied in health professions education[30,44]: Messick's sources of validity evidence and Kane's argument-based approach.[45,46] In Messick's approach, multiple sources of evidence are gathered to support the interpretations and uses of assessment data. These include evidence based on (a) test content (what construct is being assessed?); (b) response processes (how do assessors or respondents operationalize the assessment?); (c) internal structure (are the tools or items together coherently measuring the intended construct?); (d) relations to other variables (does any other triangulating information support [or not] the interpretation?); and (e) consequences of testing (is there evidence that the intended and unintended impacts of assessment decisions are acceptable?). Table 5.1 translates Messick's sources of validity evidence when using EPAs as WBAs.

Table 5.1: Questions to guide the acquisition of Messick's five sources of validity evidence.

Sources	Questions to ask	
	Individual raters	**Competency committees**
Content	Was the right activity observed or discussed and assessed? Was it a sound representation of the intended EPA?	Were all aspects of the EPA sufficiently represented in the various observations and discussions?
Response process	Did the assessor understand what to observe and how to complete the rating tool? What was taken into account when making the entrustment decision?	Have all committee members been trained to use the data? Did they review and understand the available information about the trainee? Has the assessor thought about the perspective they bring while assessing the trainee?
Internal structure	Is the entrustment decision supported by the information provided on the rating tool? Does the rating tool provide sufficient information to provide meaningful feedback on readiness for entrustment?	Were multiple different observers involved in assessing the trainee? How did the judgments converge?
Relations to other variables	Are there sources of evidence that support (or contradict) the available information?	How do the outcomes of EPA entrustment decisions compare to other assessments the trainee completed?
Consequences	Did the observer follow up after their recommendation? Are there unintended consequences of the decision? What is the impact of trainees identified as entrustable versus trainees that still need additional training and remediation?	Does the committee keep track of decisions and trainee action to justify their decisions? Were the decisions fair? Is there evidence of bias or equity concerns (e.g., gender, race)?

Kane uses an argument-based approach to validation whereby evidence is prioritized and used to support or refute a chain of inferences connecting the moment of assessment to the resulting decision or use from the assessment or, in this case, an entrustment decision. Evidence is collected to support multiple different types of inferences: scoring, generalization, extrapolation, and implication (Figure 5.1).

Inferences in validity arguments are claims drawn from available information.[47] The information is there to support the entrustment decisions. In Kane's model, each sequential inference requires additional information in support of those claims, thus making the argument in support of the decision.

Both validity frameworks can support each other with the information gathered through Messick's sources of evidence supporting Kane's inferences, as depicted in Table 5.2.

Most traditional assessments in education use supporting evidence for scoring and generalization inferences, leading to judgments about knowledge and skill, and to decisions about student progress, often as passing or failing tests and receiving grades. Summative entrustment decisions bring deliberate operational decisions that affect patient care, and are thus related to *consequences* in Messick's model and Kane's *implication inference*. In the latter model, extrapolation to determine the readiness for entrustment and autonomy is the step made in many programs using EPAs: a decision that reflects trust in the trainee, or an 'entrustment determination.' However, that is not the ultimate step. The proof of the pudding is the actual summative entrustment, reflecting the willingness to schedule a trainee for lesser supervision or unsupervised clinical service. This

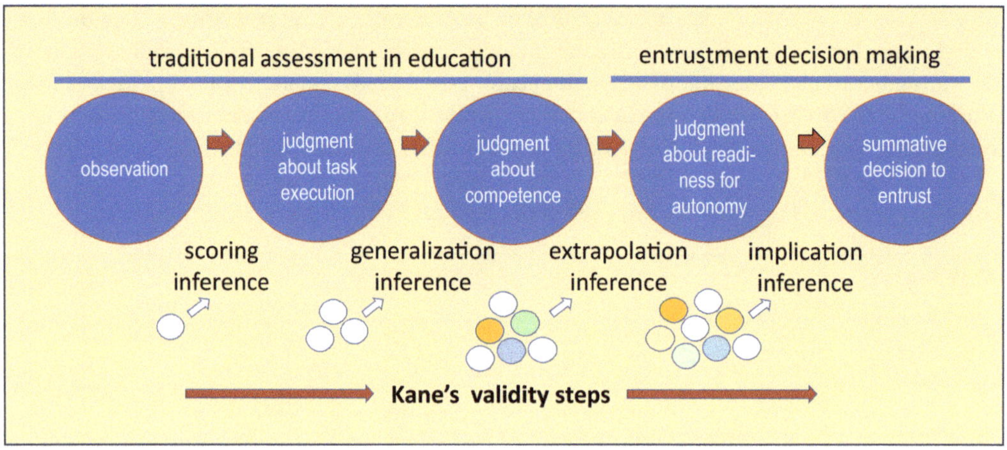

Figure 5.1: Entrustment decisions using Kane's validity argument.

step has implications for the trainee in the philosophy of EPA-based education, emphasizing assessment directing progressive autonomy and entrustment decisions. It also has implications for the patient, because of the direct relationship to patient care responsibilities. In reality, at least to date, rules and regulations often restrict true entrustment, which may explain why implication inferences and consequences evidence are not yet commonly reported.[11,48,49,50]

Table 5.2: Blending Messick's and Kane's validity models.

		Kane's validity inferences			
		Scoring	**Generalization**	**Extrapolation**	**Implication**
Messick's sources of validity evidence	Content	•	•	•	
	Response process	•			
	Internal structure		•	•	
	Relation to other variables			•	•
	Consequences				•

Defensible summative entrustment decisions

Optimizing entrustment decisions relies on sampling and gathering the right information. This may sound simple but it is not. Entrustment-based WBAs occur in authentic clinical environments. The clinical workplace is a complex, adaptive environment with many variables that cannot be controlled or standardized for the purpose of trainee assessment. Assessments thus vary across multiple facets—the time when administered, the patient or case of interest, the assessor in charge, and more. At the very least, it is much less prescribed and controlled than either written or simulated assessments. Thus the validity of entrustment within the context of WBAs warrants further exploration.

Sampling

With most assessments using written or simulated settings, trainees are assessed on a standardized set of items or scenarios representing a sampling of the universe of possible items. This sample is representative, one of convenience, and similar for a group of individuals being assessed in standardized conditions. Items are scored in a prescribed fashion and the data are analyzed and scrutinized for reliability using tried and true approaches. Quantitative methods are available to describe the level of validity evidence at every step of either or both of the Messick and Kane approaches.

In general, EPA-based data collection has been accepted to be a convenience sample of trainee performance. EPA assessments are initiated opportunistically within the daily clinical workflow. We assume the convenience sample is representative of the trainee's larger body of work. Recent research is calling this into question.[51,52,53] First, the sampling approach used can appear to be purposive rather than for convenience, generating assessment data that intentionally select certain observations and are, therefore, not producing a representative dataset. Second, the purposes for initiating the assessment of a particular encounter are highly variable depending on the motivation of the person making the initiation decision, potentially leading to bias or underrepresentation.

To avoid bias and underrepresentation in sampling, it is important for programs to have a clear blueprint for the sampling expected. It may be helpful to also gather information on context such as the complexity of the patient or case to better understand the sample upon which an entrustment decision is being made. Finally, bringing different assessments together (e.g., EPA observations, case-based discussions, multisource feedback, product evaluation) in a trainee portfolio can then be used for summative entrustment decisions.

Mitigating threats to validity

Threats to validity occur when the assessment measures something other than what is intended. Two different categories that threaten validity are (a) construct underrepresentation and (b) construct-irrelevant variance. Construct underrepresentation (CU) occurs when the assessment does not fully represent the construct intended. For example, if the construct is the care of an adult population and the trainee has only been assessed with male patients, then there is the underrepresentation (or, in this case, no representation) of female patients. Construct-irrelevant variance (CIV) is a systematic error whereby the assessment scores are affected by variables that are extraneous to the assessment's intended purpose.[31,54] CU and CIV can affect the validity argument put forth for decision-making. If significant enough, these can negatively impact decisions and refute the argument. Not attending to these can impact patient and trainee safety. Table 5.3 provides examples of threats to validity and measures to mitigate them.

Reconceptualizing reliability

Bringing together the different assessments from a trainee's portfolio is necessary to make holistic decisions. Based on this data, competence committees (CCs) consider whether the trainee is ready to act with less supervision. In order for decisions to be robust and reproducible, clear specifications about which assessments will be included and how the data will be interpreted and used should be clearly defined.[55,56]

Establishing reliability for trainee assessments requires demonstrating the reproducibility of ratings across multiple assessment occasions.[57] The greater the extent to which assessment ratings are dependent on factors external to the trainee, the more challenging it is to establish this reproducibility. Entrustment intentionally incorporates factors outside of the control of trainees, such as an authentic clinical setting and varying patient acuity/complexity, into the rating construct itself. In addition, the concept of reproducibility is problematic as individual observations are usually followed by feedback to improve performance next time, changing the conditions for reproduction. Thus, when looking at entrustment of a trainee for an EPA over time, we are

Table 5.3: Threats to validity and examples, related to Messick's sources of validity evidence.

Sources of validity evidence	Threats to validity	Measures to consider
Sampling/content	• Observed cases have been relatively simple • Too many favorable observation moments chosen by trainees	• Include 'case complexity' scores in observation ratings • Include unannounced observations
	• Trainees lack critical experiences in patient care	• Including logs of patient encounters in portfolio to evaluate experience • Carefully designing schedules and rotational experiences • Including entrustment-based discussions (with what-if probes)
Response process	• Benefit-of-the-doubt ratings given	• Faculty development and frame-of-reference training • Forcing raters to think prospectively (will you trust your next patient with this trainee?)
	• Trainee adjusts behavior, aware of observer present	• Weighing longitudinal (MSF) information more heavily
	• CC members have not absorbed relevant trainee data	• Require preparation for CC meetings • Present aggregated trainee data in highly digestible (visual) way
Internal structure	• Contradictory data at the CC table • Insufficient variety of data available	• Discuss trainee only when sufficient data available • Explore sources of contradictions
Relationship with other variables	• Variable personal experiences of CC members with individual trainees • Circumstantial information reflecting presumptive trust diverges from observational data	• Evaluate trainee data against general framework (e.g., A RICH) • Analyze and understand external source of data
Consequences	• Incidents reported about the trainee after the summative entrustment decision	• Evaluate trainees after summative decisions • Analyze incidents to disentangle competence from unusual case complexity

looking for growth or improvement, not consistency of performance. So, for a trainee performing an individual EPA over time, using growth rate reliability and growth curve reliability might be more appropriate. Park et al. used these types of reliability calculations to estimate longitudinal consistency in milestone ratings.[58] This provided reliable longitudinal data to track individual progress in a manner that would likely be appropriate for EPAs as well.

When evaluating the reliability of a portfolio for summative decisions such as transitions to practice, other forms of reliability calculations can be considered. To improve the reliability of the decisions based on multiple assessments, composite reliability of multiple data sources or assessment systems can be considered.[59] A qualitative approach can also be used. Trustworthiness of the data and triangulation with corroboration of data across assessments can be used when viewing the entire body of data for a trainee.[60] In addition, the reliability of CC decisions could be explored through decision consistency and investigating the extent to which different CCs would make similar decisions using the same trainee data. Studies such as this have yet to be done. Regardless of the approach used, the collective judgment made by experts in a CC with multiple data points should lead to decisions that are valid.[61,62]

Constructing an argument for defensible decisions

Variability of cases, contexts, and raters is inherent to WBAs. Sampling can be purposive but is always limited and assessments require a shared subjectivity or argued 'intersubjective judgment,' rather than proof of absolute objectivity. Decisions must be made with inherently incomplete data, and a prediction that this trainee will absolutely not make mistakes after summative entrustment is impossible. In a critical review, Kinnear et al. suggest that argumentation theory can help frame validity arguments over whether one chooses Messick's framework, Kane's, or both.[47] Those building the arguments and intended audiences need to develop a shared understanding of the validity argumentation process and its standards. Arguments should be tailored to the needs of, and clearly understood by, the audiences, be they trainees, teachers, programs, or credentialling agencies. Strength and cogency of argumentation should determine interpretations and inferences to arrive at best possible decisions.

Various examples are offered in the literature on how to construct a validity argument for decision-making. Touchie et al. discuss validity in the setting of summative decision-making using both Messick's and Kane's approaches.[30] Rotthoff et al. posit that assessments are not necessarily analytic or holistic but rather may be on a continuum.[63] Kinnear et al., in two different studies, offer a validity map also using both Messick and Kane to support decision-making in residency training and use theory to support time-variable training and decisions about readiness for practice.[64,65] Consistent across these examples is the reliance on established experts to review diverse sources of data, draw conclusions, and make summative decisions. Reliability evidence in this context argues that a separate set of experts would likely come to similar judgments on the adequacy of the data and decisions made.

Conclusions

Entrustment decision-making has implications for trainees and for patient care. Entrustment as a construct is complex and poses challenges when gathering validity evidence. It has validity implications that differ from other assessment formats. Using the validity frameworks of Messick and Kane, we can apply theory to gather the evidence necessary for the defensibility of decision-making. These provide a platform to reconceptualize assumptions underlying sampling, reliability, and decision-making and to understand how to mitigate threats to validity.

Competing interests

The authors declare that they have no competing interests.

References

1. Guralnick S, Yedowitz-Freeman J. Core entrustable professional activities for entry into residency: curricular gap or unrealistic expectations. *J Grad Med Educ.* 2017;9(5):593–594. DOI: https://doi.org/10.4300/JGME-D-17-00559.1
2. Krupat E. Critical thoughts about the core entrustable professional activities in undergraduate medical education. *Acad Med.* 2018;93(3):371–376. DOI: https://doi.org/10.1097/ACM.0000000000001865

3. Dijkstra J, Galbraith R, Hodges BD, et al. Expert validation of fit-for-purpose guidelines for redesigning programmes of assessment. *BMC Med Educ.* 2012;12:20. DOI: https://doi.org/10.1186/1472-6920-12-20
4. ten Cate O, Hart D, Ankel F, et al. Entrustment decision-making in clinical training. *Acad Med.* 2016:91(2):191–198. DOI: https://doi.org/10.1097/ACM.0000000000001044
5. Aulet TH, Moore JS, Callas PW, Nicholas C, Hulme M. (En)trust me: validating an assessment rubric for documenting clinical encounters during a surgery clerkship clinical skills exam. *Am J Surg.* 2020;219(2):258–262. DOI: https://doi.org/10.1016/j.amjsurg.2018.12.055
6. Brasel KJ, Lindeman B, Jones A, et al. Implementation of entrustable professional activities in general surgery: results of a national pilot study. *Ann Surg.* 2023;278(4):578–586. DOI: https://doi.org/10.1097/SLA.0000000000005991
7. McDowell L, Hamrick J, Fetterman J, Brooks K. Preceptors' perceptions of an entrustable professional activities-based community introductory pharmacy practice experience curriculum. *Curr Pharm Teach Learn.* 2024;16(2):109–118. DOI: https://doi.org/10.1016/j.cptl.2023.12.026
8. Newton WP, Magill M, Barr W, Hoekzema G, Karuppiah S, Stutzman K. Implementing competency based ABFM board eligibility. *J Am Board Fam Med.* 2023;36(4):703–707. DOI: https://doi.org/10.3122/jabfm.2023.230201R0
9. Tu CY, Huang KM, Cheng CH, Lin WJ, Liu CH, Yang CW. Development, implementation, and evaluation of entrustable professional activities (EPAs) for medical radiation technologists in Taiwan: a nationwide experience. *BMC Med Educ.* 2024;24:95. DOI: https://doi.org/10.1186/s12909-024-05088-9
10. ten Cate O, Hoff RG. From case-based to entrustment-based discussions. *Clin Teach.* 2017;14(6):385–389. DOI: https://doi.org/10.1111/tct.12710
11. Sigurdsson V, ten Cate O. Do summative entrustment decisions actually lead to entrustment? *Clin Teach.* October 10, 2023:e13668. DOI: https://doi.org/10.1111/tct.13668
12. Dubois DG, Lingley AJ, Ghatalia J, McConnell MM. Validity of entrustment scales within anesthesiology residency training. *Can J Anaesth.* 2021;68(1):53–63. DOI: https://doi.org/10.1007/s12630-020-01823-0
13. Weller JM, Castanelli DJ, Chen Y, Jolly B. Making robust assessments of specialist trainees' workplace performance. *Br J Anaesth.* 2017;118(2):207–214. DOI: https://doi.org/10.1093/bja/aew412
14. Sandhu G, Nikolian VC, Magas CP, et al. Optrust: validity of a tool assessing intraoperative entrustment behaviors. *Ann Surg.* 2018;267(4):670–676. DOI: https://doi.org/10.1097/SLA.0000000000002235
15. Liebert CA, Melcer EF, Keehl O, et al. Validity Evidence for ENTRUST as an assessment of surgical decision-making for the inguinal hernia entrustable professional activity (EPA). *J Surg Educ.* 2022;79(6):e202-e212. DOI: https://doi.org/10.1016/j.jsurg.2022.07.008
16. Li S, Qi X, Li H, Zhou W, Jiang Z, Qi J. Exploration of validity evidence for core residency entrustable professional activities in Chinese pediatric residency. *Front Med (Lausanne).* 2023;10:1301356. DOI: https://doi.org/10.3389/fmed.2023.1301356
17. Pitts S, Schwartz A, Carraccio CL, et al. Fellow entrustment for the common pediatric subspecialty entrustable professional activities across subspecialties. *Acad Pediatr.* 2022;22(6):881–886. DOI: https://doi.org/10.1016/j.acap.2021.12.019
18. Mink RB, Schwartz A, Herman BE, et al. Validity of level of supervision scales for assessing pediatric fellows on the common pediatric subspecialty entrustable professional activities. *Acad Med.* 2018;93(2):283–291. DOI: https://doi.org/10.1097/ACM.0000000000001820
19. Lau ST, Ang E, Shorey S, Lau Y. Entrustable professional activity assessment tool for clinical procedures: a psychometric study. *J Clin Nurs.* 2021;30(19–20):2822–2831. DOI: https://doi.org/10.1111/jocn.15788

20. Colbert-Getz JM, Lappe K, Gerstenberger J, Milne CK, Raaum S. Capturing growth curves of medical students' clinical skills performance. *Clin Teach.* 2023;20(6):e13623. DOI: https://doi.org/10.1111/tct.13623
21. Warm EJ, Held JD, Hellmann M, et al. Entrusting observable practice activities and milestones over the 36 months of an internal medicine residency. *Acad Med.* 2016;91(10):1398–1405. DOI: https://doi.org/10.1097/ACM.0000000000001292
22. Dewhirst S, Wood TJ, Cheung WJ, Frank JR. Assessing the utility of a novel entrustment-supervision assessment tool. *Med Educ.* 2023;57(10):949–957. DOI: https://doi.org/10.1111/medu.15156
23. Violato C, Cullen MJ, Englander R, et al. Validity evidence for assessing entrustable professional activities during undergraduate medical education. *Acad Med.* 2021;96(7S):S70-S75. DOI: https://doi.org/10.1097/ACM.0000000000004090
24. Ryan MS, Khan AR, Park YS, et al. Workplace-based entrustment scales for the core EPAs: a multisite comparison of validity evidence for two proposed instruments using structured vignettes and trained raters. *Acad Med.* 2022;97(4):544–551. DOI: https://doi.org/10.1097/ACM.0000000000004222
25. Ryan MS, Gielissen KA, Shin D, et al. How well do workplace-based assessments support summative entrustment decisions? A multi-institutional generalisability study. *Med Educ.* January 2, 2024. DOI: https://doi.org/10.1111/medu.15291
26. Brazelle M, Zmijewski P, McLeod C, Corey B, Porterfield JR, Lindeman B. Concurrent validity evidence for entrustable professional activities in general surgery residents. *J Am Coll Surg.* 2022;234(5):938–946. DOI: https://doi.org/10.1097/XCS.0000000000000168
27. Kennedy TJT, Regehr G, Baker GR, Lingard L. Point-of-care assessment of medical trainee competence for independent clinical work. *Acad Med.* 2008;83(10 Suppl):S89-S92. DOI: https://doi.org/10.1097/ACM.0b013e318183c8b7
28. Yoon MH, Kurzweil DM, Durning SJ, et al. It's a matter of trust: exploring the basis of program directors' decisions about whether to trust a resident to care for a loved one. *Adv Health Sci Educ Theory Pract.* 2020;25(3):691–709. DOI: https://doi.org/10.1007/s10459-019-09953-x
29. ten Cate O, Chen HC. The ingredients of a rich entrustment decision. *Med Teach.* 2020;42(12):1413–1420. DOI: https://doi.org/10.1080/0142159X.2020.1817348
30. Touchie C, Kinnear B, Schumacher D, et al. On the validity of summative entrustment decisions. *Med Teach.* 2021;43(7):780–787. DOI: https://doi.org/10.1080/0142159X.2021.1925642
31. American Educational Research Association, American Psychological Association, National Council on Measurement in Education (AERA). *Standards for Educational and Psychological Testing.* American Educational Research Association; 2014.
32. Hauer K, ten Cate O, Boscardin C, et al. Understanding trust as an essential element of trainee supervision and learning in the workplace. *Adv Health Sci Educ.* 2014;19(3):435–456. DOI: https://doi.org/10.1007/s10459-013-9474-4
33. Lurie S. History and practice of competency-based assessment. *Med Educ.* 2012;46:49–57. DOI: https://doi.org/10.1111/j.1365-2923.2011.04142.x
34. Norman G, Norcini J, Bordage G. Competency-based education: milestones or millstones? *J Grad Med Educ.* 2014;6(1):1–16. DOI: https://doi.org/10.4300/JGME-D-13-00445.1
35. Hodges B. Assessment in the post-psychometric era: learning to love the subjective and collective. *Med Teach.* 2013;35(7):564–568. DOI: https://doi.org/10.3109/0142159X.2013.789134
36. Gingerich A, Kogan J, Yeates P, Govaerts M, Holmboe E. Seeing the 'black box' differently: assessor cognition from three research perspectives. *Med Educ.* 2014;48(11):1055–1068. DOI: https://doi.org/10.1111/medu.12546

37. Valentine N, Durning SJ, Shanahan EM, Schuwirth L. Fairness in assessment: identifying a complex adaptive system. *Perspect Med Educ.* 2023;12(1):315–326. DOI: https://doi.org/10.5334/pme.993
38. ten Cate O, Regehr G. The power of subjectivity in the assessment of medical trainees. *Acad Med.* 2019;94(3):333–337. DOI: https://doi.org/10.1097/ACM.0000000000002495
39. Crossley J. Validity and truth in assessment. *Med Educ.* 2013;47(12):1152–1154. DOI: https://doi.org/10.1111/medu.12317
40. Virk A, Joshi A, Mahajan R, Singh T. The power of subjectivity in competency-based assessment. *J Postgrad Med.* 2020;66(4):200–205. DOI: https://doi.org/10.4103/jpgm.JPGM_591_20
41. Tavares W, Kinnear B, Schumacher DJ, Forte M. 'Rater training' re-imagined for work-based assessment in medical education. *Adv Health Sci Educ.* 2023;28(5):1697–1709. DOI: https://doi.org/10.4103/jpgm.JPGM_591_20
42. Jonker G, Ochtman A, Marty AP, et al. Would you trust your loved ones to this trainee? Certification decisions in postgraduate anaesthesia training. *Brit J of Anaesth.* 2020;125(5):e408-e410. DOI: https://doi.org/10.1016/j.bja.2020.07.009
43. Fletcher KE, O'Connor AB, Kisielewski M, Willett LL. Why do residency program directors consider resigning? A mixed-methods analysis of a national program director survey. *Amer J Med.* 2020;133(6):761–767. DOI: https://doi.org/10.1016/j.amjmed.2020.02.016
44. Schuwirth L, van der Vleuten C. Programmatic assessment and Kane's validity perspective. *Med Educ.* 2012;46(1):38–48. DOI: https://doi.org/10.1097/ACM.0000000000002495
45. Messick S. Validity. In: Linn RL, ed. *Educational Measurement.* 3rd ed. Macmillan; 1989:13–103.
46. Kane MT. Validating the interpretations and uses of test scores. *J Educ Measur.* 2013;50(1):1–73.
47. Kinnear B, Schumacher DJ, Driessen EW, Varpio L. How argumentation theory can inform assessment validity: a critical review. *Med Educ.* 2022;56:1064–1075. DOI: https://doi.org/10.1111/medu.14882
48. Beckman TJ, Cook DA, Mandrekar JN. What is the validity evidence for assessments of clinical teaching? *J Gen Int Med.* 2005;20:1159–1164. DOI: https://doi.org/10.1111/j.1525-1497.2005.0258.x
49. Cook DA, Zendejas B, Hamstra SJ, Hatala R, Brydges R. What counts as validity evidence? Examples and prevalence in a systematic review of simulation-based assessment. *Adv Health Sci Educ.* 2014;19(2):233–250. DOI: https://doi.org/10.1007/s10459-013-9458-4
50. ten Cate O, Jarrett JB, *Would* I trust or *will* I trust? The gap between entrustment determinations and entrustment decisions for trainees in pharmacy and other health professions. *Pharmacy (Basel).* 2023;11(3):107. DOI: https://doi.org/10.3390/pharmacy11030107
51. Teunissen PW, Stapel DA, van der Vleuten C, Scherpbier A, Boor K, Scheele F. Who wants feedback? An investigation of the variables influencing residents' feedback-seeking behavior in relation to night shifts. *Acad Med.* 2009;84(7):910–917. DOI: https://doi.org/10.1097/ACM.0b013e3181a858ad
52. Gaunt A, Patel A, Rusius V, Royle TJ, Markham DH, Pawlikowska T. 'Playing the game': how do surgical trainees seek feedback using workplace-based assessment? *Med Educ.* 2017;51(9):953–962. DOI: https://doi.org/10.1111/medu.13380
53. Gauthier S, Braund H, Dalgarno N, Taylor D. Assessment-seeking strategies: navigating the decision to initiate workplace-based assessment. *Teach Learn Med.* 2023, June 29:1–10. DOI: https://doi.org/10.1080/10401334.2023.2229803
54. Downing SM, Haladyna TM. Validity threats: overcoming interference with proposed interpretations of assessment data. *Med Educ.* 2004;38(3):327–333. DOI: https://doi.org/10.1046/j.1365-2923.2004.01777.x
55. Lineberry M, Park YS, Cook DA, Yudkowski R. Making the case for mastery learning assessments: key issues validation and justification. *Acad Med.* 2015;90(11):1445–1450. DOI: https://doi.org/10.1097/ACM.0000000000000860

56. Hu WCY, Dillon HCB, Wilkinson TJ. Educators as judges: applying judicial decision-making principles to high-stakes education assessment decision. *Teach Learn Med.* 2023;35(2):168–179. DOI: https://doi.org/10.1080/10401334.2022.2038176
57. Downing SM. Reliability: on the reproducibility of assessment data. *Med Educ.* 2004;38(9):1006–1012. DOI: https://doi.org/10.1111/j.1365-2929.2004.01932.x
58. Park YS, Hamstra SJ, Yamakazi K, Holmboe E. Longitudinal reliability of milestones-based learning trajectories in family medicine residents. *JAMA Network Open.* 2021;4(12):e2137179. DOI: https://doi.org/10.1001/jamanetworkopen.2021.3717
59. Park YS, Lineberry M, Hyderi A, Bordage G, Xing K, Yudkowski R. Differential weighting for sub-component measures of integrated clinical encounter scores based on the USMLE Step-2 CS examination: effects on composite score reliability and pass-fail decisions. *Acad Med.* 2016;91(10):S24-S30. DOI: https://doi.org/10.1097/ACM.0000000000001359
60. Cook DA, Brydges R, Ginsburg S, Hatala R. A contemporary approach to validity arguments: a practical guide to Kane's framework. *Med Educ.* 2015;49:560–575. DOI: https://doi.org/10.1111/medu.12678
61. Kinnear B, Warm EJ, Hauer KE. Twelve tips to maximize the value of a clinical competency committee in postgraduate medical education. *Med Teach.* 2018;40(11):1110–1115. DOI: https://doi.org/10.1080/0142159X.2018.1474191
62. Hauer KE, ten Cate O, Boscardin CK, et al. Ensuring resident competence: a narrative review of the literature on group decision-making to inform the work of clinical competence committees. *J Grad Med Educ.* 2016;8(2):156–164. DOI: https://doi.org/10.4300/JGME-D-15-00144.1
63. Rotthoff T, Kadmon M, Harendza S. It does not have to be either or! Assessing competence in medicine should be a continuum between an analytic and a holistic approach. *Adv Health Sci Educ.* 2021;26:1659–1673. DOI: https://doi.org/10.1007/s10459-021-10043-0
64. Kinnear B, Kelleher M, May B, et al. Constructing a validity map for a workplace-based assessment system: cross-walking Messick and Kane. *Acad Med.* 2021;96:S64-S69. DOI: https://doi.org/10.1097/ACM.0000000000004112
65. Kinnear B, Martini A, Varpio L, et al. How do validity experts conceptualise argumentation? It's a rhetorical question. *Med Educ.* 2024, January 18. DOI: https://doi.org/10.1111/medu.15311

CHAPTER 6

Integrating key concepts in workplace-based assessment: entrustable professional activities, programmatic assessment, and milestones

Harold G.J. Bok, Gersten Jonker, Stanley J. Hamstra, Christy K. Boscardin, Olle ten Cate, Marije P. Hennus

Abstract

Despite their independent origins, entrustable professional activities, Milestones, and programmatic assessment are interconnected concepts within the domain of competency-based education. While some organizations prioritize the use of entrustable professional activities, others prefer using Milestones. Simultaneously, competency-based education in health professions has embraced programmatic assessment as a core concept. A question raised regularly is how the three relate and whether they can be used in combination when designing an assessment system. This chapter aims to offer definitions of the three concepts and explore their mutual reinforcement, benefiting the quality of health professions education and, ultimately, patient care. To facilitate health professions trainees' progression along their educational path and enhance their autonomy through entrustment with specific clinical tasks, every curriculum needs a program of assessment. This chapter illustrates the alignment of the three concepts and provides practical examples on how they come together in a program of assessment. In summary, the seemingly distinct concepts share more common ground than previously acknowledged. By integrating the concepts, growth in context-dependent performance from novice to expert levels can be fostered, all while promoting learning in conjunction with high-stakes entrustment decision-making.

How to cite this book chapter:

Bok HGJ, Jonker G, Hamstra SJ, Boscardin CK, ten Cate O, Hennus MP. Integrating key concepts in workplace-based assessment: entrustable professional activities, programmatic assessment, and milestones. In: ten Cate O, Burch VC, Chen HC, Chou FC, Hennus MP. (Eds). *Entrustable Professional Activities and Entrustment Decision-Making in Health Professions Education*, Chapter 6, pp. 65–73. [2024] London: Ubiquity Press. DOI: https://doi.org/10.5334/bdc.f

This chapter uses cross-references to other chapters of the same book. For those who read this chapter as a standalone publication: all cross-references can be found at: https://doi.org/10.5334/bdc

Authors

- Harold G.J. Bok, DVM, PhD. Faculty of Veterinary Medicine, Utrecht University, the Netherlands. Correspondence: g.j.bok@uu.nl
- Gersten Jonker, MD, PhD. University Medical Center Utrecht, the Netherlands.
- Stanley J. Hamstra, PhD. University of Toronto, and Sunnybrook Research Institute, Toronto, Canada.
- Christy K. Boscardin, PhD. University of California San Francisco, San Francisco, USA.
- Olle ten Cate, PhD. University Medical Center Utrecht, Utrecht, the Netherlands and University of California, San Francisco, USA.
- Marije P. Hennus, MD, PhD, MSc Clin Ed. University Medical Center Utrecht, Utrecht, the Netherlands.

Introduction

Entrustable professional activities (EPAs),[1] Milestones,[a] and programmatic assessment (PA)[2,3] were introduced during a period in which competency frameworks[4–6] and workplace-based assessment (WBA)[7,8] were gaining much attention. All three concepts are related to competency-based education (CBE) but have originated independently, and in different jurisdictions. The key concept behind CBE is to ensure that trainees achieve competencies essential to providing high-quality patient care. EPAs, Milestones, and PA, with their emphasis on developmental trajectories and continuous feedback, are critical to operationalizing CBE. These three interconnected concepts contribute to ensuring comprehensive and continuous evaluation of a trainee's development toward meeting required competencies. A program of assessment (PofA) is integral to CBE as it provides a framework for health professions trainees to successfully progress through their educational trajectory and acquire increasing autonomy through entrustment with concrete units of clinical work. As a foundation for the PofA, some organizations mandate the use of Milestones, others the use of EPAs to inform trainees' developmental trajectories. CBE in the health professions has embraced PA as a core component.[9] Accreditation bodies generally endorse all three concepts but there is a lack of clear guidelines on how to integrate them cohesively and collaboratively. Considering that WBAs form the cornerstone of PA in health professions education and serve as the practical embodiment of its core concepts, our discussion will be specifically framed within the context of WBA. General principles of WBA include:

1. contextual relevance: assessment needs to be integrated into the actual performance and work of the health professions;
2. developmentally focused and continuous feedback: informative, frequent, continual, and longitudinal feedback are critical aspects of WBA; and
3. reflecting professional standards: aligned with competencies of the profession.[9]

This chapter sets out to provide clear definitions of EPA, Milestones, and PA and explore where the three augment each other for the benefit of the quality of clinical education and, eventually, of patient care. We will show how the concepts align and provide some practical examples in the context of WBA in health professions education.

Entrustable professional activities and entrustment

EPAs are the units of professional practice that constitute what clinicians do as daily work. They can be conceived of responsibilities or tasks that must be done in patient care, i.e., the work that trainees must be prepared to assume when they commence with unsupervised patient care practice. Trainees must gain experience and must grow into a professional role in the workplace phase of health professions training. Entrustment decisions about professional tasks have always been part of clinical training. What the concept of EPAs adds is a structure to build a curriculum and operationalize a PofA that allows a gradual and safe increase in responsibilities. EPAs' focus on the progression toward autonomy and unsupervised care provides a way to conceptualize developmental trajectory within health professions education. This requires assessments with an eye on both proficiency and risk. Assessment as entrustment does not *primarily* regard deci-

[a] In this chapter we use Milestones (with a capital M) as defined for US postgraduate medical programs. The US Accreditation Council for Graduate Medical Education (ACGME) requires programs to report every six months on the progress of all residents on predefined Milestones for all competencies.

sions of progression but refers to decisions about quality and safety of care and, *indirectly*, about trainee progression.

The process of mastering EPAs may be regarded as 'milestones' toward full professional responsibility. While those 'milestones' are not the same Milestones in the specific sense of an accrediting body such as ACGME, the purpose of EPAs and Milestones aligns. Similarly, the literature on PA may not elaborate on EPAs but the two concepts also align well in their purpose to visualize and support trainee development and progression.

Programmatic assessment principles

PA in health professions education, after its inception in 2005,[2] has been elaborated in various sets of principles.[10,11] As we interpret these principles, three core elements stand out:

1. Assessment of clinical competence in the workplace based on any single moment (one 'data point') is unreliable. In PA, a single assessment data point however should yield meaningful feedback to promote a dialogue or learning conversation with the learner (i.e., informative and low-stakes).
2. Multiple assessment data points from multiple occasions, raters, and methods, based on the educational justification for using that method and each with their own weight, are documented and aggregated to inform high-stakes decision-making. By shifting the focus to multiple assessments, a PofA based on the principles of PA can increase authenticity and construct validity without compromising reliability.
3. Equitable and credible high-stakes decisions on trainee progress or permission to practice are made by a team or committee, based on sufficient data, in a process of justifiable expert consensus.[12,13]

In PA, the traditional distinction between formative and summative assessment is replaced by a continuum of stakes. A single data point in WBA is usually a low-stakes assessment that does not result in a pass/fail decision, which separates data collection from decision-making. Decisions based on assessment and the number of data points required should be proportional to the stakes involved; the higher the stakes, the more data points are required. The trainee typically collects data points in an electronic portfolio that includes an outcome framework, usually with competencies or EPAs or both, to enable high-stakes decision-making. Since the portfolio contains both quantitative and qualitative data, decisions cannot be based on just numbers; holistic decisions must be made by a team of experts, such as a *competency committee* or *entrustment committee*. Workplace information sources to be aggregated to support high-stakes decision-making are summarized below. The committee oversees the aggregated data, assesses sufficiency of information, weighs data, and makes a decision about summative entrustment and trainee progress. EPAs and Milestones provide a way to conceptualize and operationalize the necessary components for making holistic decisions around advancement and entrustment.

Milestones

Milestones are concrete behavioral descriptions following the five developmental stages proposed by Dreyfus and Dreyfus (i.e., novice, advanced beginner, competent, proficient, expert) and adopted by health professions education scholars to conceptualize developmental trajectories toward meeting competencies.[14,15] Linking progression to the attainment of specific Milestones and the entrustment of EPAs ensures that learners advance based on their demonstrated competence rather than time spent in training. Central to Milestones is the concept of developmental

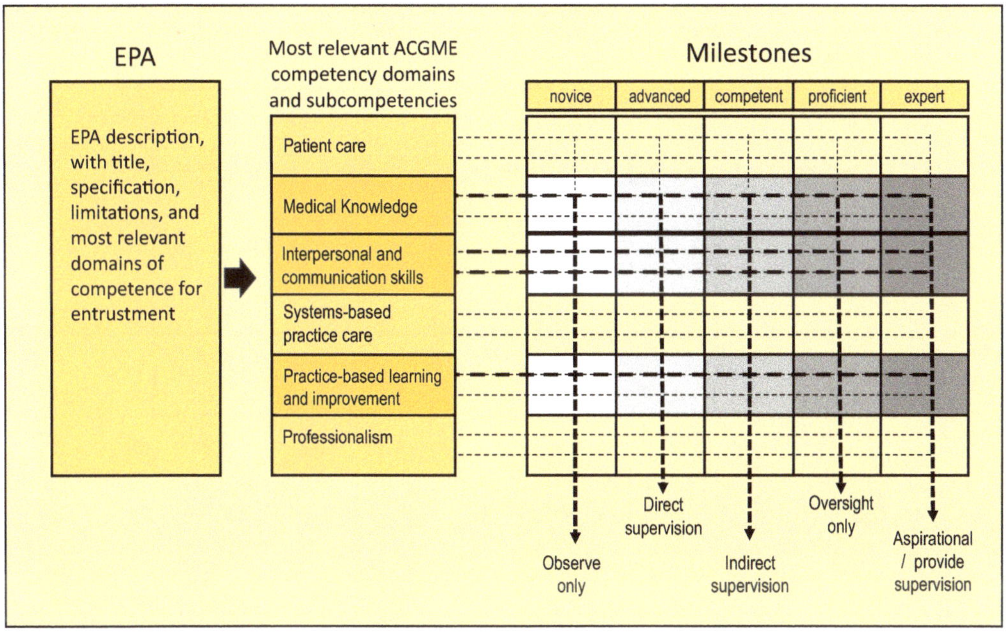

Figure 6.1: EPAs and Milestones combined.

trajectories and the focus on multiple assessment data that align with the key principles of PA. Reporting the Milestones for each competency for all residents every half year has been mandated in the US by the ACGME.[16] Milestones have subsequently been adopted for Canadian residencies[17] and in a number of other countries that aim to meet North American standards for postgraduate medical training. Milestones map the developmental path a trainee takes toward achieving the competence needed for unsupervised practice following graduation. With an increasing number of US residency specialties exploring the use of EPAs, several educators have posed the question of how to reconcile the two approaches and how to avoid overdocumentation.

Inspired by Warm's semi-annual ACGME reports using the five-point entrustment–supervision (ES) scale for the internal medicine residency at the University of Cincinnati, normalized to the nine-point Next Accreditation System (NAS) Milestone rating form,[18] Figure 6.1 was created, adapted from earlier publications.[19]

Figure 6.1 shows how for each EPA various competencies within the ACGME competency domains can be evaluated using the Dreyfus developmental stages, supported by behavioral descriptions for these stages. These descriptions for each Milestone are available for all ACGME competencies in all US residency programs. In Figure 6.1, competencies and subcompetencies are depicted as horizontal dotted lines; the black arrow represents a section of the full description of an EPA: the mapping of competencies to this EPA.[20] These developmental Milestones align reasonably well with the five generic ES levels used in entrustment decision-making. Mink et al. recently confirmed such a correlation in a study among over 2,000 fellows in pediatrics.[21] For a high-stakes entrustment decision for an EPA, all relevant competencies should be evaluated. Only when all available observational data meet the previously defined standards (i.e., the set of Milestones within a given level) can a conclusion be drawn about a justified level of supervision.[b]

[b] One detail is somewhat inconsistent. As elaborated in Chapter 1, 'competent' was suggested to qualify a trainee for unsupervised practice. In Figure 6.1 this aligns with indirect supervision. We prefer to use 'competent' for having passed the threshold to allow for unsupervised practice.

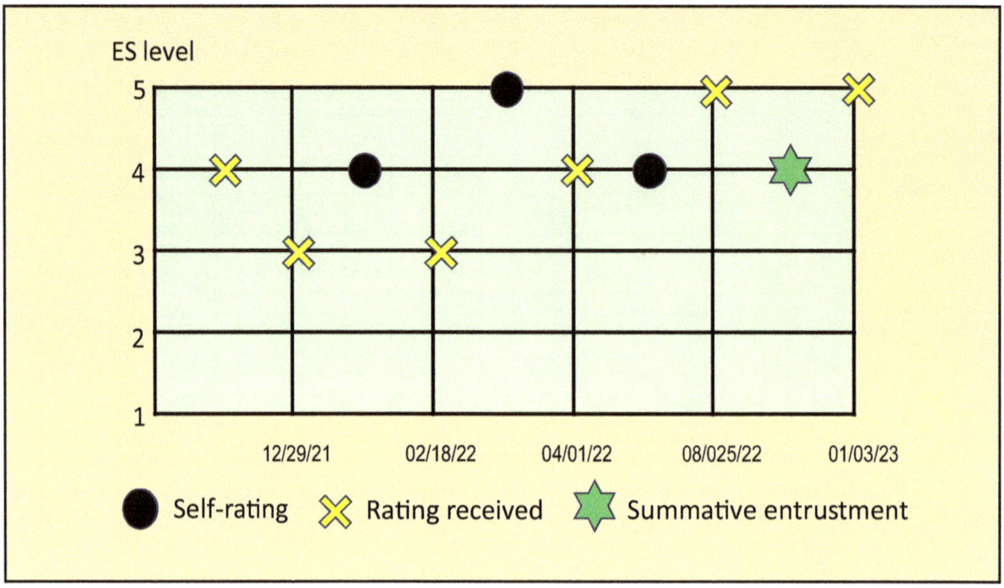

Figure 6.2: Simple dashboard visualization for a single trainee, including multiple individual data points on an ES scale, across a year.

Sources of information for workplace-based assessment

A PofA requires a definition of the data points that are included. A reasonable summary of current WBA approaches is the categorization of *sources of information* to ground major decisions about trainee progress and about high-stakes entrustment decisions with tasks in patient care. These sources can arguably be summarized in the following four categories: (a) direct observation, (b) conversation, (c) longitudinal observation, and (d) product evaluation (see Chapter 17 for a more extensive discussion).[22] Drawing from these four sources, a PofA can be designed to inform on competency development (i.e., through Milestones evaluations) and entrustment decisions. To that end, data from these sources are aggregated in a concise and informative format to support clinical competency committees to make decisions. These four WBA information sources are often not the only information available. Written tests and skills tests may be required for trainees during their training. While we do not consider these workplace-based information sources, they can contribute as a meaningful information source.

Examples of program of assessment visualizations

Figure 6.2, a simple dashboard visualization, was adapted from a portfolio system for veterinary practitioners.[c] It is a visualization of the monitoring and self-monitoring of a recently graduated veterinarian who started as a postgraduate trainee in an emergency clinic for companion animals. The yellow marks in this example of an individual's record over a year are individual, low-stakes, WBA data points pertaining to one EPA illustrating at what level of entrustment–supervision the person has been rated at ad hoc moments for that EPA; the black marks are self-assessments of the same ES level and the green star represents a high-stakes entrustment decision. This decision is made by a committee based on aggregate information derived from the low-stakes data points

[c] Courtesy of Dr. Robert Favier and Theo van den Herik, Evidensia, the Netherlands.

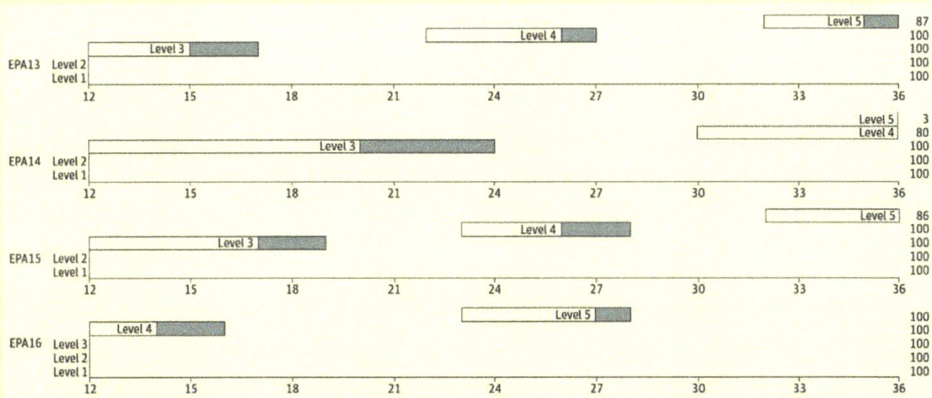

Percentages (right) of residents who have reached level 3, 4 or 5 of entrustment, after 12-36 months in training. Beginning of the white bar =25%; beginning of shaded bar =75%; end of shaded bar =90% (Schumacher et al 2020)

Figure 6.3: Example of aggregated cohort data of residents across two training years.

(i.e., yellow and black marks). Figure 6.2 is similar to the illustration that emphasizes the assessment for learning function of high-stakes decision-making committees in PA.[13] By tailoring the educational process to individual learning priorities and visualizing meaningful performance-relevant information collected through WBA, PA fosters ownership and accountability. When trainees fall short of expected outcomes, predefined thresholds and historical data guide the identification of targeted support strategies. These interventions can be effectively coordinated through the competency committee responsible for high-stakes entrustment decision-making.

Figure 6.3 shows aggregated data of the development of a cohort of medical residents across 24 months, regarding four EPAs. It is just one example of how visualization can aid a competency committee in the deliberations about a program and about an individual trainee. It provides information of how an individual's performance projects against the cohort. The example is adapted from Schumacher et al. (2020).[23]

Conclusion

In summary, EPAs, Milestones, and PA appear to be complementary and to have more in common than initially conceived. The three concepts pertain to the same principles of increasing responsibility, continuous feedback, using an outcomes framework as a foundation for the curriculum, and allowing high-stakes decision-making for certifying purposes. In this chapter we have argued that educational programs do not have to choose between these concepts but can instead 'have the best of three worlds.' By applying the foundational principles as a starting point, PA provides an operational framework for a CBE using both EPAs and Milestones. EPAs and Milestones are foundational to operationalizing and conceptualizing the evaluation of trainees' development toward entrustment and competence. Both EPAs and Milestones operationalize the principles of PA by ensuring that assessments are frequent, varied, and integrated over time to provide a comprehensive picture of a trainee's competence. PA ensures decision-making based on cumulative evidence rather than isolated assessments, emphasizing the development of competence through continuous learning and improvement, which are central to CBE. By integrating the three concepts, growth in context-dependent performance from novice to expert levels is fostered, and aimed at promoting learning in conjunction with high-stakes entrustment decision-making.

Competing interests

The authors declare that they have no competing interests.

Figure justification

Figure 6.3 is adapted from Schumacher et al. (2020).[23]

References

1. ten Cate O. Entrustability of professional activities and competency-based training. *Med Educ.* 2005;39(12):1176–1177. DOI: https://doi.org/10.1111/j.1365-2929.2005.02341.x
2. van der Vleuten CPM, Schuwirth LWT. Assessing professional competence: from methods to programmes. *Med Educ.* 2005;39(3):309–317. DOI: https://doi.org/10.1111/j.1365-2929.2005.02094.x
3. van der Vleuten CPM, Schuwirth LWT, Driessen EW, et al. A model for programmatic assessment fit for purpose. *Med Teach.* 2012;34(3):205–214. DOI: https://doi.org/10.3109/0142159X.2012.652239
4. Frank JR, Jabbour M. *Skills for the New Millennium: Report of the Societal Needs Working Group CanMEDS 2000 Project.* Royal College of Physicians and Surgeons of Canada.; 1996:1–21.
5. Batalden P, Leach D, Swing S, Dreyfus H, Dreyfus S. General competencies and accreditation in graduate medical education. *Health Aff (Millwood).* 2002;21(5):103–111. DOI: https://doi.org/10.1377/hlthaff.21.5.103
6. ten Cate O. Competency-based medical education and its competency frameworks. In: Mulder M, ed. *Competence-Based Vocational and Professional Education. Bridging the Worlds of Work and Education.* 1st ed. Springer International Publishing Switzerland 2017; 2017:903–929.
7. Norcini JJ, Holmboe ES, Hawkins RE. Evaluation challenges in the era of outcomes-based education. In: Holmboe ES, Hawkins RE, eds. *Practical Guide to the Evaluation of Clinical Competence.* 1st ed. Mosby Elsevier; 2008:1–9.
8. Norcini J, Burch V. Workplace-based assessment as an educational tool: AMEE Guide No. 31. *Med Teach.* 2007;29(9):855–871. DOI: https://doi.org/10.1080/01421590701775453
9. Van Melle E, Frank JR, Holmboe ES, et al. A core components framework for evaluating implementation of competency-based medical education programs. *Acad Med.* 2019;94(7):1002–1009. DOI: https://doi.org/10.1097/ACM.0000000000002743
10. Torre D, Rice NE, Ryan A, et al. Ottawa 2020 consensus statements for programmatic assessment - 2. Implementation and practice. *Med Teach.* 2021;43(10):1149–1160. DOI: https://doi.org/10.1080/0142159X.2021.1956681
11. Heeneman S, de Jong LH, Dawson LJ, et al. Ottawa 2020 consensus statement for programmatic assessment – 1. Agreement on the principles. *Med Teach.* 2021;43(10):1139–1148. DOI: https://doi.org/10.1080/0142159X.2021.1957088
12. Hauer KE, Chesluk B, Iobst W, et al. Reviewing residents' competence: a qualitative study of the role of clinical competency committees in performance assessment. *Acad Med.* 2015;90(8):1084–1092. DOI: https://doi.org/10.1097/ACM.0000000000000736
13. Bok HGJ, van der Vleuten CPM, de Jong LH. 'Prevention is better than cure': a plea to emphasize the learning function of competence committees in programmatic assessment. *Front Vet Sci.* 2021;8:638455. DOI: https://doi.org/10.3389/fvets.2021.638455
14. Dreyfus HL, Dreyfus SE. *Mind over Machine.* Free Press; 1986.

15. Carraccio CL, Benson BJ, Nixon LJ, Derstine PL. From the educational bench to the clinical bedside: translating the Dreyfus clinical skills. *Academic Medicine*. 2008;83(8):761–767.
16. Nasca TJ, Philibert I, Brigham T, Flynn TC. The next GME accreditation system—rationale and benefits. *N Engl J Med*. 2012;366(11):1051–1056. DOI: https://doi.org/10.1056/NEJMsr1200117
17. Harris K, Frank J. *Competence by Design*. Royal College of Physicians and Surgeons of Canada; 2014.
18. Warm EJ, Mathis BR, Held JD, et al. Entrustment and mapping of observable practice activities for resident assessment. *J Gen Intern Med*. 2014;29(8):1177–1182. DOI: https://doi.org/10.1007/s11606-014-2801-5
19. Touchie C, ten Cate O. The promise, perils, problems and progress of competency-based medical education. *Med Educ*. 2016;50(1):93–100. DOI: https://doi.org/10.1111/medu.12839
20. ten Cate O, Taylor DR. The recommended description of an entrustable professional activity: AMEE Guide No. 140. *Med Teach*. 2021;43(10):1106–1114. DOI: https://doi.org/10.1080/0142159X.2020.1838465
21. Mink RB, Carraccio CL, Herman BE, et al. Relationship between EPA level of supervision with their associated subcompetency milestone levels in pediatric fellow assessment. *BMC Med Educ*. 2023;23(1):720. DOI: https://doi.org/10.1186/s12909-023-04689-0
22. ten Cate O, Chen HC, Hoff RG, Peters H, Bok H, van der Schaaf M. Curriculum development for the workplace using entrustable professional activities (EPAs): AMEE Guide No. 99. *Med Teach*. 2015;37(11):983–1002. DOI: https://doi.org/10.3109/0142159X.2015.1060308
23. Schumacher DJ, West DC, Schwartz A, et al. Longitudinal assessment of resident performance using entrustable professional activities. *JAMA Netw Open*. 2020;3(1):e1919316. DOI: https://doi.org/10.1001/jamanetworkopen.2019.19316

CHAPTER 7

Entrustable professional activities: addressing confusions and controversies

Daniel J. Schumacher, Benjamin Kinnear,
Natasha Khursigara-Slattery, Jennie B. Jarrett, Olle ten Cate

Abstract

In this chapter, we address common confusions and controversies with entrustable professional activities (EPAs). With an eye toward practicality, we seek to offer resolutions or advice for these controversies where possible. We detail the differences between competencies and EPAs and discuss how they are complimentary approaches to health professions education that employ different lenses (individuals for competencies, and activities for EPAs). We next detail how EPAs should not be treated as an 'assessment tool' but rather as an approach to education that facilitates a stepwise decrease in supervision within the philosophy of competency-based education. Many terms related to EPAs and entrustment are conflated or poorly understood. This chapter disentangles many of these terms, including entrustment, supervision, trustworthiness, competence, supervision, autonomy, and independent practice. With precise definitions for these terms, it becomes clear how entrustment decisions are a forward-looking decision for the future rather than a report of past performance or supervision provided. Finally, we explore how EPAs and entrustment can support time variability and also how approaches to entrustment vary between contexts and cultures.

How to cite this book chapter:
Schumacher DJ, Kinnear B, Khursigara-Slattery N, Jarrett JB, ten Cate O. Entrustable professional activities: addressing confusions and controversies. In: ten Cate O, Burch VC, Chen HC, Chou FC, Hennus MP. (Eds). *Entrustable Professional Activities and Entrustment Decision-Making in Health Professions Education*, Chapter 7, pp. 75–83. [2024] London: Ubiquity Press. DOI: https://doi.org/10.5334/bdc.g

This chapter uses cross-references to other chapters of the same book. For those who read this chapter as a standalone publication: all cross-references can be found at: https://doi.org/10.5334/bdc

Authors

- Daniel J. Schumacher, MD, PhD, MEd. Cincinnati Children's Hospital Medical Center/ University of Cincinnati College of Medicine, Cincinnati, Ohio, USA. Correspondence: Daniel.Schumacher@cchmc.org0000-
- Benjamin Kinnear, MD, MEd. Cincinnati Children's Hospital Medical Center/University of Cincinnati College of Medicine, Cincinnati, Ohio, USA. 0000-0003-0052-4130
- Natasha Khursigara-Slattery, MD, MEHP. Mid-West Intern Network, University of Limerick, Limerick, Ireland.
- Jennie B. Jarrett, PharmD, MHPE. University of Illinois Chicago College of Pharmacy, Chicago, Illinois, USA. 0000-0003-0583-308X
- Olle ten Cate, PhD. University Medical Center Utrecht, Utrecht, the Netherlands and University of California, San Francisco, USA.

In this chapter, we address common confusions and controversies with entrustable professional activities (EPAs). With an eye toward practicality, we seek to offer resolutions or advice for these controversies where possible.

Contrasting EPAs and competencies

The prevailing approaches to competency-based education are grounded in defining competencies, entrustable professional activities (EPAs), or both. While some may think competencies and EPAs are similar or alternatives to choose from, this is not the case. Competencies define the abilities of people. A competency integrates knowledge, skills, and attitudes and is specific, durable, focused on performance, and learnable.[1,2] EPAs, however, are activities in a workplace. If a competency is 'the ability to do something successfully' (an Oxford Dictionary definition), then the activity is that 'something.' Execution of an activity requires specific competencies but that activity in and of itself is not a competency.

EPAs are sometimes depicted as large domains of competence, which in turn are composed of select competencies from those domains, in turn composed of milestone stages of development for each of those competencies (Figure 7.1, left). However, the relationship between EPAs and competencies depicted this way can lead to confusions, as EPAs thus seem to represent (large) competencies. EPAs are just the work-units trainees must be prepared to take on. The dimension of health care requirements and the dimension of competencies that professionals bring with them may be better viewed as perpendicular. In addition, EPAs do not need to be large. The contributions of a junior medical student to patient care can be relevant but small, and will, at later stages, be nested with the much broader EPAs of senior students and residents. Thus, EPAs related to competencies can better be visualized two axes or dimensions—one focused on features of individuals and the other focused on features of work, i.e., the activities that those individuals could do (Figure 7.1, right). EPAs are context-specific by definition. The reason that 'interprofessional collaboration,' as an example, can be a desired competency or skill but not an EPA is that it is not a concrete activity with a beginning and end that can be assigned at a specific time to a health professional or trainee.[3] However, it is a required skill for most EPAs. However, if a contextual specification (e.g., chairing an interprofessional session or committee) can be provided, it might be an activity that meets EPA criteria.[4] Finally, Figure 7.1 (right) also shows that the requirements to allow a trainee to be entrusted with the responsibility for an EPA can be specified to include not only specific competencies but also other skills, attitudes, and experiences.

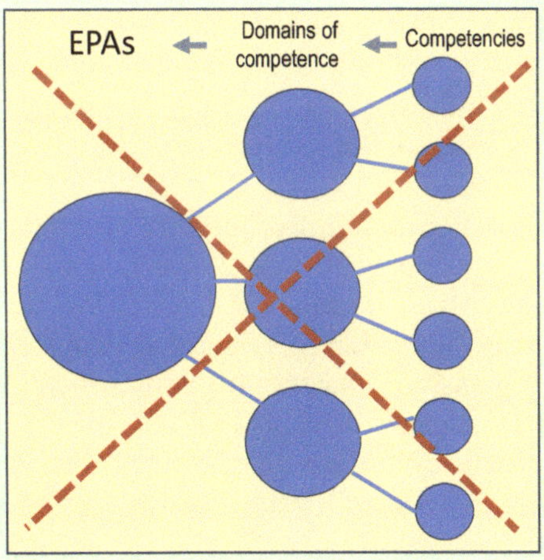

Competency requirements to allow for EPA entrustment	EPA 1	EPA 2	EPA 3	EPA 4
Competency A	X		X	
Competency B		X		
Competency C	X		X	X
Skill A		X	X	
Skill B				
Skill C				
Attitude A	X	X	X	X
Attitude B		X	X	
Experience A	X			X
Experience B	X	X		X

Figure 7.1: Not recommended (left) and recommended (right) representations of competencies, skill, and abilities versus EPAs.

The term 'EPA'

As units of professional practice, EPAs were introduced to facilitate a stepwise decrease in supervision for trainees executing activities that are germane to their profession. Because entrustment with these activities requires assessment of trainees, EPAs are often presented as an assessment method or framework. However, they are not an approach to assessment but rather a philosophical approach to health professions education, encompassing curriculum and assessment. Viewing EPAs simply as an approach to assessment fails to recognize their importance in defining the work of a profession and thus the requisite curriculum to be able to prepare individuals to execute the EPAs as well as develop their professional identity over time. When trainees are asked to secure supervisor observations of the performance on an EPA, they may say things like: 'if we don't have enough EPAs, we're going to fail.'[5] When they say this, trainees may actually be referring to observations rather than EPAs, expressing sentiments that reflect the experience of seeking a quantity of assessments rather than feelings about the EPAs themselves.

What is 'competent'?

The word 'competent' is often interpreted in multiple ways. For some, the word defines a comfortably acceptable level for physicians who no longer require supervision. However, for others, 'competent' is considered a level barely meeting standards ('all our graduates should be excellent, not competent'). Still others would regard a medical student as 'competent' in an area *for their stage of training*, while a resident with identical skills would be deemed not competent. The Dreyfus developmental model (novice–advanced beginner–competent–proficient–expert),[6] extensively applied in health professions training, places 'competent' in the middle of the trajectory. To escape such confusions, most of the EPA literature defines 'competent' as the threshold level in the development of a trainee when they are entrusted to act unsupervised.[7] That is not a moving target but rather fixed and defined for EPAs. It includes the primary meaning of competent, that is, '[p]ossessing the requisite qualifications for, or to [something]; properly qualified' (Oxford Dictionary), thus being entitled to act. This also implies that an individual cannot be competent in general but only in relation to particular EPAs.

Entrustable, trustworthiness, and trust

Scholars and educators have spoken of trainees being 'entrustable' and even 'pre-entrustable.'[8] However, entrustable was never intended to refer to individuals but rather to activities. Thus, an activity is entrustable when it can be entrusted to someone.

Rather than 'entrustable,' individuals should be described in terms of their trustworthiness. Trustworthiness itself is a complex construct that has been explored in medical education. ten Cate and Chen have summarized varying components of trainee trustworthiness with regard to entrustment decision-making: agency (proactive toward work, team, safety, personal development), reliability (conscientious, predictable, accountable, responsible), integrity (truthful, benevolent, patient-centered), capability (specific knowledge, skills, experience, situational awareness), and humility (recognizes limits, asks for help, receptive to feedback).[9] Although entrustment decisions are context-dependent (dependent on the assessor, context, task, etc.), trainee trustworthiness is a central component of all entrustment decisions.[10,11]

In common parlance, trustworthiness is spoken of as a moral character trait ('we can always rely on that person's word'). However, in connection with EPAs, it should be applied to specific entrustment decisions. To draw a parallel: a parent may deem their 15-year-old daughter more trustworthy than their 19-year-old son, yet would allow him but not her to drive their car because he has a driver's license and she does not.

Trustworthiness is different from trust. Trust has been defined in medical education as 'the willingness of a party to be vulnerable to the actions of another party on the basis of the expectation that the other will perform a particular action, irrespective of the trustor's ability to monitor or control that other party.'[12] Trust is the expected response from a person when they determine another individual to be trustworthy. However, trustors vary in their baseline propensity to trust.[13] Thus, trust is situationally determined based on: (a) the trainee's trustworthiness, (b) the trustor's trust propensity, and (c) the context and risk for the task at hand.[14]

Because entrustment does not follow solely from the trustworthiness of an individual, we believe it is best to avoid using potentially harmful phrasing such as 'not trusting' trainees. Rather, we suggest using language such as 'not yet ready' to practice a task at a given level of supervision in a particular context. This phrasing not only avoids language that could be harmful but also anchors conversations with trainees in the task at hand. A trustworthy trainee may simply not be ready for a particular task. The use of the word 'yet' also implies that they can be determined ready in the future.

Entrustment decisions versus entrustment determinations

Trust is future-facing. One individual can only entrust another with tasks that will occur in the (uncertain) future (e.g., whichever patient comes through the door next). Past experiences with the trainee matter, as predictions for what will happen in the future are often based on past events.[15] Trust, however, focuses on what might happen next. Entrustment is, therefore, a prospective *decision* about a future task.

In practice, entrustment in health professions education programs is often framed only as a score on a retrospective-oriented scale. That score is informed by a completed activity performance and assigning an entrustment–supervision level score reflecting what the supervisor in fact chose to allow at that time. This summary of past performance can be called an entrustment *determination*[16] but should not be confused with an entrustment *decision*.[17] In the context of entrustment, decisions are determinations that have real-world consequences in terms of advancement or granting of more responsibilities for trainees. Entrustment decisions operationalize the stepwise, graduated autonomy and responsibility to move trainees from legitimate peripheral participation[18] in patient care toward the center of the professional team. Failure to decrease supervision when warranted deprives trainees of the opportunity to execute work with full responsibility, including the psychological weight of being the individual ultimately responsible, during training. This blunts trainee growth and development and may risk patient safety once a trainee graduates.[19]

Disentangling supervision, autonomy, and independent practice

The decision to entrust another individual with unsupervised practice requires further consideration as it pertains to what being unsupervised means in terms of autonomy. Supervision and autonomy are often presented as opposite ends of the same spectrum with an inverse relationship—an individual can either have full autonomy or require full supervision. However, we prefer the definition of autonomy that Ryan and Deci present in self-determination theory: the ability to 'self-regulate one's experiences and actions.'[20] Framed this way, autonomy is more than just unfettered agency. Even an individual requiring full supervision can be allowed to self-regulate. For example, a medical student on the first day of a new clinical rotation can be allowed to choose which patients to care for or which clinic to attend.

'Unsupervised' and 'independent' practice are also often conflated. True independent practice is exceedingly rare in modern health care, and 'unsupervised' practice should therefore be the preferred term. Independent practice connotes that an individual works without any support from others. This is simply not consistent with the realities of working in nearly all health systems, where individual health professionals are a part of a team and where help is always available in person, over the phone, or over email.

How an EPA-based model aligns with flexibility and time variability in training

A basic tenet of competency-based education is the idea of time variability,[21] that is, moving from a fixed training time with variable trainee outcomes to fixed outcomes (i.e., minimum competence standards) and variable training time.[22–24] Yet time-variable training has proven challenging to implement. Many health profession educators acknowledge that some trainees complete training while not meeting all critical objectives; however, the provision of more time, or conversely graduating others earlier, frequently leads to practical problems. One cause of the concern is a fixed transition point in the year. The annual North American selection or match procedure (resulting in a start date of July 1 for all residents) differs significantly from other countries, where graduation from medical school and entry into residency programs is more flexible in terms of timing.[25] Importantly, time variability should not lead to unexpected surprises at the end of training. Extensions and reductions in training time should be foreseen by programs, and communicated to trainees, months or semesters ahead.

In theory, EPAs could facilitate more granular time variability, as the EPAs for which one is not ready to practice should be definable at any point of time in training. Owing to logistical or other challenges, if time variability is not a potential option, entrustment decisions run a substantial risk of remaining a theoretical construct, relying on the presumption that a PGY-4 (postgraduate year four) can be entrusted with an activity just because they are a PGY-4.

International and cultural differences in entrustment

How trainees and educators think and behave with respect to particular tasks and environments is socially, culturally, and historically contingent.[26] Controversy and confusion can arise during international discussions about entrustment and consequent responsibilities for trainees in health care. Differences in entrustment practices are affected by the nature of the educational continuum (for an overview, see Chapter 16), by regulatory and legislative differences, by differences in resources for health care and training in countries in the Global North and Global South, and by historically rooted differences in culture and hierarchy. We could not locate useful references, even though we felt these differences exist. In preparation for this chapter, a subset of authors convened a discussion group of medical educators with backgrounds in India, the Philippines, Taiwan, China, Malaysia, Ireland, the Netherlands, and Canada to obtain an impression of differences. In some countries (e.g., India, Malaysia), interns are entrusted with a wide range of responsibilities (e.g., lumbar puncture, chest tube insertion, pericardiocentesis, uncomplicated deliveries) in public medical colleges that predominantly supply graduates for rural areas. In this scenario, supervision is formalized as countersigning histories and procedures done by trainees in task-oriented logbooks. In contrast, in private medical colleges, where high numbers of supervisory teaching faculty are employed, trainee responsibilities are much more restricted and supervised. Paradoxically, although graduates from private medical colleges receive more teaching, they may be far less prepared for practical patient care responsibilities than graduates from government-sponsored public academic hospitals that frequently rely on interns to meet the health care needs of large rural populations.

Timelines for licensure can also differ vastly. For example, the Philippines allows some unsupervised practice prior to licensure, while China delays that fully until after licensure. Politico-historical developments within a country can also affect hierarchical permissions of autonomy. Until 1945, during the period of Japanese rule, a strong Prussian-styled hierarchy (originally derived from German medical education culture) determined the roles of professors, attendings, and trainees in Taiwan. Physicians had significant autonomy to perform procedures owing to an elevated societal respect for the profession. The SARS epidemic in 2003 became a turning point, with an emphasis on patient safety outweighing the cultural respect for physicians. As a result, direct supervision increased and North American influence became more dominant in medical education.

Conclusion

In this chapter, we have attempted to resolve confusion and debate around EPAs and entrustment decision-making, addressing both conceptual and practical issues. Undoubtedly, such debates will continue; however, this book may serve as a supportive resource to provide reference for the implementation of educational innovations. Educational improvement is a continuous endeavor, with the path to inventive and productive progress often charged/infused with dialogue, debate, clarification, and argumentation aiming for a shared mental model and common terminology.

Acknowledgments

We wish to thank well-informed HPE educators Drs. Reshma Kini (Father Muller College, Mangalore, India), Patrick Tan (from the Philippines, currently working at Shantou University Medical College, Shantou, China), Fremen Chihchen Chou (China Medical University, Taichung, Taiwan), and Sylvia Sushila Samuel (RCSI and UCD Malaysia Campus, Malaysia) for a rich discussion in February 2024 on international and cultural differences in entrustment practices, as well as Dr. Zhongfang Zhang (Shantou University Medical College, Shantou, China), who added to Dr Patrick Tan's knowledge of the Chinese context.

Competing interests

The authors declare that they have no competing interests.

References

1. ten Cate O. Competency-based medical education. In: Cockerham WC, Dingwall R, Quah S, eds. *The Wiley-Blackwell Encyclopedia of Health, Illness, Behavior, and Society*. John Wiley & Sons; 2014:1329–1335.
2. van Merriënboer JJG, van der Klink MR, Hendriks M. *Competencies: From Complications Toward Agreement (Dutch)*. Educational Council of The Netherlands; 2002.
3. ten Cate O, Pool IA. The viability of interprofessional entrustable professional activities. *Adv Health Sci Educ Theory Pract*. 2020;25(5):1255–1262. DOI: https://doi.org/10.1007/s10459-019-09950-0
4. ten Cate O, Taylor DR. The recommended description of an entrustable professional activity: AMEE Guide No. 140. *Med Teach*. 2020:1–9.

5. Ahn EA-O, LaDonna KA-O, Landreville JA-O, McHeimech R, Cheung WA-O. *Only as Strong as the Weakest Link: Resident Perspectives on Entrustable Professional Activities and Their Impact on Learning.* (1949–8357 (Electronic)).
6. Dreyfus SE. The five-stage model of adult skill acquisition. *B Sci Technol Soc.* 2004/06/01 2004;24(3):177–181. DOI: https://doi.org/10.1177/0270467604264992
7. ten Cate O SL, Carraccio C. Medical competence: The interplay between individual ability and the health care environment. *Med Teach.* 2010;32:669–675.
8. Curran VR, Deacon D, Schulz H, et al. Evaluation of the characteristics of a workplace assessment form to assess entrustable professional activities (EPAs) in an undergraduate surgery core clerkship. *J Surg Educ.* 2018;75(5):1211–1222.
9. ten Cate O, Chen HC. The ingredients of a rich entrustment decision. *Med Teach.* 2020;42(12):1413–1420. DOI: https://doi.org/10.1080/0142159X.2020.1817348
10. Schumacher DJ, Michelson C, Winn AS, Turner DA, Martini A, Kinnear B. A realist synthesis of prospective entrustment decision making by entrustment or clinical competency committees. *Med Educ.* 2023; https://doi.org/doi:10.1111/medu.15296
11. Schumacher DJ, Michelson C, Winn AS, Turner DA, Elshoff E, Kinnear B. Making prospective entrustment decisions: knowing limits, seeking help and defaulting. *Med Educ.* 2022;56(9):892–900. DOI: https://doi.org/10.1111/medu.14797
12. Mayer RC, Davis JH, Schoorman FD. An integrative model of organizational trust. *Acad Manag Rev.* 1995;20(3):709–734.
13. ten Cate O. Entrustability of professional activities and competency-based training. *Med Educ.* 2005;39:1176–1177.
14. Hauer KE, ten Cate O, Boscardin C, Irby DM, Iobst W, O'Sullivan PS. Understanding trust as an essential element of trainee supervision and learning in the workplace. *Adv Health Sci Educ Theory Pract.* 2014;19(3):435–456. DOI: https://doi.org/10.1007/s10459-013-9474-4
15. Schumacher DJ, ten Cate O, Damodaran A, et al. Clarifying essential terminology in entrustment. *Med Teach.* 2021;43(7):737–744.
16. Brown DR, Moeller JJ, Grbic D, et al. Comparing entrustment decision-making outcomes of the Core Entrustable Professional Activities Pilot, 2019–2020. *JAMA Netw Open.* 2022;5(9):e2233342. DOI: https://doi.org/10.1001/jamanetworkopen.2022.33342
17. ten Cate O, Jarrett JB. *Would* I trust or *will* I trust? The gap between entrustment determinations and entrustment decisions for trainees in pharmacy and other health professions. *Pharmacy (Basel).* 2023;11(3). DOI: https://doi.org/10.3390/pharmacy11030107
18. Lave J, Wenger E. *Situated Learning: Legitimate Peripheral Participation.* Cambridge University Press; 1991.
19. Dacey RG, Nasca TJ. Seniorization of tasks in the academic medical center: a worrisome trend. *J Am Coll Surg.* 2019;228(3):299–302. DOI: https://doi.org/10.1016/j.jamcollsurg.2018.11.009
20. Deci EL, Ryan RM, Williams GC. Need satisfaction and the self-regulation of learning. *Learn and Individ Differ.* 1996;8(3):165–183.
21. ten Cate O, Gruppen LD, Kogan JR, Lingard LA, Teunissen PW. Time-variable training in medicine: theoretical considerations. *Acad Med.* 2018;93(3S):S6-S11. DOI: https://doi.org/10.1097/ACM.0000000000002065
22. Carraccio C, Wolfsthal SD, Englander R, Ferentz K, Martin C. Shifting paradigms: from Flexner to competencies. *Acad Med.* 2002;77(5).
23. Lucey CR, Thibault GE, ten Cate O. Competency-based, time-variable education in the health professions: crossroads. *Acad Med.* 2018;93(3S):S1-S5. DOI: https://doi.org/10.1097/ACM.0000000000002080

24. Carraccio C, Lentz A, Schumacher DJ. Dismantling fixed time, variable outcome education: abandoning 'ready or not, here they come' is overdue. *Perspect Med Educ.* 2023;12(1):68–75. DOI: https://doi.org/10.5334/pme.10
25. Hoff RG, Frenkel J, Imhof SM, ten Cate O. Flexibility in postgraduate medical training in the Netherlands. *Acad Med.* Mar 2018;93(3S):S32-S36. DOI: https://doi.org/10.1097/ACM.0000000000002078
26. Cong-Lem N. Vygotsky's, Leontiev's and Engeström's cultural-historical (activity) theories: overview, clarifications and implications. *Integr Psychol Behav Sci.* 2022;56(4):1091–1112. DOI: https://doi.org/10.1007/s12124-022-09703-6

SECTION B

Entrustable professional activities defined

CHAPTER 8

Entrustable professional activities and EPA frameworks defined

David R. Taylor, Siobhan Fitzpatrick, María José López, Marije P. Hennus, Adrian P. Marty, Olle ten Cate

Abstract

Entrustable professional activities (EPAs) serve important purposes in health professions education. These purposes include supporting curriculum development and delivery and guiding trainee assessment, as well as grounding high-stakes decisions to allow trainees to practice in unsupervised settings. These purposes require more than a succinct and recognizable title of an EPA. For their full potential, descriptions of EPAs must be fully elaborated with the detailed information required to deliver on each of these purposes. Elaborating EPAs also requires a clear understanding of the relationships between other educational and professional constructs such as knowledge and competencies. This chapter discusses the distinction and relationship between knowledge, skills, and attitudes (KSAs), competencies, and EPAs, discusses the components of a fully elaborated EPA and why these components are important to implementing EPAs in educational programs, and examines how EPAs are assembled into frameworks of EPAs to serve a profession or discipline. The chapter concludes with a brief discussion of transdisciplinary EPAs.

How to cite this book chapter:

Taylor DR, Fitzpatrick S, López MJ, Hennus MP, Marty AP, ten Cate O. Entrustable professional activities and EPA frameworks defined. In: ten Cate O, Burch VC, Chen HC, Chou FC, Hennus MP. (Eds). *Entrustable Professional Activities and Entrustment Decision-Making in Health Professions Education*, Chapter 8, pp. 87–100. [2024] London: Ubiquity Press. DOI: https://doi.org/10.5334/bdc.h

This chapter uses cross-references to other chapters of the same book. For those who read this chapter as a standalone publication: all cross-references can be found at: https://doi.org/10.5334/bdc

Authors

- David R. Taylor, MD, MHPE. Queen's University, Kingston, Ontario, Canada. Correspondence: taylord@queensu.ca
- Siobhan Fitzpatrick, MA. World Health Organization, Geneva, Switzerland.
- María José López, MSc. Facultad de Ciencias Médicas, Universidad Nacional de Cuyo, Mendoza, Argentina.
- Marije P. Hennus, MD, PhD, MSc. Clin Ed. University Medical Center Utrecht, the Netherlands.
- Adrian P. Marty, MD, MME. University Hospital Balgrist, University of Zurich, Zurich, Switzerland.
- Olle ten Cate, PhD. University Medical Center Utrecht, Utrecht, the Netherlands and University of California, San Francisco, USA.

Introduction

Many schools, programs, professional bodies, and curriculum committees in the health professions are currently involved in the implementation of entrustable professional activity (EPA)-based education,[1–4] but not all conceptualizations are equally helpful.[5] A risk of new educational curricular concepts and frameworks, such as an EPA model, is the ease with which the focus of educational leaders shifts from *why is this framework important?* to *how do I adopt this new framework?* Developing EPAs and building EPA-based curricula requires that curricular leaders have an in-depth understanding of the rationale for the curricular change. This requires a rich understanding of EPA construction and its application within competency-based training, as well as limitations and opportunities of EPAs in areas of curriculum, assessment, and the local professional workplace. This chapter begins with a description of the essential characteristics of EPAs, followed by a discussion of three related but distinct constructs used in competency-based education (CBE)—EPAs; knowledge, skills, and attitudes (KSAs); and competencies. Building on these concepts, the chapter then focuses on designing a coherent framework of EPAs as part of a competency-based curriculum that is suitable for assessment decisions that capture grounded trust in trainees' readiness for unsupervised professional practice.

Essential characteristics of EPAs

As described in earlier chapters, an EPA is a *unit of work in professional practice*—it could be a bundle of tasks, it could be big or small, it could be an early activity, later nested within a broader EPA, but in all cases it should be an observable, standalone activity. If speaking a second language were the skill a person possessed, acting as a translator would be an example of an entrusted activity.[6] Therefore, EPAs are *not* 'possessed' by a trainee (like knowledge or skills), but rather 'owned' by the profession and may be 'delegated' or 'given' to a practitioner, or one in training, to execute, which makes the activity 'entrustable.'

This draws on employment literature, which generally defines scopes of practice and role responsibilities using the activities of professional practice.[7,8] In health care, EPAs are the work done in caring for patients. They constitute the task list for which KSAs and competencies are needed.

Understanding EPAs as units of work is an important starting point. Those embarking on developing EPAs must go beyond this, building a rich understanding of the purposes of developing and implementing EPAs.[9] How one approaches elaborating descriptions of work naturally depends on the intended purpose(s) of developing the description.[7] For CBE, identifying and elaborating EPAs supports decision-making related to education progression and professional certification, and supports curriculum planning within programs. More specifically, EPAs:

- operationalize competencies into observable units of work;
- support determinations of readiness for trainees to enter unsupervised practice, i.e., to allow for entrustment decisions and subsequent transfer of responsibility;
- guide the organization of learning and assessment within an education program;
- reflect what professionals do in practice.

Building on these core purposes of EPAs, the health professions literature has established eight defining characteristics of EPAs—characteristics considered essential to these purposes.[9–11] (Table 1).

Table 8.1: Entrustable professional activity characteristics.

Defining characteristics of an EPA
• Is essential professional work in a given context • Leads to a recognized output of professional labor • Requires adequate knowledge, skill, and attitudes that are generally acquired through training to perform successfully • Is confined to qualified personnel • Is executable independent of other EPAs • Is executable within a defined time frame • Is observable and measurable in process and outcome (well done or not well done) • Requires integration of multiple competencies

It follows that EPAs developed for health professions education need to align with these characteristics in order to achieve their purposes. This sounds straightforward, but several EPA initiatives have produced EPAs that failed to achieve this alignment.[12–15] These problematic outcomes may stem from a variety of mistakes during development including confusion in distinguishing between learning objectives, KSAs, competencies, and EPAs, or failing to develop a robust shared mental model among project team members.[15] To help EPA development teams evaluate EPA quality and ensure this important alignment, Taylor et al. generated the EQual Rubric tool to evaluate EPA quality (see Chapter 11 for details).[16] Organizing these defining characteristics into three, practical categories, the rubric structures the evaluation of EPAs as: (1) discrete units of work; (2) entrustable and essential to the profession; (3) described in a way that aligns with educational principles. Additionally, a faculty development video associated with the rubric can be used for educational purposes in addition to preparing people to use the rubric.[17] Readers should also be aware of several articles useful in helping build a rich understanding of EPAs and their application in CBE.[9,11,15]

KSAs, competencies, and entrustable professional activities

To understand the defining characteristics of EPAs, it is also important to understand the distinctions and relationships between KSAs, competencies, and EPAs. Although the lines between these often seem to blur,[6,18–20] the underlying principles used to distinguish them are crucial. Hasty attempts to adopt CBE without the development of the prerequisite understanding of these related but distinct concepts have frequently undermined the goals and benefits of pursuing competency-based curricular design.[6,15,21] Figure 8.1, adapted from the Royal Australian College of Physicians and the World Health Organization, demonstrates the relationship between KSAs, competencies, and EPAs using the 'knowing, being, doing' curricular model. Arrows show the dependencies between these domains,[22,23] highlighting the ultimate goal of caring for patients through clinical work.

KSAs represent the foundational building blocks in curricula acquired in preparation for professional practice. Although sometimes broad, they are often more granular abilities—ones that generalize across contexts and settings. Examples of KSAs include: the ability to examine an ECG and identify rate, rhythm, axis, and intervals; non-verbal communication skills; and knowing the complications of compartment syndrome. Importantly, KSAs are abilities possessed by a trainee—something they either have or do not have when entering a clinical situation.

Like KSAs, competencies are also possessed by a trainee, but competencies represent higher-order abilities that integrate multiple KSAs. Building on the above examples, competencies might include: interpretation of ECGs for clinical decision-making; communication in emotionally charged situations; and examining limbs for neurovascular compromise. In contrast to singular KSAs, competencies require integration of multiple foundational KSAs to produce a clinically

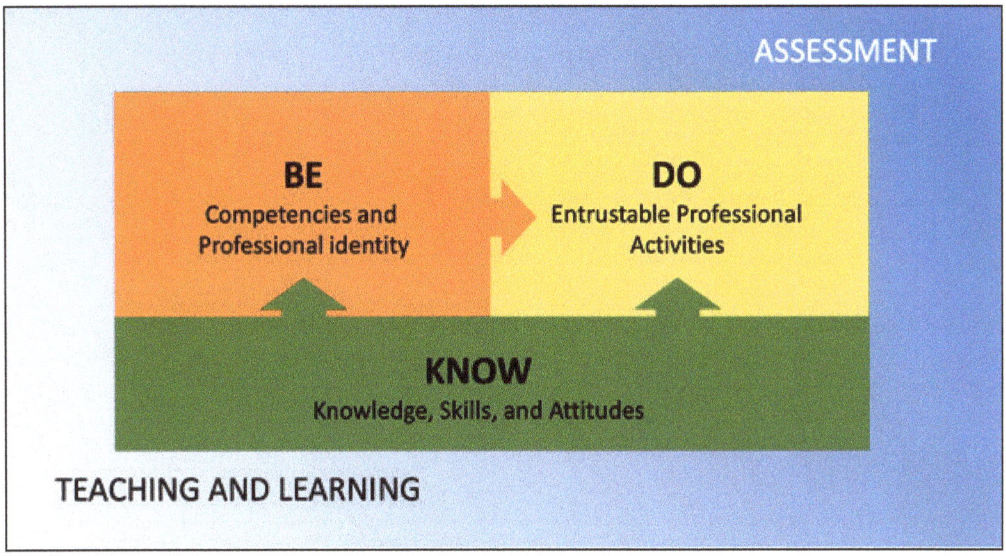

Figure 8.1: Relationships between KSAs, competencies, identity, and EPAs in the know-do-be curricular model.

usable ability that is recognizable within a profession or discipline. One cannot see the competencies trainees possess simply by looking at them. Instead, you can observe the *application* of competencies when trainees use them to perform the *tasks* of patient care as required for the context.

As described earlier, EPAs are the activities done in caring for patients. Performing an EPA requires trainees to draw from the KSAs and competencies that they bring with them to the clinical encounter—selecting those they recognize as necessary to deliver the care required for that patient. Performing an EPA is therefore specific to the clinical context and not something that is possessed by a trainee. Returning to our examples used for KSAs and competencies above, an example of an EPA would be 'Managing trauma care,' comprising numerous competencies (including the example competencies identified above), and foundational KSAs.

	EPA 1	EPA 2	EPA 3	EPA 4
Competency A	+	+		+
Competency B		+	+	
Competency C			+	

Figure 8.2: Relationship of EPAs and competencies as two dimensions of a grid.

This 'knowing, being, doing' model shows how KSAs, competencies, and a professional identity are prerequisites for practice, and EPAs representing that practice. The relationship between competencies and EPAs becomes clear when examining the construction of a framework of EPAs as two dimensions of a grid. Figure 8.2 shows how the competencies required for a profession relate to the EPAs performed in providing health care. A matrix such as the one in Figure 8.2 can provide a start to a useful blueprint for curricula and guide the organization of learning content.

Not all important curricular components should fit the EPA construct

The definition of an EPA presented here can raise concerns around important areas in health professions education that do not fit the EPA construct. Lifelong learning, collaboration, and cultural safety are all essential competencies in health professions education but are in themselves not units of work that can be simply entrusted. With an emerging construct such as EPAs, there is often pressure to make everything fit the novel construct. By exclusively emphasizing EPAs, education programs can paradoxically diminish the value of these competencies by attempting to make them into EPAs. 'Interprofessional collaboration,' for example, is sometimes proposed as one EPA within an EPA framework; this disregards the need for interprofessional skills as a prerequisite for almost all entrustable activities in health care.[24] Curricula, programs, credentialling bodies, and others must ensure that such domains are taught and assessed as competencies—in addition, of course, to ensuring trainees synthesize these competencies into their clinical work, i.e., in EPAs, when appropriate.

Fully elaborated description of entrustable professional activities

An EPA is more than a succinct label of a clinical activity. A fully elaborated EPA should include the eight recommended components (Table 8.2) in order to provide transparency, robustness, validity, and applicability.[11] Each of these components provides information important to key stakeholders in health professions education. For curricular leaders it clarifies what students

Table 8.2: Components of a fully elaborated EPA, their purpose, and relevant stakeholders.

Component	Purpose	Most relevant persons
1. Title	Succinctly and clearly identifies the task	Trainees, clinical supervisors
2. Specification and limitations	Describes the task in detail to make clear what the qualification for this EPA includes	Trainees, clinical supervisors
3. Potential risks in case of failure	Identifies possible adverse outcomes from inadequate performance of the EPA	Trainees, supervisors, academic advisers/coaches
4. Most relevant competency domains	Identifies the key competency domains required to perform the EPA	Curriculum developers
5. Required KSAs and experiences	Maps the activity to relevant competencies and/or KSAs and identifies relevant learning experiences	Curriculum developers
6. Information sources to assess progress and support summative entrustment	Identifies sources of assessment data important to making summative entrustment decisions for the EPA	Curriculum developers, competence committees
7. Entrustment/supervision level expected at which stage of training	Provides a map of expected trainee progression toward readiness for unsupervised practice	Trainees, academic advisers/coaches
8. Time period to expiration if not practiced	Sets a timeline for which the skills needed to perform the task safely are likely to extinguish if not practiced	Regulators, practitioners

must learn (domains of competence and KSAs); for medical regulators it defines what exactly the clinician is certified to do without supervision and for what period of time (specifications, limitations, and time to expiration if not practiced). Each component serves a specific purpose in operationalizing EPA-based education in today's highly regulated health care and other professional fields. It is also important to recognize that not all components are relevant to all people. Table 8.2 highlights key stakeholders to whom components are most relevant. The appendix at the end of the chapter provides tips for elaborating EPAs in the eight-component format, with examples.

When developing EPAs, it is important to recognize that development teams do not need to (and in fact should not) define all components of an EPA from the outset. *EPA title, specifications and limitations*, and *most relevant competency domains* should be the first priority. These three components establish the shared mental model for performing the EPA in practice. If consensus is achieved on these components, elaborating the other components will be much easier and more meaningful. If there is not consensus on these priority components, it will be very difficult, if not impossible, to build consensus on the rest.

Beyond its application within professional training programs, this recommended approach to describing EPAs opens the possibility of microcredentialling for new or specialized clinical activities. Bedside ultrasound is a task that is increasingly becoming standard of care in many medical specialties. Yet many practicing physicians were trained prior to its widespread availability. Developing a fully elaborated EPA for such an activity provides opportunities for physicians to learn new skills and establish certification for their use.

EPA frameworks

Beyond elaboration of individual EPAs, it is important to consider how a discipline, profession, service area, or specialty is represented by a set (or framework) of EPAs. A framework of EPAs is a coherent and reasonably comprehensive set of EPAs that define the core activities of a discipline, generally arrived at through consensus methods.[9,25] If a single EPA describes a single unit of work, then a framework of EPAs should capture all of the essential, entrustable work performed for the goals and scope of the profession or discipline. The framework (or core set) of EPAs allows for a certification, diploma, even a title (job title or professional title), and/or license. In essence, it constitutes the activities that would be listed in the job description of a profession—the activities entrusted and regulated in that profession. But a framework of EPAs for a specific profession is more than simply an aggregate of EPAs. The term 'framework' reflects the need for adaptability to the heterogeneity of practice that may be seen across a professional jurisdiction. Consider how a framework of EPAs for family medicine might include the same defined outcomes. In practice, the application of 'Managing chronic disease, referring for specialized care, managing urgent presentations' will look very different in a local urban setting than in a national context that includes rural and remote regions. It is the context that changes, not the EPA.[26]

It is also important to recognize that there is not a single approach to developing a framework of EPAs. Frameworks can be composed of small activities with many identified, or broad and few.[27] Each of these approaches offers advantages and trade-offs (discussed in Chapter 9). In considering the use of EPAs within education programs and for professional certification, highly granular EPA frameworks often become unwieldy, and risk venturing into sets of skills rather than activities or tasks. For programs leading to professional certification, experience suggests a total of no more than 20 is ideal.[28–30] Professions with a narrow scope of practice may have fewer; those with a broad scope of practice, such as family medicine, may require more. Regardless, operational feasibility is a critical consideration in planning.

Table 8.3: Features of an EPA framework to guide EPA development.

Features of a cohesive EPA framework
• It identifies the groups of tasks that graduates will be certified to perform[9,23] • It demonstrates congruent logic(s) across the EPAs[27] • It clearly distinguishes each EPA from the others[15,16] • It supports structural entrustment decisions for EPAs (i.e., STARs*)[9] • It describes EPAs broadly with limited numbers[28] • It requires contextualization in how activities are realized in different clinical contexts—case to case and setting to setting[23,25] • It shows alignment between EPAs in the framework and the competencies expected in practice[9,15,23,28]

Ensuring an EPA framework is cohesive is another important consideration. Seven described features of EPA frameworks can be helpful to consider when envisioning or preparing to develop EPAs (Table 8.3).

*STAR or statement of awarded responsibility, is a certificate awarded to a trainee granting them permission to perform an EPA at a specified level of supervision (see Chapter 10).

One quality that warrants further explanation is the use of logics in developing EPAs.[27] While more extensively elaborated in Chapter 9, EPAs can be organized as procedures ('Colonoscopy'), as functions ('Consulting on inpatients'), or in relation to diseases ('Managing patients with acute kidney injury'). It is easy to see each of these EPAs as a discrete, observable, and entrustable activity for that discipline. Although procedural EPAs combine well in frameworks with either of the other logics, blending function- and disease-oriented EPAs within a framework can be problematic. Considering the examples 'Consulting on inpatients' and 'Managing patients with acute kidney injury,' these EPAs create areas of overlap that introduce confusion. It is difficult to see how a trainee could be awarded the former EPA and not the latter. Attention to logics employed is important for developing a coherent framework.

Completeness of a framework

A final consideration with frameworks of EPAs surrounds professional certification decisions linked to licensing. As has been previously highlighted, summative entrustment decisions for EPAs are intended to enable authorization to perform those EPAs in unsupervised practice. However, certification for unsupervised practice is a regulatory decision generally made comprehensively for the full scope of practice in a given discipline. In most jurisdictions, it is impractical to routinely customize professional practice licenses from one individual to the next. The implication is that, if EPAs are adopted in a discipline and intended to inform high-stakes certification decisions, it is important that there is a complete framework of EPAs that represent the full scope of practice in that discipline. Microcredentialling, as described above, could in future be linked to certifications and permissions for individual EPAs, which could in turn enable a responsive workforce—as evidenced during the COVID-19 pandemic response. However, current practices are associated with whole qualifications linked to licensing. For that purpose, and for the EPA framework to provide the bridge between education, practice, and regulation, there must be a core set of EPAs providing a reasonably comprehensive description of professional practice.

Similar EPAs across different disciplines

There is increasing interest in examining aspects of overlap in clinical practice between disciplines and professions. In some cases, multiple disciplines may perform the same task, in the same context, for the same purpose. For example, both gastroenterologists and general surgeons may perform a colonoscopy to identify the source of gastrointestinal bleeding in a patient with iron-deficient anemia. It seems reasonable that an EPA awarded in one discipline could be carried over to practice in the other discipline. More commonly, different disciplines or professions perform similar tasks, but for distinguishably different purposes and in different contexts. Patient handover is a common activity in most (if not all) health professions, but it is often performed differently in different contexts and for different purposes. Most would argue the handover EPA is not simply interchangeable across professions.

Increasingly, health professionals are being asked to work beyond their scope of practice or even provide aspects of care that are typically provided by another different health profession. This was perhaps most evident at the height of the COVID pandemic. Constructing the certification for health professions and design of health care systems with adaptability to shift work across disciplines in times of crisis is now understood to be of important value. Transdisciplinary EPAs, those EPAs that apply to multiple disciplines or specialties, provide an attractive approach to delivering on this need.[31] But it should be noted that there remains significant debate around how this would and could be implemented, because the context in which an EPA is performed is crucial to its portability. Research into understanding how a transdisciplinary EPA awarded in one discipline can be safely transported by a specialist into a new context or discipline will be important in advancing this promising concept. Additional discussion of transdisciplinary EPAs can be found in Chapter 10.

Conclusion

EPAs and frameworks of EPAs constitute an attractive approach to clarify the core of health disciplines and their activities. Defining and identifying EPAs to be truly useful for the purpose of the training for these health professions requires thoughtful deliberation, consensus among educators, and careful planning.

References

1. O'Dowd E, Lydon S, O'Connor P, Madden C, Byrne D. A systematic review of 7 years of research on entrustable professional activities in graduate medical education, 2011–2018. *Med Educ.* 2019;78(1):39. DOI: https://doi.org/10.1111/medu.13792
2. Shorey S, Lau TC, Lau ST, Ang E. Entrustable professional activities in health care education: a scoping review. *Med Educ.* 2019;53(8):766–777. DOI: https://doi.org/10.1111/medu.13879
3. Bramley AL, McKenna L. Entrustable professional activities in entry-level health professional education: a scoping review. *Med Educ.* 2021;55(9):1011–1032. DOI: https://doi.org/10.1111/medu.14539
4. Pinilla S, Lenouvel E, Cantisani A, et al. Working with entrustable professional activities in clinical education in undergraduate medical education: a scoping review. *BMC Med Educ.* 2021;21(1):172. DOI: https://doi.org/10.1186/s12909-021-02608-9
5. Moore SJ, Egerton T, Merolli M, Lees J, Scala NL, Parry SM. Inconsistently reporting post-licensure EPA specifications in different clinical professions hampers fidelity and practice translation: a scoping review. *BMC Med Educ.* 2023;23(1):372. DOI: https://doi.org/10.1186/s12909-023-04364-4
6. ten Cate O, Schumacher DJ. Entrustable professional activities versus competencies and skills: exploring why different concepts are often conflated. *Adv Heal Sci Educ.* 2022;27(2):491–499. DOI: https://doi.org/10.1007/s10459-022-10098-7
7. Morgeson FP, Brannick MT, Levine EL. *Job and Work Analysis.* 3rd ed. SAGE Publishing; 2019.

8. International Labour Organization. ISCO International Standard Classification of Occupations. Published June 21, 2016. Accessed March 25, 2024. https://www.ilo.org/public/english/bureau/stat/isco/isco08/
9. ten Cate O, Scheele F. Competency-based postgraduate training: can we bridge the gap between theory and clinical practice? *Acad Med.* 2007;82(6):542–547. DOI: https://doi.org/10.1097/acm.0b013e31805559c7
10. ten Cate O. Entrustability of professional activities and competency-based training. *Med Educ.* 2005;39(12):1176–1177. DOI: https://doi.org/10.1111/j.1365-2929.2005.02341.x
11. ten Cate O, Taylor DR. The recommended description of an entrustable professional activity: AMEE guide no. 140. *Med Teach.* 2021;43(10):1106–1114. DOI: https://doi.org/10.1080/0142159x.2020.1838465
12. Taylor DR, Park YS, Smith CA, Karpinski J, Coke W, Tekian A. Creating entrustable professional activities to assess internal medicine residents in training: a mixed-methods approach. *Ann Internal Med.* 2018;168(10):724–729. DOI: https://doi.org/10.7326/m17-1680
13. Meyer EG, Taylor DR, Uijtdehaage S, Durning SJ. EQual rubric evaluation of the Association of American Medical Colleges' core entrustable professional activities for entering residency. *Acad Med.* 2020;95(11):1755–1762. DOI: https://doi.org/10.1097/acm.0000000000003504
14. Tekian A. Are all EPAs really EPAs? *Med Teach.* 2016;39(3):232–233. DOI: https://doi.org/10.1080/0142159x.2016.1230665
15. ten Cate O, Chen HC, Hoff RG, Peters H, Bok H, van der Schaaf M. Curriculum development for the workplace using entrustable professional activities (EPAs): AMEE guide no. 99. *Med Teach.* 2015;37(11):983–1002. DOI: https://doi.org/10.3109/0142159x.2015.1060308
16. Taylor DR, Park YS, Egan R, et al. EQual, a novel rubric to evaluate entrustable professional activities for quality and structure. *Acad Med.* 2017;92(11S):S110-S117. DOI: https://doi.org/10.1097/acm.0000000000001908
17. Taylor DR, Park YS, Tekian A. *Queen's EPA Quality (EQual) rubric training.* Vol 17:41; 2016. Accessed March 26, 2024. https://youtu.be/yQZuWdzkQKM
18. ten Cate O. Competency-based education, entrustable professional activities, and the power of language. *J Grad Med Educ.* 2013;5(1):6–7. DOI: https://doi.org/10.4300/jgme-d-12-00381.1
19. Englander R, Frank JR, Carraccio C, et al. Toward a shared language for competency-based medical education. *Med Teach.* 2017;39(6):582–587. DOI: https://doi.org/10.1080/0142159x.2017.1315066
20. Mills JA, Middleton JW, Schafer A, Fitzpatrick S, Short S, Cieza A. Proposing a re-conceptualisation of competency framework terminology for health: a scoping review. *Hum Resour Health.* 2020;18(1):15. DOI: https://doi.org/10.1186/s12960-019-0443-8
21. Broussenko M, Burns S, Leung FH, Toubassi D. Can teachers distinguish competencies from entrustable professional activities? *PRiMER.* 2019;3:19. DOI: https://doi.org/10.22454/primer.2019.433736
22. Royal Australasian College of Physicians. RACP Curriculum Model. Published online October 2017:1–8. https://www.racp.edu.au//docs/default-source/default-document-library/racp-curriculum-model.pdf?sfvrsn=75bd3c1a_17
23. World Health Organization. *Global Competency and Outcomes Framework for Universal Health Coverage.* World Health Organization; 2022. Accessed April 2, 2024. https://www.who.int/publications/i/item/9789240034662
24. ten Cate O, Pool IA. The viability of interprofessional entrustable professional activities. *Adv Heal Sci Educ.* 2020;25(5):1255–1262. DOI: https://doi.org/10.1007/s10459-019-09950-0
25. Taylor D, Park YS, Smith C, ten Cate O, Tekian A. Constructing approaches to entrustable professional activity development that deliver valid descriptions of professional practice. *TLM.* 2020;2(3):1–9. DOI: https://doi.org/10.1080/10401334.2020.1784740

26. Association of Family Medicine Residency Directors. *Entrustable Professional Activities: Overview*. 2017. Accessed March 26, 2024. https://www.afmrd.org/d/do/P1887
27. Hennus MP, Dam M, Gauthier S, Taylor DR, ten Cate O. The logic behind entrustable professional activity frameworks: a scoping review of the literature. *Med Educ*. 2022;56(9):881–891. DOI: https://doi.org/10.1111/medu.14806
28. ten Cate O. Nuts and bolts of entrustable professional activities. *J Grad Med Educ*. 2013;5(1):157–158. DOI: https://doi.org/10.4300/jgme-d-12-00380.1
29. ten Cate O. How can entrustable professional activities serve the quality of health care provision through licensing and certification? *Can Med Educ J*. 2022;13(4):8–14. DOI: https://doi.org/10.36834/cmej.73974
30. de Graaf J, Bolk M, Dijkstra A, van der Horst M, Hoff RG, ten Cate O. The implementation of entrustable professional activities in postgraduate medical education in the Netherlands: rationale, process, and current status. *Acad Med*. 2021;96(7S):S29-S35. DOI: https://doi.org/10.1097/acm.0000000000004110
31. Pool I, Hofstra S, van der Horst M, ten Cate O. Transdisciplinary entrustable professional activities. *Med Teach*. 2023;45(9):1019-1024. DOI: https://doi.org/10.1080/0142159x.2023.2170778

Appendix: Relevant components of the EPA description.

	Rationale	Tips for writing	Example 1	Example 2
1. Title	A concise title that that rings a bell with all relevant parties	• The shorter the better. EPAs should stick in the minds, as a single unit of practice. Details go into the specification, unless the title requires it to distinguish between EPAs • Avoid trainee performance qualifiers (e.g., effectively) • For verbs, use continuous tense (i.e., -ing); for the object of the verb, use plural (e.g., patients) to stress the generalized nature of the qualification	• *Managing acutely ill, unstable, high complexity patients in the pediatric ICU* [last words can be left out if the full EPA framework regards PICU]	• *Colonoscopy* [if clear, no other words are needed]
2. Specification and limitations	A specification and limitations are inextricable components of EPAs, together with the title (a title alone confuses). What is included and what is excluded? For what (exceptional) conditions does qualification for this EPA *not* hold?	• Add heading: 'Qualification for this EPA includes: …' • A bulleted list of components of the activity, not too long but enough for all relevant parties (trainees, supervisors, nursing) to grasp what the qualification includes • Avoid 'ability to …': specify the activity, not the trainee • Settings where the EPA can be practiced may be added (inpatient, outpatient, urban, rural setting) • For limitations: 'Qualification for the EPA does not include: …' include only items that might lead to confusion if not specified	*Qualification for this EPA includes:* • *Assessing the patient's condition* • *Interpreting diagnostic studies and monitoring data* • *Identifying leading and alternative diagnoses* • *Establishing patient's treatment goals* • *Implementing patient-centered testing and treatment strategies* • *Documenting encounter* *Setting: Pediatric ICU* *Limitations: Qualification for this EPA does not include extracorporeal membrane oxygenation (ECMO).*	*Qualification for this EPA includes:* • *Identifying relevant indication(s) and contraindications* • *Completing informed consent* • *Performing technical components of colonoscopy* • *Recognizing and responding to findings and complications during and after the procedure* • *Documenting procedure* *Setting: Endoscopy suite, ICU* *Limitations: None*

(Continued)

Appendix: Continued.

	Rationale	Tips for writing	Example 1	Example 2
3. Risks	All EPAs that require entrustment decisions to practice bear risks. Critical risks need to be reasonably clear	• This section can be difficult to specify, as 'patient death' or 'inadequate care' are not very informative. Try to think of specific, prevalent adverse events and present these as 'examples'	Irreversible end-organ damage including the central nervous system, heart, kidneys, and other systems	Bowel perforation, immediate and delayed bleeding, oversedation
4. Relevant broad competency domains	Which broad domains (CanMEDs, ACGME or other) apply and should serve for feedback in assessment?	• Avoid including all competency domains of a framework, but the most prominent ones, useful for feedback • Use + and ++ to distinguish between 'relevant' and 'highly relevant'	Medical expert ++ Communication + Collaboration + Professionalism +	Medical expert ++ Collaboration ++ Health advocate + Professionalism +

5. KSAs and experiences	Specific knowledge, skills attitudes and specific experiences that must be present to allow for a summative entrustment decision	• This may potentially lead to unwieldy long lists or uninformative short statements. Key is to guide trainees and curriculum developers in how trainees should become prepared to this responsibility.
		• In part this may be curriculum specific, e.g., having passed specific tests, having had specific rotations, having practiced something X times, having the general knowledge level of book Y
			• Recognition of patient instability and acuity
			• Interpretation of clinical findings in unstable patients
			• Knowledge of differential diagnosis
			• Test selection in unstable patient presentations
			• Identification of focused treatment strategies
			  ∘ CPR
			  ∘ Intubation
			  ∘ Management of hemodynamics
			• Closed loop communication
			
			Minimum of 40 cases managed prior to consideration. Should include experiences in ICU, emergency department, and neonatal ICU.
				• Knowledge of indications and contraindications and complications of procedure
				• Positioning of patient throughout the procedure
				• Manipulation of the endoscope
				• Recognition of pathologic and normal findings
				• Recognition of complications during and after the procedure
				• Collaboration with endoscopy suite nurses and staff
				• Communication and documentation of results
				
				Minimum of 150 colonoscopies before consideration. Experiences should include screening colonoscopies, patients with suspected IBD, and acute gastrointestinal bleeding.

(Continued)

Appendix: Continued.

	Rationale	Tips for writing	Example 1	Example 2
6. Information sources to support summative entrustment	Summary of the *program of assessment* that is needed to confirm the (structural) readiness for summative entrustment and that allows for decisions for a STAR	• Think of four information sources (see Chapter 17) 1. Direct observation (clinical encounters, procedures) 2. Conversations (case-based or entrustment-based discussions) 3. Longitudinal observation (multi-source feedback) 4. Product evaluation (products of trainee activity not requiring their presence for evaluation, e.g., EHR entries) • State how many *satisfactory* datapoints are needed	Requires **minimum** of 15 satisfactory assessments. Must include: • Direct observation (min 8) • Entrustment-based discussion (min 1) • Longitudinal assessment (min 3) Assessors should include supervisors, trauma team members, other nursing staff.	Requires **minimum** of 20 assessed procedures, all by direct observation. Must include presentations of: • Screening colonoscopies • Assessment of diarrhea • Acute GI bleeding • Inflammatory bowel disease Assessors should include supervisors, endoscopy suite staff, and patients.
7. Expected levels of supervision	When should trainees generally be ready for which level of supervision (1–5) at which stage of training?	Include when level 3 ('indirect supervision') or 4 ('unsupervised practice' or 'oversight only') are expected to be attained. Level 1, 2, and 5 are less relevant	Level 3 expected end of second year of training Level 4 expected by end of fourth year of training	Level 3 expected after six months of training Level 4 expected after 24 months of training
8. Expiry date	How long after qualification for unsupervised practice should this summative entrustment hold if never practiced? When should supervision be reinstalled?	• Some EPAs may not be very critical for patient safety and expiry may never be indicated • Other EPAs may be highly critical for patient safety and may require renewed supervision after one or more years of non-practice • Some EPAs may become outdated and should cease to be practiced when better alternatives arise	One year EPA can be reinstalled within four years of expiration. Reinstallation requires satisfactory performance, supervised by a qualified pediatric intensivist for minimum of five encounters. After four years, EPA requires full recertification.	Two years EPA can be reinstalled within three years of expiration. Reinstallation requires satisfactory performance, supervised by a qualified pediatric intensivist for minimum of 10 colonoscopies. After three years, EPA requires full recertification.
Title with specification and limitations are always needed to understand the EPA. Items 3, 4, and 8 may be regarded as general features; items 5, 6, and 7 may be program-specific.				

CHAPTER 9

Approaches to identifying and elaborating entrustable professional activities

Marije P. Hennus, Ylva Holzhausen, Roberta I. Ladenheim, Daniel Nel, Severin Pinilla

Abstract

In the evolving landscape of health care education, entrustable professional activities (EPAs), as units of professional practice, provide educators with an authentic means of connecting curricular design with professional practice. This chapter provides health professions educators with a comprehensive and practical guide to EPA development. Navigating the complexities of EPA development demands a nuanced understanding of the underlying constructs. This chapter sequentially tackles fundamental challenges: where to start, identifying key activities, shaping them into EPAs, building consensus on the framework, and piloting. By offering actionable insights, it empowers readers to navigate this challenging process effectively. Whether you are at the outset of a new EPA initiative or seeking refinement of previously developed EPAs, this chapter provides a practical roadmap for establishing purposeful EPAs that contribute to robust and relevant curricula.

Authors

- Marije P. Hennus, MD, PhD, MSc Clin Ed. University Medical Center Utrecht, Utrecht, the Netherlands. Correspondence: M.P.Hennus@umcutrecht.nl
- Ylva Holzhausen, MSc, PhD. Charité – Universitätsmedizin Berlin, Germany.
- Roberta I. Ladenheim, MD. Instituto Universitario Hospital Italiano de Buenos Aires, Argentina.
- Daniel Nel, Groote Schuur Hospital and University of Cape Town, South Africa.
- Severin Pinilla, MD, PhD, MEd, MPH. University of Bern, Bern, Switzerland.

How to cite this book chapter:

Hennus MP, Holzhausen Y, Ladenheim RI, Nel D, Pinilla, S. Approaches to identifying and elaborating entrustable professional activities. In: ten Cate O, Burch VC, Chen HC, Chou FC, Hennus MP. (Eds). *Entrustable Professional Activities and Entrustment Decision-Making in Health Professions Education*, Chapter 9, pp. 101–110. [2024] London: Ubiquity Press. DOI: https://doi.org/10.5334/bdc.i

This chapter uses cross-references to other chapters of the same book. For those who read this chapter as a standalone publication: all cross-references can be found at: https://doi.org/10.5334/bdc

Introduction

When identifying and defining entrustable professional activities (EPAs), it is essential to remain focused on their intended purpose—describing the core work performed in the practice of that profession. Numerous publications have elaborated on the definition of EPAs and highlighted distinctions between EPAs and competencies, which are abilities acquired by learners through training.[1–3] In addition to being an philosophical approach to health professions education, EPAs operationally describe a profession.[3] While EPAs have mainly found use in developing curricula and establishing workplace assessment procedures for specialized training, the work of identifying, elaborating, and building consensus for EPAs focuses on the profession itself. Developing EPAs demands a significant investment of time and resources. Therefore, prioritizing the development of specialty-specific or national EPAs is preferable over local initiatives. This not only emphasizes the need for a robust formulation of units of professional practice that can be recognized, entrusted, and certified as a credential but also nurtures a unified vision within a specialty or profession. Individual programs working on EPA development locally can still find value in their frameworks but run the risk of missing out on broader collaborative opportunities and may face potential redundancy or contradiction with national or specialty-wide endeavors in the future.

Effective implementation of EPAs in health professions curricula requires that EPA development adheres to various quality standards, consensus norms, and validity criteria (see Chapters 5 and 11); the goal is to ensure alignment between EPA construction and intended purpose in education. These include considerations of content validity, stakeholder endorsement, EPA quality, feedback from sounding boards within a professional society, and inclusion in continuing education programs.[4] In essence, the greater the attention given to these details, the greater the likelihood that the EPAs will 'work' as intended. This chapter aims to provide a practical and comprehensive overview of various approaches to identifying and elaborating EPAs that are fit for purpose. It sequentially tackles the following fundamental questions: where to start, how to identify key activities and shape them into EPAs, how to build consensus on the framework, and finally why and how the drafted EPAs should be piloted (Figure 9.1).

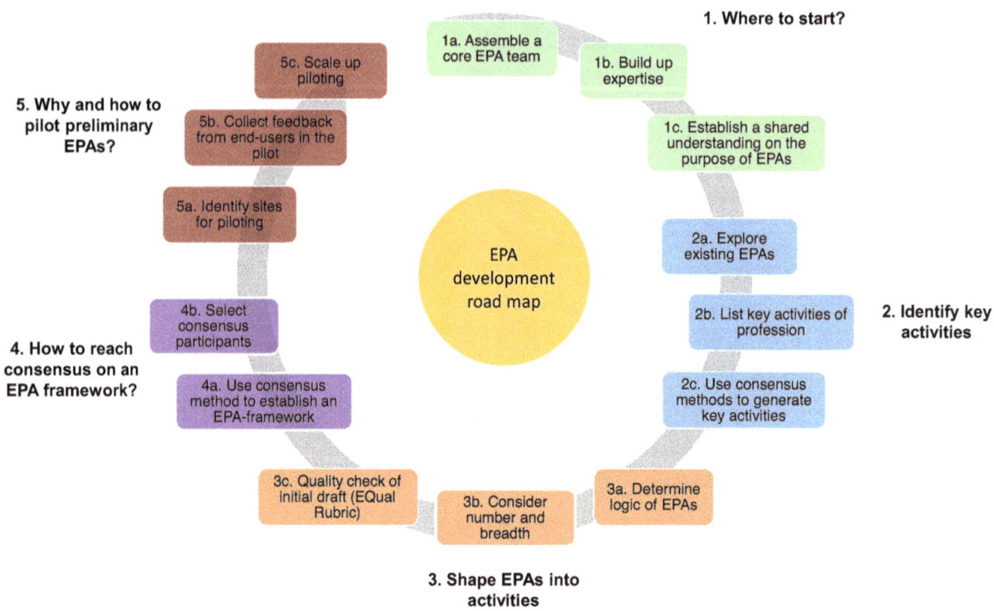

Figure 9.1: Road map to identifying and elaborating EPAs.

Where to start?

Embarking on the process of developing EPAs may initially seem overwhelming but it does not need to be. The following steps (1a through 5c; see Figure 9.1) will help establish a solid foundation for this journey.

Assemble a core team (1a)

Identifying and elaborating EPA descriptions is a team effort and often based on an official mandate, e.g., from a specialist society, government, or institutional leadership. One of the first tasks is to put together a core working group to perform this task. It is recommended that the members of the EPA core team are diverse in many ways: e.g., different (clinical) experience and hierarchical levels (e.g., from trainees to supervisors to heads of departments), varying educational expertise, and from different training centers and practice settings, as relevant.[5] The number of core team members depends on several factors, such as whether the EPAs are being developed for a single institution or a (national) specialty group; as a general rule, core teams typically include five to six members.[6] It is important to note that this core EPA team will play a central role throughout the process from development of EPAs to their implementation, necessitating broad stakeholder support for the group.

Build up expertise (1b)

Once the core team is established, identifying helpful resources to build and expand their expertise on EPAs is crucial. The existing literature offers a strong theoretical foundation.[1,7,8] and provides guidelines on EPA development in general.[2,3,5,9] EPAs have now been adopted in various professions and disciplines, providing a wealth of profession- and specialty-specific examples[10–13] and an excellent starting point. Additionally, seeking guidance from educational experts or colleagues with experience in EPA development can offer the team valuable insights. Lastly, online resources, as well as national and international workshops and courses, provide not only a theoretical background but also hands-on experience and tools for conducting workshops and courses focused on EPAs at one's institution.

Establish a shared understanding on the purpose of EPAs (1c)

Beyond building individual expertise, establishing a common vision and fostering a shared understanding of EPAs within the core team are crucial, as they significantly enhance team performance.[14] It is essential to clarify, at an early stage, the purpose and planned implementation of the EPAs in the curriculum. Important questions to address include whether EPAs will be designed for a local, regional, or national training program; the level of training expected from participants (with experienced learners typically undertaking more challenging and broader tasks); how EPAs will be used by regulators and certifying bodies; and how EPAs will be implemented within the curriculum (e.g., whether they are to be integrated longitudinally throughout the curriculum or defined for a specific training period). The responses to these inquiries will shape the number and breadth of EPAs to be developed.

Furthermore, addressing potential causes for confusion regarding EPAs is pivotal when constructing this shared mental model. Key points to consider in this regard include:

- Distinguishing competencies as abilities possessed by learners (e.g., 'conducting clinical interviews with a patient-centered approach') from EPAs, which represent units of professional work (e.g., 'assessing and treating a patient with chronic medical disease'—see Chapter 8).[15]

- Recognizing that not all competencies and objectives should or can be operationalized as EPAs. For example, essential competencies like 'lifelong learning' and 'interprofessional collaboration' are integral but do not involve discrete tasks to be mastered and performed.[16]
- Understanding that EPAs are tasks entrusted by society to professionals in a given field, requiring them to perform these tasks safely and at an accepted professional standard. Entrustment goes beyond clinical abilities, necessitating professionals to possess features described by the 'A RICH' mnemonic, namely: Agency, Reliability, Integrity, Capability, and Humility.[17]

Building this shared understanding among the EPA development team will strengthen and clarify the purpose of EPA development work being undertaken.

Identify key essential activities of a profession

A range of methods can be used, often in combination, to clearly articulate the daily activities integral to a profession, ultimately shaping an EPA framework.

Explore existing EPAs (2a)

Getting an overview of the existing EPA landscape in the field of interest can be helpful as it is certainly easier to shape the wheel than to reinvent it. However, caution is advised when adopting established EPAs. EPAs previously published may not consistently adhere to current quality standards. Furthermore, they were developed for a specific educational and clinical context that may differ in significant ways. Consequently, it is essential to adapt these EPAs to ensure their validity and feasibility within one's own context, ensuring they accurately reflect the activities undertaken by professionals in that setting. Making them fit for purpose is imperative.

List key activities of daily practice (2b)

Another approach involves retrospective reflection by a representative group within the profession, where they describe their work. Importantly, the representativeness and competence of these health professionals, particularly when aiming for broad-scale implementation, are pivotal factors influencing both the process and outcomes. In addition to focusing on activities in practice, listing key activities of trainees, according to training phase (i.e., nested EPAs), may also provide valuable insights. However, it is essential to view this process through the lens of defining end-of-training EPAs. Both approaches can be augmented with additional data from logbooks, workplace observations, or published literature, including cognitive task analysis studies. Finally, seeking expert advice from colleagues in different disciplines or countries where EPAs have already been implemented may prove highly beneficial. For instance, it can help in avoiding pitfalls, identifying areas of disagreement, and pinpointing problems that arose during implementation due to EPA construction.

Use of consensus methods to generate key activities (2c)

Using established consensus methods, such as the nominal group technique (NGT) or Delphi method, may also aid the identification and prioritization of key tasks for one's profession. The

NGT, a structured face-to-face interaction, is a particularly useful brainstorming and consensus method for this purpose.[18] It provides significant benefits by fostering equal participation among team members and mitigating power differentials among participants. NGT is very useful when groups are first identifying and prioritizing EPAs for consideration. For those less familiar with NGT, literature on its use in health professions, including curriculum development, provides an excellent introduction[19]. The Delphi method is an iterative, survey-based, decision-making process that involves a panel of experts providing anonymous feedback on a series of questions or statements. Facilitated by a moderator, participants revise the statements or responses to questions based on group feedback in successive survey rounds. This iterative process continues until consensus is reached (generally three rounds). The Delphi method is well-suited for revising preliminary EPAs into a more refined and broadly accepted framework of EPAs.[20]

The selection and use of different consensus methods will depend on a variety of factors, such as differences in power and experience among participants, the scope of the project, and the breadth of professional practice. Typically, formal consensus methodologies like the Delphi method are used for multi-institution projects, where they have the additional advantage of achieving buy-in from multiple stakeholders. However, such processes are more complex to set up and are time-consuming. Regardless of the chosen identification methods, careful selection of data sources and experts in the developmental process is crucial to ensure that the collected key activities represent the work of that profession and will inform the development of valid EPAs that are fit for purpose.

Shape key activities into EPAs

Navigating the process of identifying and describing the key activities of a clinical specialty to build a framework of well-constructed EPAs can be challenging. The following steps offer guidance in accomplishing this:

Determine the logic of EPAs (3a)

Three primary logics, the perspectives used by developers in medical education to break down the practice of their profession into units of professional work, are commonly employed in EPA frameworks.[9] These are: 'service provision,' 'procedures,' and 'disease or patient categories,' with many programs adopting a combination of at least two of these logics. Each logic (or approach) comes with its own set of advantages and limitations. The 'service provision' logic defines EPAs as broadly described tasks, for example 'assessing and treating acute patients.' While this approach results in a smaller number of EPAs, it lacks case-specificity when applied to patient encounters. In contrast, the 'disease and patient categories' logic involves crafting EPA descriptions that capture the specifics of patient encounters within a specialty, such as 'assessing and treating canine weight loss.' However, this logic may lead to an excessive number of EPAs, especially in broad-based professions and specialties with diverse patient presentations. Consequently, when selecting the logic(s) to be used in drafting EPAs, it is crucial to consider the profession's scope of practice. Profession-specific challenges related to feasibility and case-specificity help identify the logic(s) that best align with the actual work being done. Nevertheless, it is important to remain flexible and open to revisiting this decision when progressing in the EPA development process.

Consider the number and breadth of EPAs (3b)

The granularity of the EPAs is also an important point of discussion, as the breadth or scope of EPAs is directly linked to their total number. Opting for a few large or many small EPAs comes with both advantages and disadvantages. For instance, if only a handful of EPAs covers an entire specialty, they inherently become broad. This risks having EPAs that are only partially observable, draw on long lists of competencies, and are only generally recognizable in everyday clinical practice or less functional in early training stage. In such cases, breaking down these larger EPAs into subordinate EPAs, known as 'nested EPAs,' can be beneficial. Nested EPAs allow for more focused assessment of a particular application in an earlier training stage or for specific contexts (clinical/educational) of the broader parent EPA. On the other hand, defining many smaller EPAs brings specificity and observability and facilitates rich feedback discussions. However, concerns arise regarding the potential atomization of EPAs and the logistical and administrative burden associated with managing a large number of them. High assessment quotas may threaten the feasibility and sustainability of EPA implementation, leading to a tick-box mentality that lacks formative value and creates low-quality data of little use in making high-stakes decisions. Consequently, a guideline value of a *maximum* 10 EPAs per year of continuing education or approximately 30 for a whole education program is recommended.[21] Increasingly, programs are using 10 or fewer EPAs for an entire program, which allows for greater feasibility and inclusivity of diverse (clinical) situations and contexts. During the process of identifying and selecting preliminary EPAs, careful consideration should be given to the possibility of combining or splitting certain EPAs with this general number in mind. Subsequently, the establishment of core EPAs that all graduates must master, along with optional or 'elective' EPAs available for those who have the capacity to tackle more, may enhance the flexibility and effectiveness of the educational framework.

Discuss the pros and cons of logics, numbers, and breadth of EPAs with panel members at the outset, before employing the NGT. This will help shape a shared mental model for the target product to be developed. Such deliberations significantly contribute to refining EPA development strategies and can prevent problems that are difficult to address later in the process.

Quality-check initial draft of EPAs (3c)

Ensuring high-quality construction of the initial EPAs early in the process is crucial to avoid unnecessary use of resources and the need to correct problems later. To support the development of EPAs, there is a quality benchmark—the EQual Rubric tool—that should be applied right from the start to check whether a proposal for an EPA is really an EPA (see the section on the EQual Rubric tool in Chapter B11).[22] Every correction of a poor-quality EPA in a later phase of the development process involves additional effort.

How to reach consensus on an EPA framework?

Once a preliminary set of EPAs is established and refined and has passed quality assurance, the next crucial step is to build broad consensus on that set.[23] At this stage, the focus shifts toward engaging the ultimate end users of the EPAs. Feedback from end users that is gathered during the consensus process allows for refinement of the elaborated components of the EPAs to better align EPA descriptions with their use in curriculum, assessment, and entrustment decisions. Additionally, consensus facilitates collaboration and buy-in from educators, supervisors, trainees, and accrediting bodies, promoting a unified approach to EPAs.

Use a consensus method to establish an EPA framework (4a)

Consensus may be achieved by simple methods like expert meetings, with the involvement of discipline-specific leadership committees, or by more formal consensus methods such as the

Delphi technique.[11] A common modification of the Delphi approach in EPA development provides respondents with a set of partially elaborated EPAs from the outset.[24] EPA descriptions provided, at a minimum, include the EPA title, specifications and limitations, and domains of competence.[3] These core components establish the groundwork for understanding how to execute the EPA effectively in real-world scenarios. Once consensus is reached on these essential components, it becomes simpler and more impactful to expand and elaborate upon the other aspects of the EPA. Finally, it is important to allow respondents the opportunity to provide commentary on the entire, preliminary set of EPAs and be given the opportunity to suggest potential additional EPAs.

Participant selection for consensus methods (4b)

As respondents play a pivotal role in the Delphi process, it is essential to establish criteria for the expertise required and determine the desired number of respondents thoughtfully. A range of 10 to 50 respondents is considered adequate.[25] They should possess knowledge not only about the EPA concept but also about the specific (health) profession content. It is important to note that Delphi respondents may be aware that they will be working with the resulting EPAs. This can enhance their interest in participating but may also introduce bias as responses will not only reflect content expertise but also consider feasibility, implementation, and political acceptability. By contrast, involving Delphi respondents with limited understanding of EPAs or only a modest level of interest may lead to high consensus scores for EPAs with questionable validity. This can create the illusion of a high-quality product, which in turn influences the adoption and implementation of potentially problematic EPAs. EPA developers should be cautious about this potential trap when selecting Delphi respondents.[18]

Why and how should a preliminary EPA framework be piloted?

Once the quality of the preliminary EPAs is ensured (see Chapter 11) and broad consensus is obtained, the next step involves testing their suitability and feasibility for use in programs. Pilot-testing offers a low-risk, high-return opportunity and can be viewed as the final rehearsal for drafted EPAs.

Identify sites for piloting (5a)

Pilot-testing is typically conducted with a small sample of intended users in real-world conditions to assess the feasibility of implementing a new initiative and gauge its potential benefits on a larger scale. If a set of national EPAs has been developed, consider piloting at two to four institutions, ones that would be anticipated to have distinct implementation challenges. For local EPAs, pilot-testing with five to 10 local users (supervisors and trainees) will likely suffice.

Collect feedback from end users (5b)

Pilot-testing should also begin with a selected subset of the EPAs that can guide decisions on the feasibility of rolling out the full list of EPAs, ensuring that manageable assessment quotas are implemented.[26] During pilot-testing, it is crucial to go beyond simply deploying EPA-based assessment tools and reviewing assessment data collected. It is essential to conduct interviews with learners and supervisors to gather feedback on the EPAs themselves, the assessment tools used, the impact on workflow, and any barriers identified.

Scale up piloting (5c)

Scaling up the piloting of EPAs, if needed, from one to more sites and more EPAs iteratively allows for the evaluation and refinement in diverse clinical settings, ensuring they are adaptable and effective across different contexts. This approach facilitates the collection of broad feedback on practical implementation issues and the integration into various workflows, crucial for identifying and resolving barriers early.

Conclusion

Successfully navigating the development of EPAs hinges on a clear understanding of their purpose. This chapter offers a practical and thorough guide to identifying and elaborating EPAs. Key considerations include assembling a diverse core team, building expertise through literature and expert guidance, and fostering a shared understanding of EPA purpose. Methods for identifying key activities range from exploring existing EPAs to reflecting on daily practice and employing consensus-building techniques. Shaping these activities into EPAs necessitates selecting a (combination of) logic(s) and striking a balance in EPA granularity and total number of EPAs. The attainment of consensus, which may be facilitated by methods like Delphi, is paramount, while pilot-testing ensures feasibility. This comprehensive overview is designed to equip (future) developers with the tools needed to create effective and purposeful EPAs within their professional contexts.

Acknowledgments

This chapter draws substantially from a paper published in *Medical Education*[9] and in *Medical Teacher*.[5] ChatGPT 3.5 aided in sentence editing.

Competing interests

The authors declare that they have no competing interests.

References

1. ten Cate O. Entrustability of professional activities and competency-based training. *Med Educ.* 2005;39(12):1176–1177.
2. ten Cate O, Chen HC, Hoff RG, Peters H, Bok H, Van Der Schaaf M. Curriculum development for the workplace using entrustable professional activities (EPAs): AMEE Guide No. 99. *Med Teach.* 2015;37(11):983–1002. DOI: https://doi.org/10.3109/0142159X.2015.1060308
3. ten Cate O, Taylor DR. The recommended description of an entrustable professional activity: AMEE Guide No. 140. *Med Teach.* 2021;43(10):1106–1114. DOI: https://doi.org/10.1080/0142159X.2020.1838465
4. Taylor D, Park YS, Smith C, ten Cate O, Tekian A. Constructing approaches to entrustable professional activity development that deliver valid descriptions of professional practice. *Teach Learn Med.* 2021;33:1, 89–97 DOI: https://doi.org/10.1080/10401334.2020.1784740
5. Hennus MP, Jarrett JB, Taylor DR, ten Cate O. Twelve tips to develop entrustable professional activities. *Med Teach.* 2023;45(7):701–707. DOI: https://doi.org/10.1080/0142159X.2023.2197137

6. Klein K. Is your team too big? Too small? What's the right number? Knowledge@Wharton. Published 2006. Accessed May 16, 2022. https://knowledge.wharton.upenn.edu/article/is-your-team-too-big-too-small-whats-the-right-number-2/
7. ten Cate O. Nuts and bolts of entrustable professional activities. *J Grad Med Educ*. 2013;5(1): 157–158. DOI: https://doi.org/10.4300/JGME-D-12-00380.1
8. ten Cate O. Trust, competence, and the supervisor's role in postgraduate training. *Br Med J*. 2006;333(7571):746–748. DOI: https://doi.org/10.1136/bmj.38961.475718.68
9. Hennus MP, Dam M, Gauthier S, Taylor DR, Cate O. The logic behind EPA-frameworks: a scoping review of the literature. *Med Educ*. 2022;56(9):881–891. DOI: https://doi.org/10.1111/medu.14806
10. Meyer EG, Chen HC, Uijtdehaage S, Durning SJ, Maggio LA. Scoping review of entrustable professional activities in undergraduate medical education. *Acad Med*. 2019;94(7):1040–1049. DOI: https://doi.org/10.1097/ACM.0000000000002735
11. O'Dowd E, Lydon S, O'Connor P, Madden C, Byrne D. A systematic review of 7 years of research on entrustable professional activities in graduate medical education, 2011–2018. *Med Educ*. 2019;53(3):234–249. DOI: https://doi.org/10.1111/medu.13792
12. Shorey S, Lau TC, Lau ST, Ang E. Entrustable professional activities in health care education: a scoping review. *Med Educ*. 2019;53(8):766–777. DOI: https://doi.org/10.1111/medu.13879
13. Abeyaratne C, Galbraith K. A review of entrustable professional activities in pharmacy education. *Am J Pharm Educ*. 2023;87(3):ajpe8872
14. Mathieu JE, Goodwin GF, Heffner TS, Salas E, Cannon-Bowers JA. The influence of shared mental models on team process and performance. *Journal of Applied Psychology*. 2000;85(2):273–283. DOI: https://doi.org/10.1037/0021-9010.85.2.273
15. ten Cate O, Schumacher DJ. Entrustable professional activities versus competencies and skills: exploring why different concepts are often conflated. *Advances in Health Sciences Education*. 2022;27(2):491–499.
16. ten Cate O, Pool IA. The viability of interprofessional entrustable professional activities. *Advances in Health Sciences Education*. 2019;25(5):1255–1262. DOI: https://doi.org/10.1007/s10459-019-09950-0
17. ten Cate O, Chen HC. The ingredients of a rich entrustment decision. *Med Teach*. 2020;42(12):1413–1420. DOI: https://doi.org/10.1080/0142159X.2020.1817348
18. Humphrey-Murto S, Varpio L, Gonsalves C, Wood TJ. Using consensus group methods such as Delphi and Nominal Group in medical education research. *Med Teach*. 2017;39(1):14–19. DOI: https://doi.org/10.1080/0142159X.2017.1245856
19. Harvey N, Holmes CA. Nominal group technique: an effective method for obtaining group consensus. *Int J Nurs Pract*. 2012;18:188–194. DOI: https://doi.org/10.1111/j.1440-172X.2012.02017.x
20. Keeney S, Hasson F, McKenna HP. A critical review of the Delphi technique as a research methodology for nursing. *Int J Nurs Stud*. 2001;38(2):195–200. DOI: https://doi.org/10.1016/S0020-7489(00)00044-4
21. ten Cate O. An updated primer on entrustable professional activities (EPAs). *Rev Bras Educ Med*. 2019;43:712–720.
22. Taylor DR, Park YS, Egan R, et al. EQual, a novel rubric to evaluate entrustable professional activities for quality and structure. *Acad Med*. 2017;92(11):S110-S117. DOI: https://doi.org/10.1097/ACM.0000000000001908
23. Englander R, Flynn T, Call S, et al. Toward defining the foundation of the MD degree: core entrustable professional activities for entering residency. *Academic Medicine*. 2016;91(10):1352–1358.
24. Custer RL, Scarcella JA, Stewart BR. The modified Delphi technique – a rotational modification. *Journal of Vocational and Technical Education*. 1999;15(2):50–58. https://files.eric.ed.gov/fulltext/EJ590767.pdf

25. Turoff M. The Delphi method: techniques and applications. In: Linstone HA, Turoff M, eds. *The Delphi Method. Techniques and Applications.* Vol 13. 2002:80–96. DOI: https://doi.org/10.2307/3150755
26. Lindeman B, Brasel K, Minter RM, Buyske J, Grambau M, Sarosi G. A phased approach: the general surgery experience adopting entrustable professional activities in the United States. *Acad Med.* 2021;96(7):S9-S13. DOI: https://doi.org/10.1097/ACM.0000000000004107

CHAPTER 10

Clarifying terminologies related to entrustable professional activities and entrustment decision-making

Olle ten Cate, Eric J. Warm, Adrian P. Marty, Inge A. Pool

Abstract

Entrustable professional activities (EPAs) and entrustment decision-making have become common language in competency-based education in the health professions. Since its introduction, several other related concepts have been introduced, which has made it more complex to get an overview of the domain. This chapter sets out to discuss OPAs (observable practice activities), EPA specifications, nested EPAs, core EPAs versus elective EPAs, transdisciplinary EPAs, Practice Activities as used by the WHO, retrospective versus prospective entrustment–supervision scales, STARs (statements of awarded responsibility), microcredentials, and hospital privileging. The concepts are defined and elaborated with examples.

Authors

- Olle ten Cate, PhD. University Medical Center Utrecht, Utrecht, the Netherlands and University of California, San Francisco, USA. Correspondence: t.j.tencate@umcutrecht.nl
- Eric J. Warm, MD. University of Cincinnati College of Medicine, Cincinnati, Ohio, USA.
- Adrian P. Marty, MD, MME. University Hospital Balgrist, University of Zurich, Zurich, Switzerland.
- Inge A. Pool, PhD. Isala Academy, Isala Hospitals, the Netherlands.

How to cite this book chapter:

ten Cate O, Warm EJ, Marty AP, Pool IA. Clarifying terminologies related to entrustable professional activities and entrustment decision-making. In: ten Cate O, Burch VC, Chen HC, Chou FC, Hennus MP. (Eds). *Entrustable Professional Activities and Entrustment Decision-Making in Health Professions Education*, Chapter 10, pp. 111–120. [2024] London: Ubiquity Press. DOI: https://doi.org/10.5334/bdc.j

Introduction

Despite the wide uptake of the concept of entrustable professional activities (EPAs) in many health professions education programs, and the seemingly simple and intuitive nature of the concept (an activity one would trust a trainee or professional to do), translating it into practice has been less straightforward and has led to questions about what an EPA is and how one can use it. In addition, the language around EPAs has expanded with the addition of new, related concepts. This chapter aims to help the reader see the forest for the trees' by explaining several of these related concepts and providing guidance on how to use them in health professions education. We distinguish between concepts directly related to EPAs and those related to entrustment decision-making. This chapter is not exhaustive and every chapter in this book uses and explains language for a good understanding of its content. The terminologies here stand out, as publications in the literature using these do not always provide clear explanations.

Terminology related to entrustable professional activities

EPAs are units of clinical practice that, as a whole, can be entrusted to a professional, or someone in training for that profession.[1,2] Not all daily activities of a clinician are suitable for professional entrustment (e.g., 'Creating a personal development plan'), if they are not contributions to patient care. EPAs are 'entrustable,' i.e., a decision of entrustment can be made to transfer the responsibility for the activity,[3] either ad hoc or more permanently after a summative entrustment decision. EPAs can be rather broad responsibilities, such as 'Serving on an outpatient diabetes clinic' for a resident in internal medicine or 'Perioperative care for the critically ill surgery patient' for one in surgery. Clearly, such broad EPAs can be described in more detail, and can include smaller activities (e.g., 'Obtaining informed consent'). Here is where alternative terms for units of practice arise.

OPAs, or observable practice activities

Warm and colleagues introduced the idea of multiple small and specific *observable practice activities* (OPAs), to be measured over time, leading to entrustment decisions mapped to Milestones (which, with a capital M, are significant points in the development of competencies, required in the USA to be reported semi-annually to the Accreditation Committee for Graduate Medical Education, ACGME) and to EPAs, showing developmental progression.[4] OPAs and EPAs differ in two distinct ways: in their granularity (OPAs are usually small and many) and in their suitability for a summative entrustment decision. In addition, Warm proposes distinguishing 'process OPAs' (example: 'Minimize unnecessary care including tests') from 'content OPAs' (example: 'Manage ventilator changes in the ICU').[4] Both examples would be less suitable for an EPA. The first cannot easily be envisioned as a unit of practice that can be entrusted (with direct, indirect, or no supervision). The second example would only qualify as an EPA that an ICU doctor would be hired for or scheduled to do if it were combined with other OPAs. While OPAs are not applied in many programs, the literature describes some other rationales for OPAs, such as the wish to specify established EPAs in more detail, and the wish to link observable activities to Milestones,[5] the required reporting format of the ACGME in the US.[6,7]

The emphasis in assessment of OPAs is on observation. Their purpose is twofold. The first is to assess learners' competence regarding activities that require 'discrete collections of knowledge, skills, and attitudes that can be observed and entrusted,'[8] rather than to grant an actual qualification, with a summative entrustment decision. The other purpose is to collect information that can be mapped over time to inform larger assessment collection efforts for progress or entrustment decisions (such as Milestones or EPAs).

Major decisions about granting entrustment with units of professional practice (STARs – see below) would be unwieldy if these would regard hundreds of small OPAs[8], and would lose the sense of holistic decisions. EPAs serve to provide steps toward increasingly autonomous practice in patient care, through grounded, summative entrustment decisions, shared by the educational team or competency committee of a program for each EPA. However, bundles of OPAs together can establish an EPA.[9] Here is where OPAs show overlap with the 'specification' section of an EPA description.[1]

EPA specification items as bundled small EPAs

EPA sets are frequently published and utilized in consensus processes solely based on their titles. Yet these titles rarely provide a comprehensive understanding of the qualifications and responsibilities granted to a trainee following a summative entrustment decision. It is essential for the trainee, clinical staff, interprofessional team, and others to understand well which responsibilities are included in an EPA qualification and which are not. Providing specifications and delineating limitations is a crucial aspect of defining an EPA.[1] The specification includes smaller components of this responsibility and can be listed in different ways. They could be the chronological steps of the EPA or the combined sub-activities that the EPA qualification encompasses. The specification describes the activity in necessary detail. It frequently happens that, when a new framework of EPAs is created—for instance with a nominal group technique—a long series of small activities is generated and subsequently reorganized into broader EPAs, each with component sub-activities, so items listed in the specification can often be regarded as small EPAs. Box 10.1 shows a very elaborate EPA—derived from an article under submission[10]—that was created after two nominal group procedures with experts. In many cases, specifications can be briefer: enough to inform relevant stakeholders, but not more. Our recommendation would be that developers who consider using OPAs to be small units of practice within an EPA think of writing these out as specifications of the EPAs.

In the full description of an EPA, not only is a specification included but also competency domains, knowledge, skills, attitudes (KSAs), and experiences, which are sometimes regarded

Box 10.1: EPA example.	
Title	**Providing care to non-hospitalized adult patients with a known common chronic condition**
Specification	*This EPA implies qualification for:* • History taking and physical examination • Establishing and prioritizing differential diagnoses • Requesting and interpreting common diagnostic and screening tests • Providing treatment as appropriate, including writing prescription orders, for conditions at least including hypertension, diabetes, dyslipidemia, COPD, heart failure, asthma, anxiety, depression, hypothyroidism, GI disorders, osteoarthritis, and chronic skin, infectious (HIV), and renal and neurological diseases • Counseling patients (and families) about condition and treatment, especially around medication use • Evidence-based screening, considering age and risk factors • Educating patients regarding risk factor modification and preventive care • Documenting medical notes, referral letters, and clinical evolution • Conducting home or remote monitoring regarding chronic health problems or disabilities • Referring patients to other health care practitioners and specialists as appropriate *This EPA includes a qualification to attend to patients unsupervised in the following settings:* • Outpatient setting; patient-home setting; urban setting; rural setting

as a specification. This conceptualization is not correct, as competencies and KSAs are required features of the trainee before an entrustment decision can be made to allow them to practice the activity, and 'specification' is merely the activity explained, as a list of its components.

Nested EPAs

A concept in the EPA language, somewhat related to OPAs and specifications but still distinct, is the *nesting of smaller EPAs* within broader EPAs.[11] As trainees progress through the educational continuum, their responsibilities grow over time and EPAs become broader. Nested EPAs are a developmental concept. When a student is trusted with examining a patient for a specific reason (e.g., to measure blood pressure) and their report is no longer checked or questioned but accepted and incorporated in a medical record, then an entrustment decision has been made for a small EPA. However, further in training, that small EPA is no longer a useful entity because it becomes too small and should be incorporated (nested) within a full physical examination. Subsequently, measuring blood pressure becomes part of a full consultation, then full management of a patient and finally a whole clinic (Figure 10.1).[11] Nested EPAs can thus be defined as true EPAs (stand-alone contributions to patient care), to be entrusted often up to the level of indirect supervision, and to become part of a broader EPA at a later stage of training.

This way, the number of EPAs at a particular stage of training can be limited to the relevant activities for *that* stage. At the end of postgraduate and fellowship training it is no longer useful to talk about nesting, as the EPAs will reflect actual units of professional practice.

Nested EPAs have not been used frequently, but the Utrecht undergraduate medical program employs them. Five broad EPAs are defined for the final year, which includes an advanced 12-week clerkship, akin to a subinternship. 'The clinical consult' is one of the broad EPAs that includes a full history and physical examination. In prior years, specialty-specific basic history and physical examination EPAs have been defined for internal medicine, surgery, neurology, pediatrics, obstetrics/gynecology, and psychiatry, as these are not identical. Students are first trained and qualified

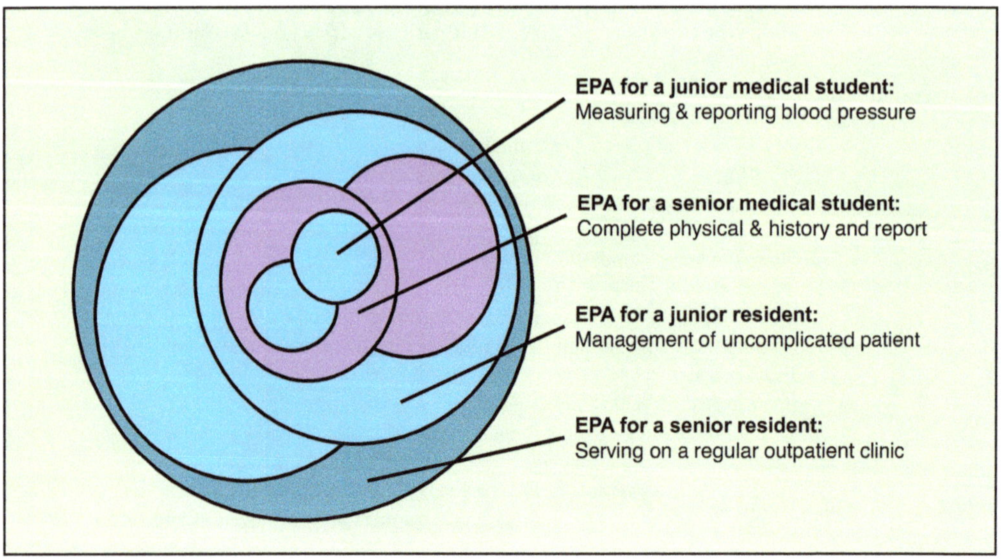

Figure 10.1: Examples of nested EPAs.

for specialty-specific clinical-consult EPAs, which are subsequently all considered to be nested in the overarching final-year EPA 'The Clinical Consult.'[12] Nested EPAs may also serve in postgraduate programs, such as when complex surgeries are broken down into components that can be entrusted to junior surgical residents. A nested surgical EPA (e.g., 'Open entry into the abdomen') can occur in multiple different types of surgical procedures.

Core EPAs and elective EPAs

Many programs have defined core EPAs.[13,14] Few, however, have defined elective EPAs. Core EPAs can be defined as EPAs that every graduate should be prepared to do. Training and summative entrustment for elective EPAs can be offered to trainees who develop faster than predicted and have the space and capacity to master additional, noncore EPAs. Offering elective EPAs is one way to respond to wishes of time-variability. Elective EPAs can, for example, be rare procedures, only trained and executed in specialized centers, offered to residents with a special interest.

If a curriculum focuses on the target of having trainees be ready for all core EPAs a half year before the end of training, then there is space for those who need more time, and training and qualification in elective EPAs can be offered to those who do not need more time. This requires flexibility[15,16] that not all jurisdictions can easily offer. Alternatively, elective EPAs are being used in Dutch postgraduate nursing training when a hospital offers training for employment in specific and restricted areas of care, without requiring full training in that specialty.[17,18]

Transdisciplinary and transprofessional EPAs

EPAs are generally designed for a program. That can be a general program, such as for undergraduate medical education,[13] for specific programs such as a pediatric ICU fellowship,[19] or even personalized, such as for physician assistant training.[20] However, EPAs do not need to apply to only one program or discipline, or even one health profession. Advanced trauma life support, for instance, can be regarded as an EPA for which several health care workers may be qualified, either as a core EPA in their program or as an elective EPA to be added.

Transdisciplinary EPAs (sometimes called 'common EPAs') apply to multiple disciplines, and transprofessional EPAs to multiple professions. The terminology originated during the comprehensive reorganization of postgraduate nursing education in the Netherlands in 2019–2022. This transition shifted from isolated educational programs to training focused on EPAs as foundational components (Figure 10.2). This shift aimed to create a more tailored career trajectory and to enhance responsiveness of the workforce to health care needs.[17] An example from this work is 'Providing care for adult patients with imminent risk for cardiac arrest' in the domain of emergency nursing. The national project offers a library of EPAs from which registered nurses can choose to advance their skills and meet their needs, all with appropriate restrictions and regulations.[18]

Figure 10.2 shows the example of the restructured Dutch postgraduate nursing programs, from fully parallel, siloed programs to a highly flexible model with hexagonal icons representing EPAs, which includes core EPAs and elective EPAs (darker and lighter hexagons, respectively), some of which are transdisciplinary (two-colored hexagons).

The WHO's practice activities

In 2022, the World Health Organization (WHO) launched a competency framework for non-medical-health professionals worldwide as a component of its universal health coverage aim[21], with a

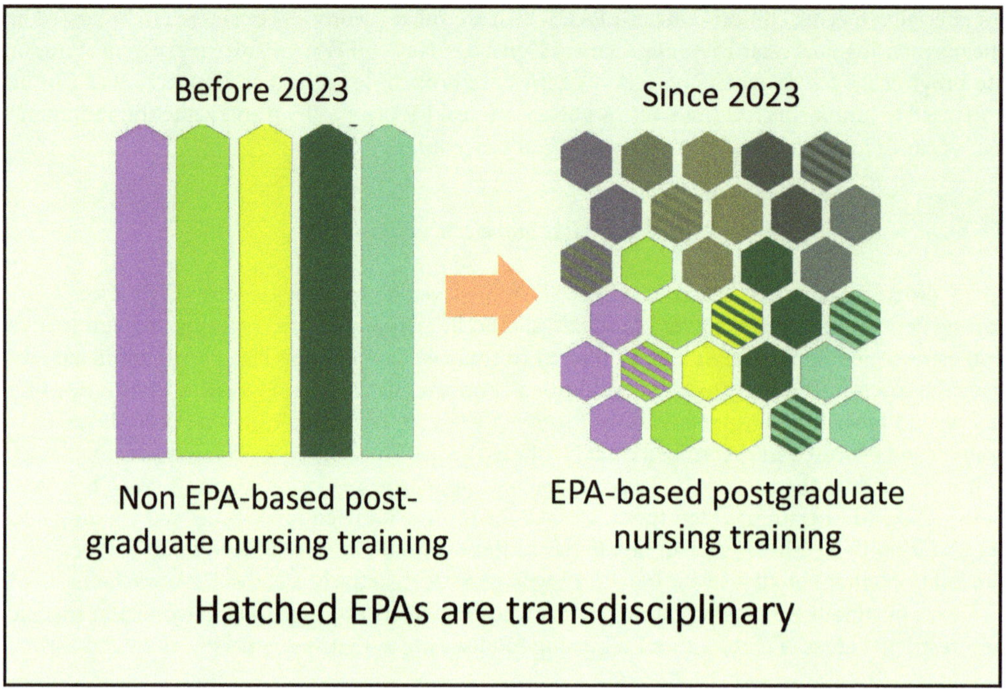

Figure 10.2: Transdisciplinary EPAs (graphics from the Dutch national CZO-Flex Level project).

competency model that has subsequently been adopted across the organization. The framework extensively elaborates on three key elements: KSAs, competencies, and the *practice activities* for which these are required. In principle, *practice activities* mirror and draw their inspiration from EPAs. However, to align with the language used by the International Labour Organization, a distinct terminology was adopted that reserves 'professional' for a narrower category of workers than the broad scope that the WHO's competency framework targets. Further, the framework offers a menu of different practice activities for the health and care team as a whole; they require specification to the occupational scope of practice, level of supervision (equivalent to the EPA scale), and context such as tools, specific health services, teams or language to be used for a specific curriculum.

Terminologies related to entrustment decision-making

EPAs derive their value from entrustment decision-making, i.e., the gradual transfer of responsibility to trainees for units of practice, either in the moment ('ad hoc') or summatively. Ad hoc decisions hold for the moment during daily practice in a teaching hospital. Summative decisions are more permanent; they require a serious evaluation of the trainee by an educational team or clinical competency committee, they must be grounded in sufficient observations, and they must follow the principles of programmatic assessment.[22] Summative entrustment decisions are not just decisions of trainee progress but deliberate decisions to entrust trainees with responsibilities they did not have before.

Retrospective versus prospective views on entrustment as assessment

In traditional approaches to assessment in education, what the student or trainee *has done* determines their score, be it in an examination or assignment or as observed performance, which implies a retrospective evaluation. Entrustment decision-making evolves around estimation of readiness for future practice with less supervision, which is a prospective endeavor. Entrustment–supervision (ES) scales[23] focus on an estimated or recommended level of supervision for this trainee and this EPA. A retrospective ES scale reports how much help or supervision a trainee needed when observed; a prospective ES scale goes a step further and includes a recommended level of supervision for future cases.

Statement of awarded responsibility

A less frequently used but not unimportant concept is Statements of Awarded Responsibility (STARs).[24] A STAR is a formal acknowledgment that a trainee is ready *and* allowed to execute an EPA, basically autonomously but with distant supervision if still formally in training.[25] A STAR can be seen as a microcredential for an EPA after a summative entrustment decision; it has been suggested that they can be translated to digital badges.[26] STARs can populate a trainee's personal portfolio to reflect what they are qualified to do at any moment during training, and during practice after training.[27,28]

EPAs versus hospital privileges and microcredentials

EPAs for which trainees are qualified resemble the units of practice for which hospitals 'privilege' physicians, nurses, midwives, and other health professions. Privileges are the permissions granted to enter premises and provide clinical care in a hospital. Privileges can be determined by state laws or hospital accrediting bodies. They include admission and discharge of patients under a physician's name and allow physicians to perform specific procedures like surgery. Privileges must be awarded by the hospital where a health professional wants to practice. Privileging also regulates supervision of some health professions by others, as well as the supervision of trainees, often specified in levels of direct and indirect supervision, and the parallel with supervision levels for EPAs (or OPAs) is striking. See examples of 51 lists for various disciplines and professions at the University of California San Francisco Health System (https://medicalaffairs.ucsf.edu/privileges).

Microcredentials, embraced by the European Council to enhance flexible, life-long learning pathways,[29] are records of small-volume learning outcomes, assessed against transparent, well-defined criteria, to be offered in addition to diplomas. Norcini envisions microcredentials to be useful for the future of medical education[30] for specific areas of practice (also referred to as microcertifications or badges) and provides the example of a US university offering 215 microcredentials in licensure-related areas such as accounting, education, engineering, health care, and veterinary sciences, and references the American Board of Internal Medicine Foundation's Institute for Clinical Evaluation, which offers credentials in areas like electrocardiogram reading skills.[30] Microcredentialing aligns well with the concept of EPAs and may operationalize the permission to practice in new areas, after completion of postgraduate training.[31,32]

Summary

Table 10.1 summarizes the EPA-related concepts as discussed in this chapter.

Figure justifications

Figure 10.1 was adapted from ten Cate et al. 2015.[11] Figure 10.2 was derived from Dutch national CZO-Flex Level project (https://www.czoflexlevel.nl).

Table 10.1: EPA-related entrustment-related terminologies explained.

Concept	Definition	Example
EPAs	Entrustable professional activities are units of professional practice that can be entrusted to a trainee who has demonstrated to possess the competencies to execute the activity unsupervised	Run a diabetes clinic; perform an anesthesia induction
OPAs	Observable practice activities are specific, small observable activities, measured over time to inform entrustment decisions. They differ from EPAs in granularity and being less suitable for summative entrustment decisions	Manage ventilator changes in the ICU
Nested EPAs	Small EPAs to be entrusted to junior trainees (often up to the level of indirect supervision), to become part of a broader EPA at a later stage of training	Measure blood pressure, become part of a full physical examination, and then caring for patients on a unit
Core EPAs	EPAs that every graduate should be prepared to do for a given profession	Recommend and interpret common diagnostic and screening tests
Elective EPAs	EPAs offered to individuals who develop faster and have the capacity to master additional, noncore EPAs	Point of care ultrasound in family medicine
Transdisciplinary EPAs	EPAs that apply to multiple disciplines	Provide care for adult patients with imminent risk for cardiac arrest in emergency medicine, anesthesia, and intensive care medicine
Transprofessional EPAs	EPAs that apply to multiple professions	Colonoscopy by gastroenterologists and advanced nursing practitioners
WHO practice activities	Inspired by EPAs, activities for which knowledge, skills, and attitudes are required (launched by the World Health Organization)	Manage a vaccination program; coordinate transfer to another care environment
Retrospective ES scale	Scales that focus on how much support a trainee required during an observed performance	The trainee needed (a) show and tell (b) active help (c) passive help (d) no help ('supervision only')
Prospective ES scale	Scales that state how much supervision a trainee is recommended to receive in a future case	Based on my observations, I estimate that this trainee is ready (a) to only observe (b) to act with direct supervision (c) to act with indirect supervision (d) to act unsupervised, (e) to act as supervisor for juniors
STAR	Statement of awarded responsibility, a formal acknowledgment that a trainee is ready and allowed to execute an EPA autonomously while still formally under supervision	Attestation that a trainee is ready to provide postoperative care unsupervised (or any other EPA)
Hospital privileges	Permissions granted to provide clinical care in a hospital; akin to EPAs but determined by state laws or hospital accrediting bodies	Admission and discharge of patients, perform specific procedures like surgery
Microcredentials	Specific areas of practice entailing shorter educational experiences followed by assessments, aligned well with the concept of EPAs	Formalized acknowledgment for any core or elective EPA

Competing interests

The authors declare that they have no competing interests.

References

1. ten Cate O, Taylor DR. The recommended description of an entrustable professional activity: AMEE Guide No. 140. *Med Teach.* 2021;43(10):1106–1114. DOI: https://doi.org/10.1080/0142159X.2020.1838465
2. ten Cate O. Entrustability of professional activities and competency-based training. *Med Educ.* 2005;39(12):1176–1177. DOI: https://doi.org/10.1111/j.1365-2929.2005.02341.x
3. ten Cate O. When I say … entrustability. *Med Educ.* 2020;54(2):103–104. DOI: https://doi.org/10.1111/medu.14005
4. Warm EJ, Mathis BR, Held JD, et al. Entrustment and mapping of observable practice activities for resident assessment. *J Gen Intern Med.* 2014;29(8):1177–1182. DOI: https://doi.org/10.1007/s11606-014-2801-5
5. Ahuja S, Tanveer N, Arora V. Defining observable practice activities for postgraduate residents in cytopathology. *CHRISMED J Health Res.* 2022;9(3):198. DOI: https://doi.org/10.4103/cjhr.cjhr_118_21
6. Nasca TJ, Philibert I, Brigham T, Flynn TC. The next GME accreditation system—rationale and benefits. *N Engl J Med.* 2012;366(11):1051–1056. DOI: https://doi.org/10.1056/NEJMsr1200117
7. Jones LK, Dimberg EL, Boes CJ, et al. Milestone-compatible neurology resident assessments: a role for observable practice activities. *Neurology.* 2015;84(22):2279–2283. DOI: https://doi.org/10.1212/WNL.0000000000001641
8. Warm EJ, Held JD, Hellmann M, et al. Entrusting observable practice activities and milestones over the 36 months of an internal medicine residency. *Acad Med.* 2016;91(10):1398–1405. DOI: https://doi.org/10.1097/ACM.0000000000001292
9. Mink R. A fellow assessment tool for the pediatric gastroenterology entrustable professional activities: a great start! *J Pediatr Gastroenterol Nutr.* 2020;71(1):4–5. DOI: https://doi.org/10.1097/MPG.0000000000002765
10. ten Cate O, Nel D, Hennus M, Peters S, Romao GS. For which entrustable professional activities must medical students be prepared if unsupervised patient care without further training is an expectation? An international Global South study. *(Submitted).* 2024.
11. ten Cate O, Chen HC, Hoff RG, Peters H, Bok H, van der Schaaf M. Curriculum development for the workplace using entrustable professional activities (EPAs): AMEE Guide No. 99. *Med Teach.* 2015;37(11):983–1002. DOI: https://doi.org/10.3109/0142159X.2015.1060308
12. ten Cate O, Graafmans L, Posthumus I, Welink L, van Dijk M. The EPA-based Utrecht undergraduate clinical curriculum: development and implementation. *Med Teach.* 2018;40(5):506–513. DOI: https://doi.org/10.1080/0142159X.2018.1435856
13. Englander R, Flynn T, Call S, et al. Toward defining the foundation of the MD degree: core entrustable professional activities for entering residency. *Acad Med.* 2016;91(10):1352–1358. DOI: https://doi.org/10.1097/ACM.0000000000001204
14. Elmes AT, Schwartz A, Tekian A, Jarrett JB. Evaluating the quality of the core entrustable professional activities for new pharmacy graduates. *Pharmacy (Basel).* 2023;11(4). DOI: https://doi.org/10.3390/pharmacy11040126
15. Hoff RG, Frenkel J, Imhof SM, ten Cate O. Flexibility in postgraduate medical training in the Netherlands. *Acad Med.* 2018;93(3S):S32-S36. DOI: https://doi.org/10.1097/ACM.0000000000002078

16. de Graaf J, Bolk M, Dijkstra A, van der Horst M, Hoff RG, ten Cate O. The implementation of entrustable professional activities in postgraduate medical education in the Netherlands: rationale, process, and current status. *Acad Med.* 2021;96(7S):S29-S35. DOI: https://doi.org/10.1097/ACM.0000000000004110
17. Pool I, Hofstra S, van der Horst M, ten Cate O. Transdisciplinary entrustable professional activities. *Med Teach.* 2023;45(9):1019–1024. DOI: https://doi.org/10.1080/0142159X.2023.2170778
18. Pool IA, van Zundert H, ten Cate O. Facilitating flexibility in postgraduate nursing education through entrustable professional activities to address nursing shortages and career prospects. *Int Nurs Rev.* October 11, 2023. DOI: https://doi.org/10.1111/inr.12892
19. Hennus MP, Nusmeier A, van Heesch GGM, et al. Development of entrustable professional activities for paediatric intensive care fellows: a national modified Delphi study. *PLoS ONE.* 2021;16(3):e0248565. DOI: https://doi.org/10.1371/journal.pone.0248565
20. Mulder H, ten Cate O, Daalder R, Berkvens J. Building a competency-based workplace curriculum around entrustable professional activities: the case of physician assistant training. *Med Teach.* 2010;32(10):e453–459. DOI: https://doi.org/10.3109/0142159X.2010.513719
21. Fitzpatrick S, ed. *Global Competency and Outcomes Framework for Universal Health Coverage.* World Health Organization; 2022.
22. Schuwirth LWT, Van der Vleuten CPM. Programmatic assessment: from assessment of learning to assessment for learning. *Med Teach.* 2011;33(6):478–485. DOI: https://doi.org/10.3109/0142159X.2011.565828
23. ten Cate O, Schwartz A, Chen HC. Assessing trainees and making entrustment decisions: on the nature and use of entrustment-supervision scales. *Acad Med.* 2020;95(11):1662–1669. DOI: https://doi.org/10.1097/ACM.0000000000003427
24. ten Cate O, Scheele F. Competency-based postgraduate training: can we bridge the gap between theory and clinical practice? *Acad Med.* 2007;82(6):542–547. DOI: https://doi.org/10.1097/ACM.0b013e31805559c7
25. ten Cate O. Entrustment as assessment: recognizing the ability, the right, and the duty to act. *J Grad Med Educ.* 2016;8(2):261–262. DOI: https://doi.org/10.4300/JGME-D-16-00097.1
26. Mehta NB, Hull AL, Young JB, Stoller JK. Just imagine: new paradigms for medical education. *Acad Med.* 2013;88(10):1418–1423. DOI: https://doi.org/10.1097/ACM.0b013e3182a36a07
27. ten Cate O, Carraccio C. Envisioning a true continuum of competency-based medical education, training, and practice. *Acad Med.* 2019;94(9):1283–1288. DOI: https://doi.org/10.1097/ACM.0000000000002687
28. de Raad T, Wiersma F, Kuilman L, ten Cate O. The fate of entrustable professional activities after graduation: a survey study among graduated physician assistants. *J Contin Educ Health Prof.* 2023;43(1):28–33. DOI: https://doi.org/10.1097/CEH.0000000000000467
29. EU Council. 3021/0402(NLE). In: *Proposal for a Council Recommendation on a European Approach to Micro-credentials for Lifelong Learning and Employability*; 2022:1–34.
30. Norcini J. Is it time for a new model of education in the health professions? *Med Educ.* 2020;54(8):687–690. DOI: https://doi.org/10.1111/medu.14036
31. Ma T, ten Cate O. Entrustable professional activities: a model for job activity competency framework with microcredentials. *IJILT.* 2023;40(4):317–333. DOI: https://doi.org/10.1108/IJILT-05-2022-0108
32. ten Cate O. How can entrustable professional activities serve the quality of health care provision through licensing and certification? *Can Med Educ J.* 2022;13(4):8–14. DOI: https://doi.org/10.36834/cmej.73974

CHAPTER 11

Monitoring and evaluating EPAs and EPA frameworks

David R. Taylor, Alan Schwartz, Abigail T. Elmes-Patel, Adrian P. Marty, Marije P. Hennus

Abstract

Evaluation is essential throughout the development of entrustable professional activities (EPAs) to ensure that the resource-intensive work required in EPA development leads to a set (or framework) of EPAs that are fit for their intended purpose. This chapter draws on program evaluation literature to show how EPA core team leaders can conceptualize evaluation as part of the EPA development process. It then covers key evaluation strategies relevant to different stages in EPA development, piloting, and implementation. In addition, an in-depth discussion of the purpose and use of the EQual rubric for evaluating individual EPA quality is provided.

Authors

- David R. Taylor, MD, MHPE. Queen's University, Kingston, Ontario, Canada. Correspondence: taylord@queensu.ca
- Alan Schwartz, PhD, JD. University of Illinois at Chicago, Chicago, USA.

How to cite this book chapter:
Taylor DR, Schwartz A, Elmes AT, Marty AP, Hennus MP. Monitoring and evaluating EPAs and EPA frameworks. In: ten Cate O, Burch VC, Chen HC, Chou FC, Hennus MP. (Eds). *Entrustable Professional Activities and Entrustment Decision-Making in Health Professions Education*, Chapter 11, pp. 121–130. [2024] London: Ubiquity Press. DOI: https://doi.org/10.5334/bdc.k

This chapter uses cross-references to other chapters of the same book. For those who read this chapter as a standalone publication: all cross-references can be found at: https://doi.org/10.5334/bdc

- Abigail T. Elmes-Patel, PharmD, MHPE. University of Illinois at Chicago, Department of Pharmacy Practice, Chicago, Illinois, USA.
- Adrian P. Marty, MD, MME. University Hospital Balgrist, University of Zurich, Zurich, Switzerland.
- Marije P. Hennus, MD, PhD, MSc Clin Ed, University Medical Center Utrecht, Utrecht, the Netherlands.

Introduction

This chapter describes evaluation methods that can be used during entrustable professional activity (EPA) development initiatives to improve the quality and construction of the EPAs produced. (This is separate from evaluation of learners *performing* EPAs, which is covered in Chapters 17 to 20.) The ultimate goal in EPA development is to produce EPAs that (a) are a clear and representative description of the work of the profession or discipline, (b) are constructed in a way that facilitates teaching and assessment of learners, and (c) can be used in making decisions on readiness for unsupervised practice.[1] Achieving these aims requires an iterative approach to EPA development that adapts to information and opinions collected throughout the process. If follows that an effective evaluation plan for EPA development should go beyond simple adjudication of the quality of proposed EPAs but must also inform the process through which the EPAs are derived, consider the implications (or consequences) of adopting the collective set (or framework) of EPAs, and address ongoing needs for monitoring and revision after implementation.[1] Evaluation in this context therefore includes both formative evaluation approaches (evaluation intended to direct improvements) and summative evaluation approaches (evaluation intended to provide quality assurance for the end product).

The term EPA *framework* is frequently referenced during this chapter and warrants defining from the outset. As described in Chapter 8, a framework of EPAs is a coherent and reasonably comprehensive set of EPAs that define the core activities of a profession or discipline.[1,2] It should capture all of the essential, entrustable work within the profession's scope of practice. The specific use of the term framework reflects that the collective set of EPAs will be applied differently across different contexts but for a shared purpose and outcome. Consideration of EPA frameworks is important from an evaluation perspective as the cohesiveness and completeness of the collective set of EPAs is an important goal in development.

Conceptualizing evaluation for EPA development

Preparing an effective evaluation plan begins with answering three key questions[3]: (a) What is the purpose of the evaluation plan? (b) Who is the audience for the evaluation results? (c) What are the questions the evaluation aims to answer? These broad questions have specific considerations when applied to evaluation in EPA development (Table 11.1). It follows from these considerations that the emphasis and purpose of evaluation activities will evolve over the process. Early

Table 11.1: Considerations when creating an evaluation plan for EPAs.

Evaluation questions	Considerations in EPA development
What is the purpose of the evaluation plan?	• Direct improvements during development (formative evaluation) • Judge the quality of the product in development and the final end product (formative and summative evaluation) • Support policy decision-making (summative evaluation)
Who is the audience for the evaluation results?	• EPA core development team • End users (learners, clinical teachers and educators) • Regulators and accreditors • Public
What are the questions the evaluation aims to answer?	• Are the EPAs representative of the core work practiced in the profession? • Does the construction of the EPAs meet quality standards? • Are the EPAs suitable for adoption across programs? • Are the EPAs acceptable from a policy standpoint?

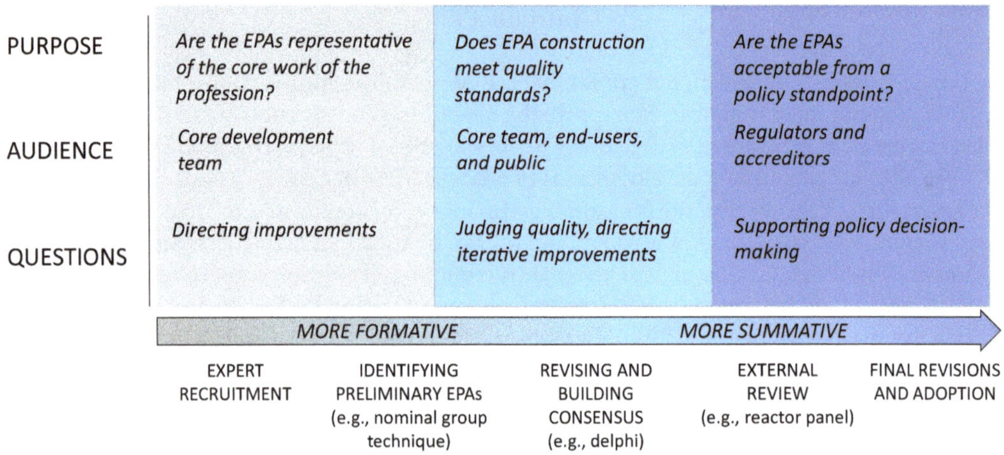

Figure 11.1: Mapping evaluation plan onto EPA development plan.

evaluation activities will be predominantly formative in nature—they aim to improve the process and support product evolution and improvement. As one nears the end of EPA development, the emphasis shifts to quality control of the end product and its suitability for use in high-stakes decisions by regulatory and certifying bodies.

Planning for evaluation starts with mapping the key considerations highlighted in Table 11.1 onto the planned EPA development methods (see Figure 11.1). At first glance, this can make evaluation appear overly complicated and intimidating. But, by taking a step back, it can be appreciated how this mapping exercise clarifies the goals of the work at each phase of the project and provides assurance of readiness for the next phase. For each phase of the project, it lays out:

- What information needs to be gathered?
- Who needs this information?
- How will they use it?

The scope of the evaluation plan should be proportional to the scope of the EPA initiative and aligned to available resources. Smaller local initiatives may choose to focus primarily on evaluating the quality of EPA construction. Initiatives at a national level with implications for licensing decisions will likely require a more comprehensive plan, potentially including an external evaluator. Each section of this chapter describes evaluation approaches useful to EPA development; it is up to project leaders to select and prioritize the most relevant to their initiative.

Evaluation strategies early in development

As the EPA development process begins, the focus of evaluation is formative. The two primary interests are ensuring the clinical content areas covered by the EPAs are representative of the profession and that EPA construction aligns with quality standards for EPAs.

Ensuring the clinical content areas of the EPAs are representative is an evaluation judgment made without prespecified metrics or tools. It aims to ensure that the final collective set (or framework) of EPAs is a cohesive and complete description of the core work done in the profession. At the early stages of EPA development, the focus is simply on establishing that the development team membership is representative of the profession or discipline for which the EPAs are being developed. There is never a perfect composition for any EPA development team, but a diversity of experts that in broad strokes represents the diversity of practice is important. This is a key checkpoint prior to starting the actual EPA development work. As the development process proceeds and candidate EPAs are proposed and revised, the evaluation questions related to content will become more specific—are there core tasks in the profession (i.e., EPAs) that have been missed? Does the collective set of EPAs over- or underrepresent certain aspects of practice? These questions are often answered through open discussion within the core development team, although they can also be worked into consensus methods such as the Delphi technique. It is important to note that content evaluation is easily overlooked at early stages of EPA development; explicitly including this in the evaluation workplan is important. Content problems in the EPA framework that are only discovered at the end of the project can be difficult to correct.

The other main evaluation interest early in development is the quality of construction for EPAs. Developing EPAs is resource-intensive, so it is important to address quality problems early in the process (see Chapter 9). If EPAs with construction problems move into and through consensus methods, the construction issues can negatively impact consensus ratings, leading to rejection of proposed EPAs that, in fact, cover important and entrustable aspects of professional practice. The consensus framework of EPAs that emerges from the process may lose the critical alignment with professional practice that is targeted.

Evaluating EPA construction requires clearly defined quality metrics for EPAs as well as a means of measuring them. Various publications have laid out the quality standards and common pitfalls in EPA construction that should anchor this work.[2,4,5] One approach is designating two to three core team members with EPA expertise as responsible for evaluating the quality of drafted EPAs and making revisions to improve their formulation. A more rigorous approach involves applying a rubric designed to measure EPA quality standards, such as the EQual rubric tool and the QUEPA instrument.[5,6] It is important to note that these rubrics were not created to rubber-stamp high-quality EPAs; instead, they provide focused feedback on the attributes of each EPA to the development team identifying areas for improvement in problematically constructed EPAs. Additionally, using a rubric may identify more systematic problems in a project. If data collected from evaluating the EPAs shows pervasive quality problems across multiple EPAs, this may be flagging faculty development needs around EPA definitions and construction.

A deeper dive into the EQual rubric

As the EPAs are the final product and purpose of the project, it is hard to overemphasize the importance of attending to the quality of each EPA being produced in any EPA development project. Assessing individual EPA quality requires a clear understanding of their purpose in the curriculum, and the quality standards for EPAs that support this purpose.[2,4] At a foundational level, the purpose of EPAs is 'operationalizing competencies to facilitate reliable assessment, which predicts future performance at a defined professional standard,' and the construction of EPAs must support this.[1,5]

In constructing the EQual rubric, Taylor et al. identified the defining features and important misconceptions of EPAs that have been published in the peer-reviewed literature.[2,4] Each feature and misconception was then reviewed to ensure its relevance to the above-described purpose of EPAs. All eight defining features clearly supported one or more elements of this purpose, and the six identified misconceptions represented potential quality threats. This provided the 14 quality standards that would be used in constructing the EQual rubric (see Table 11.2).[5] These standards are naturally organized into three domains: items describing EPAs as discrete units of work (items 1–6); items related to entrustment and professional standards (items 7–10); and items that enhance application in curriculum (items 11–14). Criterion-referenced, five-point numeric rating scales were then developed for all 14 items to enable scoring.

Table 11.2: Explanation of items in the EQual rubric.

Domain	EQual rubric item	Explanation
Units of work	**1. This EPA has a clearly defined beginning and end**	The EPA is a discrete task that has a clear beginning and end, and is completed within a discrete period of time
	2. This EPA is independently executable to achieve a defined clinical outcome	The activity does require performance of other related tasks to produce its clinical outcome
	3. This EPA is specific and focused	The task is clearly recognizable to those in the profession with the steps required to perform broadly agreed upon
	4. This EPA is observable in process	The process to performing the EPA can be observed (or directly interrogated) by a clinical supervisor
	5. This EPA is measurable in outcome	Completion of the EPA by a learner produces an outcome that can be assessed (e.g., completion of a consultation allows for a judgment of 'well done' or 'not well done')
	6. This EPA is clearly distinguished from other EPAs in the framework	The EPA does not describe clinical work that is also captured in other proposed EPAs
Entrustment and professional standards	**7. This EPA describes work that is essential and important to the profession**	EPAs should identify the core work that all individuals in the profession should be certified to perform at the end of training
	8. Performing this EPA leads to recognized output or outcome of labour	Performing the EPA should lead to a tangible product that advances clinical care (e.g., a patient treatment plan produced after a medical consultation)
	9. The performance of this EPA in clinical practice is restricted to qualified personnel	The EPA belongs within the scope of practice of the profession and is not performed by unqualified individuals without appropriate supervision
	10. This EPA addresses professional work that is suitable for entrustment	These are tasks that require specific expertise to perform safely and competently that society has entrusted to the profession
Curriculum application	**11. This EPA requires the application of knowledge, skills, and/or attitudes (KSAs) acquired through training**	To perform the EPA, learners must acquire knowledge, skills, and/or attitudes that inform the competencies required of the task
	12. This EPA involves application and integration of multiple domains of competence	The EPA does not reflect abilities from a single domain of competence (e.g., communication), but is a task that requires integration of multiple competencies to perform (e.g., history and physical examination)
	13. The EPA title describes a task, not qualities or competencies of a learner	The EPA should be work done in caring for a patient (e.g., taking a history), not an ability possessed by a learner (e.g., patient-centred communication skills)
	14. This EPA describes a task and avoids adjectives (or adverbs) that refer to proficiency	Adjectives may be included in EPAs (e.g., '...common medical presentations') but should not reference effectiveness of the learner's performance (e.g., '... obtaining an appropriate history and physical exam')

More than offering a single, summative score, grouping the 14 items into the three domains allows for more nuanced and formative evaluation of EPAs. Ratings within domains provide important information about areas for revision and improvement. Well-constructed EPAs may have items with lower scores that are offset by items with higher scores. When lower ratings occur, it is up to users to determine their significance—does a low score identify a need for revision, or does it represent acceptable variation in scoring within an otherwise acceptably scored domain? Application of EQual was not intended to provide definitive, summative judgment on EPAs; instead, it was meant to direct revisions and improvements to EPAs in an evidence-based manner. The overall cutscore for the rubric (an average item rating of 4.07, which was determined using a modified Angoff approach) is used primarily as a screening test to effectively distinguish EPAs that need major revisions from those that may need only minor revision or no revisions at all.[5,7]

This leads to the question of when to use EQual in EPA development. Although there is some value in using it at or near the end of EPA development (in advance of formally adopting a framework of EPAs), its formative value advocates for employing it early in the development process. In addition, training project team members to use the EQual rubric helps build a shared understanding around the standards for EPAs, something that is important to establish early. Ideally, EQual should be used early enough in the process that it can impact the quality of material prior to entering consensus methods such as Delphi. This needs to be balanced against the time required for its use; if there are more than 30 or 40 preliminary EPAs under consideration at this stage, the time required to apply the rubric may become prohibitive. In many cases, it may be beneficial for project leaders to revise preliminary EPAs down to a reasonable number prior to deploying EQual.

There are several principles to using EQual that are important to ensure you get the most out of it. A minimum of four EPA experts should rate the EPAs with the rubric. Studies in both undergraduate and postgraduate medical education suggest that having four expert raters provides excellent reliability.[5,7] That being said, involving five or six experts will increase the number of perspectives and enrich the feedback being collected on the EPAs. Keep in mind, applying EQual is more about collecting high-quality feedback to direct revisions than it is about getting a reliable quantitative judgment on EPA quality.

Defining what constitutes expertise for those recruited for the EQual exercise is also important. These individuals should have a background in CBME with expertise in EPAs. Evidence of expertise might come from attendance at courses and workshops, or scholarly publications in the field. Even with established experts, it is important to provide training on using the EQual rubric to ensure a shared mental model for the task. The EQual training video was designed for this purpose and is readily available on YouTube.[8] See Chapter 25 for an EQual Rubric tool.

Finally, it is important to have EPAs developed to a point that they are suitable for evaluation by the rubric. It is not expected that EPAs will be fully elaborated prior to using EQual; however, having only a title is inadequate. At a minimum, EPAs descriptions must include the title and the specifications and limitations that clearly describe the steps to performing the EPA. These descriptions should be provided to those evaluating the EPAs using EQual.

Results from using EQual (both comments and quantitative evaluation) should be reviewed by the development team. These can then direct revisions to EPAs. Teams may also consider eliminating EPAs that are fundamentally flawed and not amenable to revision to an acceptable EPA.

Evaluation strategies for EPA revision and refinement

Once an initial set of EPAs has been proposed and the construction of the EPAs evaluated and deemed appropriate, consensus methods are then typically used to direct further revision and determine suitability for inclusion in the final EPA framework. Delphi techniques are commonly used survey methods for this purpose. As described in Chapter 9, Delphi iteratively builds consensus for proposed EPAs by surveying participants through multiple rounds, revising and refining the EPA descriptions based on feedback collected after each round. Survey rounds repeat until a designated measure of agreement is achieved for the EPAs (or no further progress toward consensus is reasonably expected with additional rounds). In Delphi, the development method and the evaluation method are integrated.

Delphi can be used early in the process in a more formative manner to direct EPA development and revision.[9] The method can also be used later in a more summative manner to solicit broad, frontline clinician feedback on a proposed framework of EPAs and to identify gaps (in this context it is often referred to as a reactor panel).[10] Whenever Delphi is used, it is important to monitor for known problems that can emerge with it. There are several publications that outline approaches to monitoring for problems in use of Delphi for this context.[1,11,12]

It can be appreciated that this phase of the project requires a transition in evaluation focus. Early on, the focus is formative. However, by the end of this phase it becomes more summative, with the aim of having a defensible framework of EPAs ready for field testing. This requires a shift in evaluation from focusing on quality standards directing revisions at the beginning to considering acceptability to end users and regulatory bodies by the end. Delphi methods can often provide answers to both of these questions, depending on those engaged as participants in the Delphi.

Evaluating your end product

Can these newly developed or revised EPAs achieve the assessment and quality assurance sought by regulators? Can they support the curricular purposes required by programs and accreditors? The answers to these questions are hypothetical until real-world experience is gained. During piloting, gather information from key groups including programs, frontline clinicians, and learners, to explore authentic experiences of end users. In doing so, take the time to investigate challenges experienced and how they relate to (a) implementation, (b) the EPA descriptions, and (c) curriculum. Because these areas are not independent but highly interdependent, challenges experienced during the pilot will likely relate to two or three of these areas. This exploration can provide crucial information for final adaptations and to establish feasibility for meeting the needs of accreditors and regulators.

In doing this work, it is crucial to try to discriminate between challenges associated with introducing change and challenges stemming from the quality of the EPA framework, a task that can be difficult to near impossible. Unfortunately, leaders introducing EPAs have at times been dismissive of concerns raised during implementation, often labeling concerns as operational problems and not issues with the EPAs or curricular design.[13] As projects proceed through pilot testing, evaluation should err on the side of acknowledging and responding to concerns raised about the EPAs, even when concerns might otherwise be classified as implementation problems. Chapter 22 discusses change management strategies when implementing EPAs.

Monitoring after implementation

Evaluation does not end with adoption and implementation. As implementation of EPAs proceeds to scale, unexpected challenges and new learnings inevitably emerge. Stakeholders can report on the impact of the implementation—are learners better trained? Are patients better served? Have there been other unexpected consequences to the new framework? Some of these evaluation questions may take years to answer. Prepare for this with a coordinated plan to collect and review feedback at regular intervals, allowing time (e.g., five years) to monitor implementation prior to considering major revisions. There is no one prescription for this. Instead, leaders should leverage established program evaluation infrastructure that already exists at various program sites and coordinate regular reviews of progress and challenges. For larger projects, such as with national-level curricular change, connecting different program sites to develop a network for systematically collecting data is important and can identify system-wide problems early. An iterative and deliberative approach to monitoring after evaluation, tailored to the scope and nature of the project, is fundamental to long-term success.

Conclusion

Ensuring high-quality EPAs is essential to success when introducing an EPA-based curriculum. The evaluation strategies discussed in this chapter can help teams tasked with developing EPAs to achieve this goal. There is no one-size-fits-all strategy to evaluation, and leaders must prioritize evaluation methods most relevant to their projects and in consideration of resource constraints. Thoughtful evaluation planning will not only improve the quality of the EPAs and frameworks produced but can also save time and resources.

Competing interests

The authors declare that they have no competing interests.

References

1. Taylor D, Park YS, Smith C, ten Cate O, Tekian A. Constructing approaches to entrustable professional activity development that deliver valid descriptions of professional practice. *TLM.* 2020;2(3):1–9. DOI: https://doi.org/10.1080/10401334.2020.1784740
2. ten Cate O, Scheele F. Competency-based postgraduate training: can we bridge the gap between theory and clinical practice? *Acad Med.* 2007;82(6):542–547. DOI: https://doi.org/10.1097/acm.0b013e31805559c7
3. Fitzpatrick J, Worthen B, Sanders J. *Program Evaluation Alternative Approaches and Practical Guidelines.* 4th ed. Pearson Education Inc.; 2011.
4. ten Cate O, Chen HC, Hoff RG, Peters H, Bok H, van der Schaaf M. Curriculum development for the workplace using entrustable professional activities (EPAs): AMEE guide no. 99. *Med Teach.* 2015;37(11):983–1002. DOI: https://doi.org/10.3109/0142159x.2015.1060308
5. Taylor DR, Park YS, Egan R, et al. EQual, a novel rubric to evaluate entrustable professional activities for quality and structure. *Acad Med.* 2017;92(11S):S110-S117. DOI: https://doi.org/10.1097/acm.0000000000001908
6. Post JA, Wittich CM, Thomas KG, et al. Rating the quality of entrustable professional activities: content validation and associations with the clinical context. *J Gen Intern Med.* 2016;31(5):518–523. DOI: https://doi.org/10.1007/s11606-016-3611-8
7. Meyer EG, Taylor DR, Uijtdehaage S, Durning SJ. EQual rubric evaluation of the Association of American Medical Colleges' core entrustable professional activities for entering residency. *Acad Med.* 2020;95(11):1755–1762. DOI: https://doi.org/10.1097/acm.0000000000003504
8. Taylor DR, Park YS, Tekian A. *Queen's EPA Quality (EQual) Rubric Training.* Vol 17:41.; 2016. Accessed March 26, 2024. https://youtu.be/yQZuWdzkQKM
9. Taylor DR, Park YS, Smith CA, Karpinski J, Coke W, Tekian A. Creating entrustable professional activities to assess internal medicine residents in training: a mixed-methods approach. *Ann Intern Med.* 2018;168(10):724–729. DOI: https://doi.org/10.7326/m17-1680

10. Englander R, Flynn T, Call S, et al. Toward defining the foundation of the MD degree. *Acad Med.* 2016;91(10):1352–1358. DOI: https://doi.org/10.1097/acm.0000000000001204
11. Powell C. The Delphi technique: myths and realities. *J Adv Nurs.* 2003;41(4):376–382. DOI: https://doi.org/10.1046/j.1365-2648.2003.02537.x
12. Keeney S, Hasson F, McKenna H. *The Delphi Technique in Nursing and Health Research.* 1st ed. Wiley-Blackwell; 2011. DOI: https://doi.org/10.1002/9781444392029
13. Boyd VA, Whitehead CR, Thille P, Ginsburg S, Brydges R, Kuper A. Competency-based medical education: the discourse of infallibility. *Med Educ.* 2017;32(8):638. DOI: https://doi.org/10.1111/medu.13467

SECTION C

Curriculum

CHAPTER 12

Considerations in building a curriculum using entrustable professional activities

Robert Englander, Jonathan M. Amiel, Jennie B. Jarrett, H. Carrie Chen

Abstract

Competency-based education of health professionals has been gaining momentum across the globe for the past two decades. The central tenet is to start with the outcomes that are required of a trainee to meet the health care needs of the public. These outcomes lead to the elaboration of requisite competencies, which in turn drive the curriculum and assessment programs. Educators have encountered many challenges in the development and implementation of curricula and assessment systems that effectively teach and measure performance of the requisite competencies. Entrustable professional activities (EPAs) offer an excellent framework for addressing many of those challenges.

In this chapter, we offer the unique potential of an EPA framework in promoting a competency-based curriculum. We review some of the curricular structural implications of using EPAs, including the role of sequencing of EPAs in the curriculum, describe how an EPA-based curriculum adds agency to the trainee's journey, and explore the notion of time-variability in competency-based education and training based on success stories using an EPA framework. We conclude that a well-designed curriculum and assessment system using EPAs provides an excellent foundation for ensuring health professionals' readiness to provide safe and effective care within the scope of their discipline and at the appropriate level of supervision.

How to cite this book chapter:

Englander R, Amiel J, Jarrett JB, Chen HC. Considerations in building a curriculum using entrustable professional activities. In: ten Cate O, Burch VC, Chen HC, Chou FC, Hennus MP. (Eds). *Entrustable Professional Activities and Entrustment Decision-Making in Health Professions Education*, Chapter 12, pp. 133–144. [2024] London: Ubiquity Press. DOI: https://doi.org/10.5334/bdc.l

This chapter uses cross-references to other chapters of the same book. For those who read this chapter as a standalone publication: all cross-references can be found at: https://doi.org/10.5334/bdc

Authors

- Robert Englander, MD, MPH. University of Illinois College of Medicine, Chicago, Illinois, USA. Correspondence: rengland@uic.edu
- Jonathan M. Amiel, MD. Columbia University Vagelos College of Physicians & Surgeons, New York, New York, USA.
- Jennie B. Jarrett, PharmD, MMedEd, PhD. University of Illinois Chicago College of Pharmacy, Chicago, Illinois, USA.
- H. Carrie Chen, MD, PhD. Kaiser Permanente Bernard J. Tyson School of Medicine, Pasadena, CA, USA.

Introduction

Understanding how a curriculum can be built using entrustable professional activities (EPAs) requires a general understanding of how competency-based curricula are derived and how they differ in significant ways from the traditional structure, content, and process model of medical education prevalent across the globe throughout the past century or more. The central tenet of a competency-based system of education is to start with the needs of the public served by the trainees. The defined public needs then drive the delineation of competencies required of practitioners in the field. Those competencies in turn drive the curriculum and assessment required to ensure graduates of the education or training program are prepared for their respective transitions.[1–3] Thus, all aspects of curriculum and assessment can be directly linked to one or more of the requisite competencies. This is in direct contrast to the traditional model of health professions education, in which the central driver is the curriculum. In this traditional model, assessments are derived from the curriculum and the trainee outcomes are determined by time-based exposure to the curriculum. Curriculum is defined in this chapter as the totality of the trainee's experiences within the training program.[4]

Features of a competency-based system also include de-emphasizing the hierarchical teacher–trainee structure and focusing on a teacher–trainee collaboration, empowering the trainee to determine where time is best spent to work on development of competence; and moving from calendar-based lesson plans where 'one-size-fits-all' to variable-time progression based on the development and demonstration of competence.[1] Assessment also differs in a competency-based system and is covered elsewhere in this book, in particular Chapters 17 and 18. Any curriculum that incorporates an EPA framework will need to adhere to these tenets of competency-based education. In a seminal article, Van Melle and colleagues lay out the five core components of a competency-based medical education program: *defining the outcome competencies*, which are then *sequenced progressively* through *tailored learning experiences* using *competency-focused instruction*. *Programmatic assessment* of the trainee then supports and documents the developmental acquisition of competence.[5]

In this chapter, we consider the unique potential of an EPA framework in promoting a competency-based curriculum. We review some of the structural implications of using EPAs, including the role of sequencing of EPAs in the curriculum, describe how an EPA-based curriculum adds agency to the trainee's journey, and explore the notion of time-variability in competency-based education and training based on success stories using an EPA framework.

EPAs offer a unique curricular framework

EPAs offer a unique framework for operationalizing competency-based education in the health professions by placing competencies in the context of practice in the clinical workplace.[6] EPAs are descriptions of patient care activities that a competent person may be entrusted to perform. In contrast, competencies are descriptions of the characteristics of a person who would be competent to perform patient care activities.[7] Competencies support the ability of a person to perform EPAs and can be mapped to EPAs. That is, each EPA requires a subset of the overall competencies required of the educational or training program to perform the EPA safely and effectively (see Chapter 7 for additional details regarding the differences between competencies and EPAs). As an example, an EPA for a pediatrician might be to 'care for a well newborn.' This is clearly an essential task of a pediatrician that can be observed and entrusted to a competent practitioner to perform at the unsupervised level. Performing the EPA, though, requires the integration of several competencies, such as: the ability to communicate with families, the knowledge of requisite newborn screening and nutritional recommendations, the ability to perform a newborn physical exam, and the ability to take a maternal history to understand potential risks to the newborn. EPAs thus provide a meaningful, highly practical, and feasible core for the teaching and assessment of most of the requisite competencies of a health professional trainee. This is not to say that EPAs represent the totality of a curriculum, as EPAs may not fully capture the entirety of the desired competencies. Some requisite competencies may not fall within the framework of the EPAs. For example, a training program that includes a research component would have graduate competencies in research skills that would not be covered by EPAs focused on patient care activities.

Where EPAs may not best or solely be used to teach and assess all the competencies, mitigation strategies have been suggested and employed. For example, owing to its emphasis on professional activities or tasks, some educators have voiced concerns that teachers and trainees may lose sight of the specific competencies underlying individual EPAs when teaching or assessing the EPAs.[8] For instance, important competencies related to professionalism behaviors or habits while mapped to individual EPAs may not be explicit and can be at risk of being overlooked in both the curriculum and trainee assessment. In addition, relying on observations of EPAs to assess knowledge outcomes may result in undersampling of content and inadequate evidence of knowledge.

One strategy for addressing this concern is a model adopted by the Royal Australasia College of Physicians and the Irish Internship Curriculum, which combines the use of EPAs and competencies by conceptualizing competency outcomes into three categories: Do, Know, and Be.[9] EPAs articulate the Do competencies—units of essential professional activities graduates are expected to be able to perform at the completion of a training program. The Know category represents the knowledge graduates must have to safely carry out the EPAs. The Be category describes the behaviors, values, and habits expected in health professionals. In this model, the Know and Be competencies support the Do competencies by enabling trainees to perform the EPAs. All three sets of competencies—Do, Know, and Be—drive the curriculum and the assessment program using different assessment tools to measure competence in each of the three categories.

An emerging conception of competence considers different types of competence in three layers: canonical, contextual, and personalized competence.[10] Canonical competence is the core knowledge and skills needed for a health professional. Contextual competence is the application of the core knowledge and skills in a variety of workplace- and patient-specific contexts. Personalized competence is the practitioner's personal style of practice, which becomes increasingly relevant for senior trainees and practitioners. Though not synonymous, there is overlap with the Do, Know, Be model. Canonical competence can be seen as falling primarily under the Know category and contextual competence as falling primarily under the Do category. Different aspects of the Be category could be captured in canonical, contextual, and personalized competence. Over time and with evolution in practice, the Be category becomes increasingly aligned with personalized competence. In this conception of competence, EPAs provide a focus on the contextual level of competence which can be augmented by attention to the canonical and personalized layers.

It is worth noting that the implementation of an EPA framework may be subject to national or local considerations or both, such as what EPAs might be required at the local or national level and when, in the curriculum, they can be entrusted to trainees to perform under which levels of supervision. In several countries, national bodies have defined core EPAs for an entire profession or discipline. Institutions or programs may or may not be able to adapt or add to these core EPAs based on local priorities and regulations. In such cases, in addition to the implementation of core EPAs, programs might opt to include selective or elective EPAs to signal unique program offerings or strengths. Different jurisdictions, national or local, may also have differing accreditation and patient safety regulations that impact a trainee's role in patient care and what professional activities trainees may be entrusted with and at what levels of supervision. Chapter 14 provides further exploration of the implications of nationally versus locally defined EPA-based curricula.

Longitudinal and developmental curricula may optimize use of the EPA framework

The central goal of an EPA-based curriculum is to have trainees achieve a predetermined level of entrustment for each EPA as a prerequisite for transition to less supervised practice. That level of entrustment is most commonly *indirect supervision* for trainees moving from pre-licensure or undergraduate professional education to post-licensure or postgraduate education and *unsupervised practice* for trainees moving from either pre- or post-licensure education directly into practice. The ideal curriculum, then, would build the required knowledge and skills (the 'Know' and 'Do') in a developmental and longitudinal way. From a pedagogical standpoint, this developmental progression often starts with classroom education through case-based learning and then moves into clinical education without contributions to patient care, such as simulation with standardized patients, followed by clinical education with contributions to patient care utilizing learning experiences in the authentic clinical learning environment.

Health professions education typically follows this type of curricular path, with early classroom education followed by clinical education and increasing contributions to patient care in authentic clinical environments. The 'basic science' or predominantly classroom phase of health professions education offers opportunities to introduce the EPAs and build the foundational knowledge and skills in a longitudinal fashion (see Chapter 13 for how foundational knowledge and skills can be mapped to EPAs). Clinical skills courses that are built longitudinally to parallel the basic science courses can be ideal for an EPA curriculum. An example from medical education might be the undergraduate EPA 'perform a physical examination.' This EPA exists in some form in almost all UME iterations of EPAs to date (e.g., the core EPAs for pharmacy graduates or the core EPAs for entering residency in the US).[11,12] Take as an example the physical exam of the heart and lungs. The curriculum can provide experiences to engage trainees in courses involving knowledge and case-based learning around the heart and lungs while simultaneously teaching and assessing the heart and lung exam in a clinical skills course, using standardized patients or simulation. This would prepare trainees well for the actual performance of the physical exam in the clinical learning environment, where they would be expected to reach the level of indirect supervision before advancement to residency, or to unsupervised physical examinations in localities where medical students graduate into practice.

The traditional model of clinical education can pose some challenges to an EPA-based curriculum. First, because EPAs are rooted in the concepts of trust and entrustment, longitudinal supervisor–trainee relationships over time are a critical component to assessment at large, and specifically for the development of trust that informs assessment and feedback on EPAs[13] (see Chapters 4 and 18 for an in-depth exploration of the concepts of trust and entrustment). Generally, the use of multiple assessors and multiple observations can provide aggregate reliable and valid data to inform entrustment decisions.[14] At the same time, the trust built longitudinally between a supervisor or supervisors and trainees makes for more meaningful feedback and entrustment decisions.[15] Thus, an ideal curriculum will balance the need for multiple assessments and assessors with the provision of longitudinal relationships that allow for the development of deep trust over time.

A second challenge to an EPA-based curriculum in traditional clinical training is the tension between the fractured nature of 'rotation-based' training, and the developmental, longitudinal approach to competence development. The fragmentation of the clinical curriculum and its inconsistency with the tenets of competency-based education in general has been the subject of concern for a while.[16,17] This challenge is further underscored when employing an EPA-based curriculum that is founded on longitudinal development of competence and trust between supervisors and trainees. While the fragmented rotational approach is challenging, we recognize that many curricula will continue to employ this structure. Understanding this reality, Chapters 13 and 14 discuss mapping of EPAs to a rotational curricular structure to promote development. One potential curricular change to address the fragmentation and underscore the developmental approach to an EPA-based curriculum is increasing the longitudinality and the integration of curricula. This strategy has several benefits: (a) it enhances the opportunities for supervisor–trainee relationship development over time; (b) it allows multiple observations of the EPA over time, increasing the potential richness of feedback; and (c) it is consistent with learning theory, such as interleaving (the mixing of multiple subjects simultaneously during a defined study period).[18]

One specific tactic related to improving longitudinality of the curriculum that has been employed in UME is the longitudinal integrated clerkship (LIC). This tactic has been used predominantly in Australia, Canada, South Africa, and the United States. The basic concept is that trainees in their core clerkship curriculum are assigned to a primary care clinic, which they attend several times a week, and then spend half-days throughout the better part of a year with the preceptors in the core specialties represented by the clerkships (such as surgery, psychiatry, pediatrics, emergency medicine, and obstetrics and gynecology). The trainees thus have the opportunity to develop year-long relationships with patients, peers, and preceptors. For a definitive reference on LICs, the reader is referred to *Longitudinal Integrated Clerkships: Principles, Outcomes, Practical Tools and Future Directions.*[19]

LICs create the ideal learning pathway for an EPA-based curriculum by both nurturing the trust between supervisors and trainees and allowing the development of competence, leading to entrustment over time. In fact, LICs and EPAs have been called a 'perfect match.'[20] Similar curricular tactics to address the need to increase longitudinality and employ an EPA-based curriculum in the residency space have been published, but generally on an individual program-by-program basis.[21,22]

EPAs can provide the scaffolding for a sequenced progression through a curriculum

Curriculum designers developing an EPA framework sequence the curriculum by considering how trainees develop task-specific expertise requiring decreasing supervision over time.[5]

Sequencing from simple to more complex tasks

One such sequence might go from simpler tasks to more complex tasks that include those simpler tasks. In some of these instances, the simpler EPAs have been referred to as 'nested' within the more complex EPAs.[23] An example of such a sequence might be being taught and assessed in interviewing and examining patients, followed by engaging in the provision of care as part of a team (e.g., reporting and interpreting tests), followed by having primary responsibility for elements of a patient's care (such as entering orders and writing prescriptions), and, eventually, to practicing independently and supervising others. Nested EPAs are further defined in Chapter 10 and are explored in the context of curriculum implementation in Chapters 13 and 14.

Thinking about this sequenced progression as the primary goal of the curriculum helps designers specify teaching and learning opportunities that provide for the development and demonstration of relevant skills and assessments that can yield helpful formative feedback and inform progression decisions.[24] Such sequencing might also better enable a program to recognize a trainee who is struggling and provide support and remediation earlier. In the few extreme circumstances in which a trainee is unable to achieve entrustment, earlier detection through proper sequencing may also provide a more ethical basis for offering a compassionate opportunity to leave the training program before the trainee has invested substantial time and money.[25]

Sequencing across the education–training–practice continuum

Another option for sequencing is across the education–training–practice continuum. EPAs can be useful at any part of professional training. In their applications in medical school training, for example, EPAs have been used to help trainees progress to caring for the general medical patient without direct supervision.[12,26] EPAs for postgraduate medical education (PGME) can support progression to independent practice by field of specialty and then subspecialty.[7,27] The literature is replete with examples of EPAs developed for the transition from the preclerkship to the clerkship phase of medical school, piloted as a framework for the transition from medical school to residency, and integrated into the design of a comprehensive medical school curriculum.[23,28,29] Within specialty training in medicine, EPAs have been developed as frameworks for training in many fields including internal medicine, family medicine, anesthesia, pediatrics, general surgery, and surgical subspecialties. Many of the UME EPAs can be seen as nested in the broader EPAs of those specialties. Figure 12.1 uses medical education and training to depict the way learning experiences in each phase of education can sequence EPAs to substantiate assessment and entrustment, leading progressively to more advanced EPAs requiring less and less supervision as a trainee advances from undergraduate medical education to postgraduate medical education and then to unsupervised practice.

In each phase of education and training (undergraduate, postgraduate, and unsupervised practice), EPAs can be used to guide teaching, learning, and assessment toward entrustment and associated advancement in supervisory levels. EPAs from one phase can be nested into more advanced EPAs in subsequent phases and, eventually, inform a specific scope of professional practice (Figure 12.1).

Considerations for sequencing across the education–training–practice continuum also have implications for continuing professional development and the maintenance (or expiry) of competence. As health professions using EPAs as the framework for curriculum and assessment continue to implement their programs, they have encountered several EPAs for which trainees at

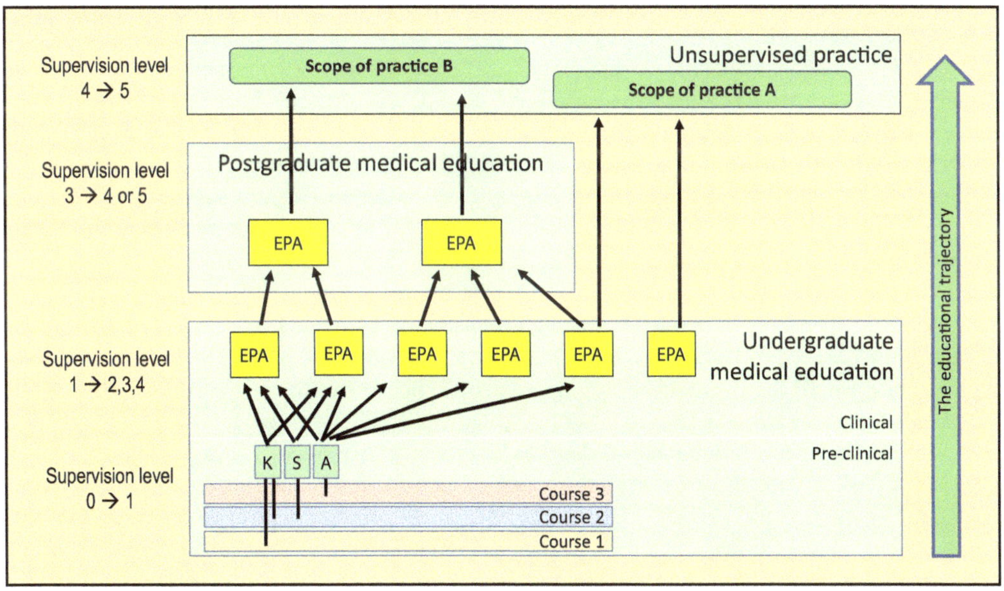

Figure 12.1: EPAs as a scaffold for sequenced progression.

the transition to practice are not uniformly gaining entrustment at the time of that transition. To overcome this challenge, two potential solutions can be considered: (a) curricula during training can adapt to ensure that trainees have the requisite learning and assessment opportunities before graduation to reach entrustment at the unsupervised level, or (b) health professions will need to provide continuing learning and assessment opportunities (continuing professional development) in practice to allow the practicing physician to be entrusted and maintain entrustment at the unsupervised level.

Trainee agency in an EPA-based curriculum

Another potential benefit to an EPA-based curriculum is the agency it affords trainees in individualizing their training experience to meet personal learning needs. The foundation of an EPA-based curriculum is direct observation of a trainee performing the EPA. Trainees have access to their EPA assessment data and thus the best knowledge of their strengths and opportunities for improvement. Further, they can actively engage the supervisor in addressing gaps by requesting the EPA to be observed during any specific clinical supervision experience. In this way the EPA-based curriculum provides boundaries for a trainee to be intentional in the selection of their learning opportunities and lean into asking for and managing feedback to build confidence in their work[30] (further discussion of the individualized learning plan opportunities afforded by an EPA-based curriculum are discussed in Chapter 14). The trainee's demonstration of agency through proactively seeking feedback builds trust with the supervisor around the trainee's self-reflection and knowledge of their limitations, while also affording the supervisor the opportunity to observe the trainee's growth.[15]

In addition to having agency around the EPAs chosen for assessment, trainee agency can take other forms in an EPA-based curriculum. For example, trainee agency can include being forthcoming with direct verbal and written communication, being engaged in their own development with curiosity and passion, and even anticipating problems and taking ownership of a patient's care.[15] An EPA-based curriculum provides a workplace-based, activities-focused mechanism for building these proactive behaviors of trainee agency, connecting the autonomous work to meaningful growth and learning.

Agency is developed over time through an iterative process where the growth of trust between the supervisor and trainee allows for increasing confidence of the trainee in their capacity to perform the EPAs, while simultaneously increasing awareness of their limitations and increasing ability to navigate discussion with supervisors about their performance.

The trainee's agency growth in an EPA- and practice-based curriculum supports a shift from identity primarily as a trainee to identity as a professional (professional identity formation). In the early stages of professional identity formation, the trainee is self-centered and externally defined, concerned with their knowledge and skills, as with an early trainee, where high-level performance on a test is the focus. However, through focusing on essential tasks of the professional in an EPA-based curriculum, trainees are able to develop their own professional identity by completing the work, where their understanding goes beyond themselves to recognize their role in the health care team (see also Chapter 13).[31] Core elements of an EPA-based curriculum that support professional identity formation include: developing confidence in practice, managing feedback on their work, dealing with supervision in the context of practice, and creating learning opportunities.[30] Trainee agency and professional identity formation produce a positive feedback loop, in which trainee agency increases as they begin to better understand the work via the EPA curriculum, and, as their agency develops and increases engagement in the work, trainees can better understand their professional role within the team.

An EPA-based curriculum as an ideal structure for time-variable advancement

An EPA-based curriculum also affords attention to one of the central tenets of competency-based education—the outcomes or competencies are fixed, while the time to achieve competence is variable. The notion of time-variability in health professions education and training has been challenged by traditional time-based models across most of the Western world. The call to move to time-variable education and training in the health professions has been gaining traction in the last decade.[32,33] Despite these calls, significant challenges remain, including: (a) calendar-based academic programs with fixed-time phases, courses, clerkships, and rotations; (b) health profession schools' accreditation requirements that mandate a minimum time in training; (c) individual practitioner certification bodies that mirror the program requirements for time in training; (d) yearly single opportunities to transition from one phase of education and training to another (such as from medical school to residency in the USA and Canada); (e) logistical challenges from off-cycle onboarding and graduations; (f) lack of clear criteria for advancement; and (g) lack of an adequate curriculum and assessment system to teach and assess the competencies in a manner that allows all stakeholders to have confidence in variable-time advancement decisions. An EPA-based curriculum offers the potential to address clear criteria and establish a curriculum and assessment system that yields defensible advancement decisions. Two programs have been published in the literature that have successfully implemented competency-based, time-variable advancement. The programs are highlighted in Boxes 12.1 and 12.2, respectively.

The difficulty of facing all the challenges to time-variable advancement was underscored in a recent publication that sought to engage any of 46 residency programs in one US health system in a competency-based, time-variable pilot.[33] Only 10 of the 46 programs originally expressed interest in the pilot, and of those only one was able to actually implement this time-variable model in their residency program. The success of the Toronto Orthopedics Program and of the Education in Pediatrics Across the Continuum (EPAC) described in Boxes 12.1 and 12.2 suggests that using EPAs as the foundation for the curriculum and assessment system offers perhaps the best hope to date for the realization of a true competency-based, time-variable system of education and training. However, it is worth noting that, even in a fixed-time program, there can be opportunities for individual trainees to advance and

Box 12.1: The Toronto Orthopedic Residency Program.[22]

One program that successfully navigated the paradigm shift to competency-based, time-variable education using an EPA framework is the University of Toronto Orthopedics Program in Toronto, Canada. In 2009, the program moved to a competency-based format that allowed the potential for time-variable advancement through the demonstration of competence within modules. Each module had a set of (a minimum of two) associated EPAs specific to the context and module. Trainees had to demonstrate competence in those EPAs to move to the subsequent module. The program leaders published the results of their first eight years of experience.[22] During that time, they went from just a proportion of residents piloting this curriculum to full-scale implementation across all residents due to its success. More than half of their residents graduated after four years, compared to the required five years in the traditional program. As of the publication, no resident had taken longer than five years to demonstrate competence. Finally, all resident graduates of the program passed their certification examination on the first attempt and had successful fellowships in orthopedic subspecialties independent of time to graduation from residency.

Box 12.2: The Education in Pediatrics Across the Continuum Pilot.[34]

A second program demonstrating successful competency-based, time-variable advancement using an EPA curriculum is a program in pediatrics in the USA that spans UME through GME. The program is called 'Education in Pediatrics Across the Continuum' (EPAC) and was specifically designed to test the feasibility of competency-based, time-variable advancement from UME to GME and GME to practice or fellowship.[34] It engaged up to four students per year at each of four medical schools from across the USA. The pilot followed four cohorts from entry in the preclerkship curriculum of the medical school through completion of pediatric residency. Upon entry into the program, students agreed to stay for residency at the program of origin in pediatrics. Advancement from UME to GME, in addition to the medical schools' graduation requirements, was determined by the student's demonstration of competence at the indirect supervision level for all the 13 core EPAs for entering residency.[35] Similarly, advancement from residency to fellowship or practice was dependent on the demonstration of competence at the unsupervised level for the 17 core EPAs for general pediatrics.[36] While all programs were able to provide the scaffolding for time-variable, competency-based advancement, only three of the four were able to advance students in a time-variable fashion. The fourth program was able to document readiness for advancement but unable to advance students owing to state education board considerations.

achieve entrustment at variable rates for different EPAs. Also, trainees advancing at a faster pace can pursue additional elective EPAs to maximize their learning within the fixed-time program. Ideas for trainee-centered variability within time-fixed programs are further explored in Chapter 14.

Conclusion

The paradigm shift to competency-based education is occurring across multiple continents and across health professions.[1-3] Competencies designed to meet the needs of the public have been delineated in many health professions, often at a national level by level of education or training (such as pre-licensure/undergraduate or post-licensure/postgraduate education), within a specialty (such as obstetrics and gynecology or pediatrics), or for an entire profession (such as physical therapy or pharmacy). Educators have encountered many challenges in the development and implementation of curricula and assessment systems to teach and measure performance of the requisite competencies. EPAs offer an excellent framework for addressing many of those challenges. A well-designed curriculum and assessment system using EPAs provides an excellent foundation for ensuring health professionals readiness to provide safe and effective care within the scope of their discipline and at the appropriate level of supervision.

Competing interests

The authors declare that they have no competing interests.

Figure justification

Figure 12.1 was adapted with permission from a presentation created for the online international Ins and Outs of Entrustable Professional Activities course (www.epa-courses.nl).

References

1. Carraccio C, Wolfsthal SD, Englander R, Ferentz K, Martin C. Shifting paradigms: from Flexner to competencies. *Acad Med.* 2002;77(5):361–367. DOI: https://doi.org/10.1097/00001888-200205000-00003
2. Frenk J, Chen L, Bhutta ZA, et al. Health professionals for a new century: transforming education to strengthen health systems in an interdependent world. *Lancet.* 2010;376(9756):1923–1958. DOI: https://doi.org/10.1016/S0140-6736(10)61854-5
3. Frank JR, Snell LS, Cate OT, et al. Competency-based medical education: theory to practice. *Med Teach.* 2010;32(8):638–645. DOI: https://doi.org/10.3109/0142159X.2010.501190
4. Kelly AV. *The Curriculum: Theory and Practice.* 6th ed. SAGE Publications Ltd; 2009.
5. Van Melle E, Frank JR, Holmboe ES, et al. A core components framework for evaluating implementation of competency-based medical education programs. *Acad Med.* 2019;94(7):1002–1009. DOI: https://doi.org/10.1097/ACM.0000000000002743
6. ten Cate O, Scheele F. Competency-based postgraduate training: can we bridge the gap between theory and clinical practice? *Acad Med.* 2007;82(6):542–547. DOI: https://doi.org/10.1097/ACM.0b013e31805559c7
7. ten Cate O. Entrustability of professional activities and competency-based training. *Med Educ.* 2005;39(12):1176–1177. DOI: https://doi.org/10.1111/j.1365-2929.2005.02341.x
8. Krupat E. Critical thoughts about the core entrustable professional activities in undergraduate medical education. *Acad Med.* 2018;93(3):371–376. DOI: https://doi.org/10.1097/ACM.0000000000001865
9. Boland J, Offiah G. *Curriculum Framework for the Internship Programme in Ireland.* Health Service Executive; 2023.
10. ten Cate O, Khursigara-Slattery N, Cruess RL, Hamstra SJ, Steinert Y, Sternszus R. Medical competence as a multilayered construct. *Med Educ.* 2024;58(1):93–104. DOI: https://doi.org/10.1111/medu.15162
11. Haines ST, Pittenger AL, Stolte SK, et al. Core entrustable professional activities for new pharmacy graduates. *Am J Pharm Educ.* 2017;81(1):S2. DOI: https://doi.org/10.5688/ajpe811S2
12. Englander R, Flynn T, Call S, et al. Toward defining the foundation of the MD degree: core entrustable professional activities for entering residency. *Acad Med.* 2016;91(10):1352–1358. DOI: https://doi.org/10.1097/ACM.0000000000001204
13. Hauer KE, ten Cate O, Boscardin C, Irby DM, Iobst W, O'Sullivan PS. Understanding trust as an essential element of trainee supervision and learning in the workplace. *Adv Health Sci Educ Theory Pract.* 2014;19(3):435–456. DOI: https://doi.org/10.1007/s10459-013-9474-4
14. Violato C, Cullen MJ, Englander R, et al. Validity evidence for assessing entrustable professional activities during undergraduate medical education. *Acad Med.* 2021;96(7S):S70-S75. DOI: https://doi.org/10.1097/ACM.0000000000004090
15. ten Cate O, Chen HC. The ingredients of a rich entrustment decision. *Med Teach.* 2020;42(12):1413–1420. DOI: https://doi.org/10.1080/0142159X.2020.1817348
16. Holmboe E, Ginsburg S, Bernabeo E. The rotational approach to medical education: time to confront our assumptions? *Med Educ.* 2011;45(1):69–80. DOI: https://doi.org/10.1111/j.1365-2923.2010.03847.x
17. Englander R, Carraccio C. A lack of continuity in education, training, and practice violates the 'do no harm' principle. *Acad Med.* 2018;93(3S):S12-S16. DOI: https://doi.org/10.1097/ACM.0000000000002071
18. Rohrer D, Pashler H. Recent research on human learning challenges conventional instructional strategies. *Educational Researcher.* 2010;39(5):406–412. DOI: https://doi.org/10.3102/0013189X10374770

19. Poncelet A, Hirsh D, eds. *Longitudinal Integrated Clerkships: Principles, Outcomes, Practical Tools and Future Directions*. Gegensatz Press; 2016.
20. Englander R, ten Cate O. LICs and entrustable professional activities: a perfect match. In: Poncelet A, Hirsh D, eds. *Longitudinal Integrated Clerkships (LICs) - Principles, Outcomes, Practical Tools and Future Directions*. 1st ed. Alliance for Clinical Education/Gegensatz Press; 2016:261–270.
21. Warm EJ, Mathis BR, Held JD, et al. Entrustment and mapping of observable practice activities for resident assessment. *J Gen Intern Med*. 2014;29(8):1177–1182. DOI: https://doi.org/10.1007/s11606-014-2801-5
22. Nousiainen MT, Mironova P, Hynes M, et al. Eight-year outcomes of a competency-based residency training program in orthopedic surgery. *Med Teach*. 2018;40(10):1042–1054. DOI: https://doi.org/10.1080/0142159X.2017.1421751
23. ten Cate O, Graafmans L, Posthumus I, Welink L, van Dijk M. The EPA-based Utrecht undergraduate clinical curriculum: development and implementation. *Med Teach*. 2018;40(5):506–513. DOI: https://doi.org/10.1080/0142159X.2018.1435856
24. Peters H, Holzhausen Y, Boscardin C, ten Cate O, Chen HC. Twelve tips for the implementation of EPAs for assessment and entrustment decisions. *Med Teach*. 2017;39(8):802–807. DOI: https://doi.org/10.1080/0142159X.2017.1331031
25. Bellini LM, Kalet A, Englander R. Providing compassionate off-ramps for medical students is a moral imperative. *Acad Med*. 2019;94(5):656–658. DOI: https://doi.org/10.1097/ACM.0000000000002568
26. Pinilla S, Lenouvel E, Cantisani A, et al. Working with entrustable professional activities in clinical education in undergraduate medical education: a scoping review. *BMC Med Educ*. 2021;21(1):172. DOI: https://doi.org/10.1186/s12909-021-02608-9
27. Liu L, Jiang Z, Qi X, et al. An update on current EPAs in graduate medical education: a scoping review. *Med Educ Online*. 2021;26(1):1981198. DOI: https://doi.org/10.1080/10872981.2021.1981198
28. Chen HC, McNamara M, Teherani A, ten Cate O, O'Sullivan P. Developing entrustable professional activities for entry into clerkship. *Acad Med*. 2016;91(2):247–255. DOI: https://doi.org/10.1097/ACM.0000000000000988
29. Amiel J, Ryan MS, Andriole DA, Whelan AJ. *Core Entrustable Professional Activities for Entering Residency Summary of the 10-School Pilot 2014–2021*. Association of American Medical Colleges; 2022.
30. Bremer AE, van de Pol MHJ, Laan RFJM, Fluit CRMG. How an EPA-based curriculum supports professional identity formation. *BMC Med Educ*. 2022;22(1):48. DOI: https://doi.org/10.1186/s12909-022-03116-0
31. Cruess RL, Cruess SR, Boudreau JD, Snell L, Steinert Y. A schematic representation of the professional identity formation and socialization of medical students and residents: a guide for medical educators. *Acad Med*. 2015;90(6):718–725. DOI: https://doi.org/10.1097/ACM.0000000000000700
32. Lucey CR, Larson T, eds. *Achieving Competency-Based, Time-Variable Health Professions Education*. Josiah Macy Jr Foundation; 2018.
33. Goldhamer MEJ, Pusic MV, Nadel ES, Co JPT, Weinstein DF. Promotion in place: A model for competency-based, time-variable graduate medical education. *Acad Med*. 2024;99(5):518–523. DOI: https://doi.org/10.1097/ACM.0000000000005652
34. Andrews JS, Bale JF, Soep JB, et al. Education in Pediatrics Across the Continuum (EPAC): first steps toward realizing the dream of competency-based education. *Acad Med*. 2018;93(3):414–420. DOI: https://doi.org/10.1097/ACM.0000000000002020
35. Englander R, Flynn T, Call S, et al. *Core Entrustable Professional Activities for Entering Residency - Curriculum Developers Guide*. AAMC; 2014:1–114.
36. Entrustable professional activities for general pediatrics. May 2023. Accessed April 8, 2024. https://www.abp.org/content/entrustable-professional-activities-general-pediatrics

CHAPTER 13

Use of entrustable professional activities in pre-licensure health professions education

Eric G. Meyer, Machelle Linsenmeyer, Ylva Holzhausen, Mabel Yap, Michael S. Ryan, H. Carrie Chen

Abstract

This chapter introduces how entrustable professional activities (EPAs) can be implemented in the pre-licensure stage of education (e.g., undergraduate health professions education), with a focus on how trainees can contribute to patient care in a legitimate participatory role prior to licensure. The relative freedom of trainees from workplace-based productivity provides pre-licensure training with a great deal of flexibility. Such flexibility allows creativity and different approaches to laying the canonical foundation for specific EPAs, preparing trainees for clinical training based on EPAs and entrustment, and establishing an appreciation for how entrustment represents an assurance of readiness for safe patient care rather than a grade. Educators can leverage the required knowledge, skills, and attitudes detailed in EPA descriptions to ensure that foundational science courses are preparing trainees for clinical care. The transition from canonical knowledge to more EPA-focused activities is ideally via a 'Z-shaped' curriculum. Factors of a trainee's trustworthiness, which underlie entrustment in later clinical stages of training, can be explicitly introduced, explored, and strengthened in pre-workplace-based settings. Lastly, the chapter delineates how early pre-licensure workplace-based learning founded on EPAs provides opportunities to introduce contextual competencies, while advanced workplace-based education further refines practice with limited supervision, preparing trainees for the transition to additional post-licensure training or licensed practice.

How to cite this book chapter:

Meyer EG, Linsenmeyer M, Holzhausen Y, Yap M, Ryan MS, Chen HC. Use of entrustable professional activities in pre-licensure health professions education. In: ten Cate O, Burch VC, Chen HC, Chou FC, Hennus MP. (Eds). *Entrustable Professional Activities and Entrustment Decision-Making in Health Professions Education*, Chapter 13, pp. 145–156. [2024] London: Ubiquity Press. DOI: https://doi.org/10.5334/bdc.m

This chapter uses cross-references to other chapters of the same book. For those who read this chapter as a standalone publication: all cross-references can be found at: https://doi.org/10.5334/bdc

Authors

- Eric G. Meyer, MD, PhD. Uniformed Services University of the Health Sciences, Bethesda, Maryland, USA. Correspondence: eric.meyer@usuhs.edu
- Machelle Linsenmeyer, EdD. West Virginia School of Osteopathic Medicine, Lewisburg, West Virginia, USA.
- Ylva Holzhausen, MSc, PhD. Dieter Scheffner Center for Medical Education and Educational Research, Charité-Universitätsmedizin Berlin, Berlin, Germany.
- Mabel Yap, MBBS, MSc, PhD. Ministry of Health Singapore and National University Health System, Singapore.
- Michael S. Ryan, MD, MEHP. University of Virginia School of Medicine, Charlottesville, Virginia, USA.
- H. Carrie Chen, MD, PhD. Kaiser Permanente Bernard J. Tyson School of Medicine, Pasadena, CA, USA.

Introduction

The entrustable professional activities (EPAs) framework has emerged as a powerful framework for implementing competency-based education.[1] EPAs define the activities that are critical to a profession, shifting the focus from characteristics of trainees to the activities trainees are required to perform upon gaining licensure (e.g., graduation, entering practice), and employing entrustment of trainees to complete the activities with increasing autonomy as a natural means of progression. EPAs as outcome expectations have been implemented across many health professions including medicine, nursing, pharmacy, psychology, veterinary medicine, allied health therapy,[a] and more.[2] EPAs were initially developed and have been primarily implemented in workplace settings with trainees who are both capable of and permitted to participate in health care delivery. This capability and permission are often recognized through licensure. In this chapter, we focus on the pre-licensure phase of education. Pre-licensure refers to the phase of training in which a health professions trainee is enrolled in their formal degree-granting education programs (e.g., medical, nursing, allied health school). The term pre-licensure is often used synonymously with *undergraduate*, particularly in the medical field—we use the term pre-licensure to offer a more inclusive frame of reference for professions that do not typically include a post-licensure or post-graduate phase. While EPAs have been predominantly described in later stages of training, this does not mean that EPAs do not also have a role in pre-licensure health professions education.[3] In fact, linking pre-licensure education to the EPAs expected of trainees in unsupervised clinical practice is critical and this linkage should be made explicit to both trainees and supervisors, to prepare trainees for professional work in clinical settings.

Notably, laws, regulations, and accepted practices vary across different regions and professions. This is true not only of supervision during training (e.g., medical trainees in Brazil are permitted to perform EPAs as part of community service without supervision)[4] but also of expectations upon completion of training. EPAs must therefore be tailored to relevant professions in their local contexts. In many regions, nurses and allied health professionals (therapists, radiographers, dietitians, etc.) transition directly from pre-licensure education into practice. Medical trainees in certain jurisdictions (e.g., South America, the Middle East) are authorized for unsupervised practice upon completing pre-licensure medical education, while those in other regions (e.g., Europe, North America, Taiwan, Singapore) must complete additional post-licensure medical education before transitioning to unsupervised practice.[5–7] While these variations necessitate customized approaches to EPA development and implementation, pre-licensure education also represents an opportunity to develop interprofessional EPAs in addition to profession-specific EPAs.[8]

This chapter delves into the implementation of EPAs in pre-licensure health professions education. Despite variations in the outcome expectations at the end of pre-licensure education, there are common principles that can be applied across professions and jurisdictions. By thoughtfully integrating EPAs into the curriculum and, as permitted, allowing pre-licensure learners to meaningfully engage in clinical workplace activities, EPAs provide a means to nurture a generation of graduates who can be entrusted to safely contribute to patient care in their transition to either further training or unsupervised practice. Moreover, because trainees in pre-licensure phases of training are not required to meet productivity targets, the pre-licensure period offers more flexibility to use creative approaches not limited by clinical workplace structures to lay the foundation for later entrustment.

---

[a] Refers to, for example, physiotherapy, occupational therapy, radiography, podiatry, dietetics, and speech therapy.

Considerations in an EPA-based pre-licensure health professions education program

The commencement of a pre-licensure health professions education program represents a major step in a trainee's journey to becoming a health professional. A key function of pre-licensure education is helping trainees broaden their attention from their own needs as a student to including the needs of their teammates and patients. Trainees need to shift their priorities from demonstrating their knowledge and skills acquisition for grades and passing courses each semester to mastering knowledge and skills in service of the patient care activities that they will perform as a health professional. The EPA framework supports this identity shift by emphasizing the patient care activities and the trust being placed on trainees to contribute to or perform those activities safely as they complete their training.[9] Trainees entering a pre-licensure education program, especially in the early preworkplace phase, may not intuit how the curriculum's content is preparing them to become a health professional. Articulating this professional identity formation as one explicit goal of an EPA-based curriculum and demonstrating how the curriculum supports trainees in achieving that goal may help trainees engage in the learner-driven elements of the programs. It also can be helpful to explicitly show trainees from the outset, and as they progress through the curriculum, the EPAs they will be expected to perform at a certain level of supervision upon graduation, henceforth referred to as core EPAs.

Additionally, mapping of the learning objectives of a curriculum to its core EPAs can help trainees understand the relationship between learning in the classroom and the activities required for clinical practice. For example, it may be helpful for trainees to realize how the theoretical content they learn in anatomy and physiology, pathophysiology and pharmacology can be applied in the management of childbirth. This represents a mindset shift from 'just in case learning' to 'just in time learning.' To further support the trainee experience of becoming a professional, smaller EPAs appropriate for practice by early trainees in different settings (simulation, workplace) may be used at different points of the curriculum. They also can be mapped to or nested within the larger core EPAs.[10] These smaller, nested EPAs allow increasing participation and contribution to patient care and ultimately prepare the trainees for the practice of the larger core EPAs. Admittedly, linking curricular components to EPAs is not easy. It often requires collaboration between clinicians and those who teach the foundational sciences. It can also painfully highlight historically prized curricular areas as potentially less relevant than previously perceived.

To actively engage with and optimize learning from an EPA-based curriculum, trainees should understand how it differs from a traditional or typical preprofessional curriculum and why these elements are beneficial to their learning. This includes the different approach to assessment (namely the use of entrustment and supervision levels versus proficiency scales), the concept of entrustment, and how trainee behaviors influence entrustment/supervision decisions. A number of trainee qualities (agency, reliability, integrity, capability, and humility), captured in the A RICH framework, have been identified as important for enabling entrustment.[11] Trainees need to be educated explicitly about these elements of 'trustworthiness' and associated behaviors and provided with opportunities to practice and receive feedback and coaching.

The implementation of EPAs in a pre-licensure health professions education program involves significant changes to traditional curriculum paradigms and requires both change management and a faculty development process (see Chapters 22 and 23).[12] Ideally, the EPA-based curriculum is an integrated, longitudinal curriculum in which the curricular content is structured with iterative and spiral opportunities for learning, application, and practice.[13] The next sections will explore in more detail how EPAs can be integrated in two distinct phases of pre-licensure education: preworkplace and workplace-based education.

Preworkplace education—education without contributions to patient care

Classroom-based learning

During pre-licensure education, a significant part of the education occurs in the classroom where foundational science content is addressed. This begs the question of how EPAs, which were developed for workplace-based training, may apply. The performance of each EPA or patient care activity requires a specific set of relevant knowledge, skills, attitudes, and experiences that are delineated in the elaborated descriptions of each EPA. This level of competence has been described as canonical competence—the standard foundational knowledge and skills, independent of context, expected of all trainees in the profession. Classroom-based learning thus provides the core knowledge and skills (canonical competence) trainees need to perform the EPAs.[1,14] In fact, the elaborated EPA descriptions should inform the selection of content and instructional methods for the classroom curriculum. As noted above, this classroom learning may be mapped to core EPAs to highlight—for both classroom educators and trainees—how foundational science knowledge and skills will support trainee ability to eventually achieve entrustment for their core EPAs and perform the work of the profession. It ensures that classroom instruction is EPA-centered, reflecting Merrill's principle of *task-/problem-centered* learning.[15] Of note, some important knowledge or attitude objectives (e.g., ethics, professionalism) may not map specifically to individual EPAs. Rather, they may support the trainee 'trustworthiness' qualities or professional values underlying all EPAs. The mapping of the classroom curriculum is also a good opportunity to introduce trainees to the concept of longitudinal and cumulative learning. Trainees, who may have been sensitized to the idea of passing 'individual courses,' can start to track their longitudinal progress in mastering and integrating increasingly complicated material as an indicator for being 'ready' to progress to future stages of training and participation in patient care activities.

More importantly, the trainee factors that enable entrustment for all EPAs (agency, reliability, integrity, capability, and humility) should be emphasized throughout pre-licensure education, including in the classroom. For instance, in team-based learning activities, trainees may be asked to demonstrate and be held accountable for agency in preparing for the sessions, reliability in the information they share based on research using valid resources, truthfulness in their interactions with peers, and willingness to ask for help and receive feedback. Role play exercises with peer-teaching activities may help make personally relevant the concept of entrustment and trustworthiness. Another often-overlooked opportunity for programs to reinforce these expectations as part of the culture is in program-supported extracurricular activities. Programs can highlight trainee capability in a leadership position, reliability in supporting a research project, or humility in a volunteer organization as authentic examples of trainee trustworthiness behaviors. Many pre-licensure programs already have expectations, hold their trainees accountable, and provide feedback and coaching for a subset of these trustworthiness qualities framed under the concept of professionalism. Making clear to trainees at the outset of pre-licensure education the expectations around agency, reliability, integrity, capability, and humility can help trainees develop these habits during classroom learning and prepare them for future entrustment with patient care activities in the workplace curriculum.

Simulated or controlled workplace-based experiences

Many pre-licensure programs offer early introductions to workplace-based experiences that are interspersed or integrated with classroom-based learning where the primary goal is exposure rather than participation in or contribution to the patient care work of the workplace. This can be considered clinical education without contribution to patient care and includes 'observerships' and practice with simulation. Here trainees begin to attend to the context in which their canonical competence will be applied and EPAs offer a helpful guide in ensuring the *task-/problem-centered* development of these experiences. They can help educators choose experiences and focus learner attention on learning points during observerships such as understanding the clinical workplace, health system, and various professional roles and specialties. Simulation activities with standardized patients, manikins, and simulated electronic health records enable early practice of communication, physical exam, and documentation skills with feedback within a safe environment without direct consequences for patient care. These experiences allow activation of canonical knowledge from the classroom, demonstration of skills in context, and application of knowledge and skills. Some programs may require that learners meet a certain level of entrustment in simulation before being allowed to progress to the workplace, where they will engage in authentic clinical activities.

Workplace-based education—education with contributions to patient care

Ideally, pre-licensure trainees enter the workplace adequately prepared by the preworkplace curriculum to join the professional community of practice and begin contributing to the patient care work of the workplace. The workplace provides a rich context in which tasks necessary for professional practice can be further demonstrated, experienced, and acquired in context. A workplace curriculum can be defined as an organized set of experiences in a real-world setting that fosters the acquisition of contextual competence tied to work that are necessary for unsupervised practice.[10,14] Here trainees practice further application of their canonical competence but also integration of their knowledge and skills for deeper problem-solving and increasingly complex tasks in the workplace to develop contextual competence.

Unique to pre-licensure trainees is the initial entry into the workplace and limitations to their readiness to engage. Their initial participation is typically heavily supervised and involves relatively low-risk peripheral yet authentic professional tasks. Programs may choose to add limitations to their EPA specifications to match the developmental expectations of an early trainee. An example would be an EPA specification that limits trainees to taking a history of a stable cognitively intact and cooperative adult patient with no emotional or physical distress with a common chief complaint.[10] As trainees progress, the limitations in the EPA specifications could be pulled back to include new developmental expectations such as taking the history of emotionally distressed patients, pediatric or geriatric patients, patients with uncommon chief complaints, patients with severe or acute illness, etc. Broadening the expectations using this spiral approach will, over time, allow trainees to be entrusted with the full specifications required at graduation. This nesting of EPAs helps support the entry of pre-licensure trainees into the real-world workplace setting and gradually prepares them for entrustment with the increased responsibility and breadth of the core EPAs.

In addition to the use of nested EPAs, the curriculum can be built using different ancillary frameworks for the developmental progression of trainees. EPAs are synthetic and holistic in their framing of competencies and early trainees may benefit from a breaking down of those competencies into more analytic or developmental steps. For instance, the RIME (reporter–interpreter–manager–educator) model often used in undergraduate medical education can allow educators and trainees to account for current ability and focus on the next level of development.[16] Regardless of the frameworks used, the curriculum must be designed to encourage developmental progression and allow the practice (with available support) of core EPAs in the final stages of training such that trainees graduate ready to practice the core EPAs with distant or no supervision.

Therefore, an EPA-based workplace curriculum should map out a route for individual trainees with summative entrustment decisions at significant moments in their training that lead to permission to engage in patient care activities with increasing responsibility and decreasing degrees of supervision. The units of professional practice that the smaller nested EPAs represent should be large enough to allow entrustment for practice under varying levels of supervision and not lose their specificity. The curriculum should account for the level of training at which trainees are expected to be able to perform nested EPAs and core EPAs with either distant supervision or unsupervised. In some training situations, achievement of a set of core EPAs may be sufficient. In others, trainees may be expected to achieve additional selective or elective EPAs that can help position them for additional post-licensure training or prepare them for transition to practice in specific workplace contexts.[17]

A challenge to workplace-based curricula in pre-licensure education is the varying rules and regulations developed around patient safety or liability concerns. Jurisdictions may limit trainee participation and/or require all patients be seen by a licensed professional. In this case, a program may not be able to build a curriculum where trainees can be entrusted with unsupervised practice for an EPA despite being ready. These requirements will be different across contexts, programs, and professions. The job of the curriculum then becomes the creation of an environment in which supervision is close enough to be safe and meet regulatory requirements, while feeling distant enough to fuel the growth in responsibility that motivates learning. Trainees demonstrating readiness for more responsibility should be allowed greater responsibility; true entrustment decisions should permit trainees to become genuine team members with legitimate roles and contributions to patient care under distant or no supervision. Education and engagement of key stakeholders, including those representing the clinical workplace and regulatory bodies, in designing the workplace-based curriculum may help the clinical setting and regulatory bodies accept and adjust expectations around trainee roles and contributions to patient care.

Entrustment decisions in pre-licensure education

Though this chapter is focused on curriculum, it is important to note considerations around assessment and entrustment decision-making in pre-licensure education. The ultimate aim of any EPA-based education program is to be able to confirm and ensure the readiness of trainees to perform the core EPAs upon graduation via summative entrustment decisions on trainees. These entrustment decisions must be valid (e.g., defensible, justifiable, and reproducible) and several principles apply to entrustment decision-making that is generalizable to all educational contexts (see Chapters 18–21). In pre-licensure education, questions about entrustment decisions arise, including: when are decisions applicable, when or how they can be used for assessment, and what is their ultimate purpose? Is the purpose of entrustment decision-making purely *for* learning or is there an advancement implication (i.e., assessment *of* learning with explicit linkage to progression, and/or remediation)?[18] Modern programmatic assessment approaches endorse the value of multiple low-stakes assessments while learning to promote the maximum growth of the trainee prior to a high-stakes decision.[19] In an EPA program, such an approach may be particularly beneficial to offer feedback throughout a trainee's growth and development.

For classroom-based education, many of the assessments, whether low- or high-stakes, will focus on the assessment of foundational knowledge, which is typically best done using traditional methods. However, as noted above, the concept of entrustment as assessment can be introduced in the context of teamwork in the classroom and entrustment of classmates for their contributions to team learning while considering agency, reliability, integrity, capability, and humility.

In workplace-based education, entrustment decisions for specific EPAs can be used to facilitate learning and trainee growth and/or to determine trainee readiness for advancement. Entrustment decisions used exclusively to facilitate learning should be driven by trainee needs. Consider the value for trainees and how the decision will inform their learning goals.

An assessment tension that is potentially unique to pre-licensure education in some health professions is the need to differentiate among trainees for the purposes of selection into post-licensure education. Epstein describes this as one of the main goals of assessment along with the other two goals of protecting public safety by ensuring trainee competence and promoting learning and optimization of trainee capabilities.[20] However, EPA-based curricula are competency-based and emphasize the latter two goals. EPA-based assessments focus on levels of supervision and readiness for unsupervised practice and do not rank trainees on levels of proficiency. Graduates are certified as having achieved readiness to perform core EPAs but are not 'graded' in relation to each other. In systems where stakeholders such as post-licensure programs and graduates seeking post-licensure training advocate strongly for grading or ranking of graduates, it can be difficult to reconcile a curriculum that uses EPA outcomes and entrustment decisions for assessment with one that grades or ranks trainees. This has led some programs to use EPAs as curricular outcomes to structure the curriculum and only operationalize entrustment for assessment in various degrees, such as for formative assessment only with a separate assessment system for grading and ranking.

Curricular design and planning

Pre-licensure education with an EPA-based curriculum faces unique design challenges, in particularly in the need to provide both pre-workplace-based and workplace-based education and transition the trainee from student to professional. An ideal curricular design is one that iteratively builds upon itself in a spiral fashion[13] and vertically integrates preworkplace-based and workplace-based education. The latter vertical integration creates what has been called a 'Z-shaped' curriculum (Figure 13.1).[21] It introduces opportunities for early application and integration of knowledge and skills to begin to build contextual competence even as initial education is primarily focused on building canonical competence. Experience with early trainees in student-run clinics show that, when given the opportunity and adequate support, they are able to apply and improve their

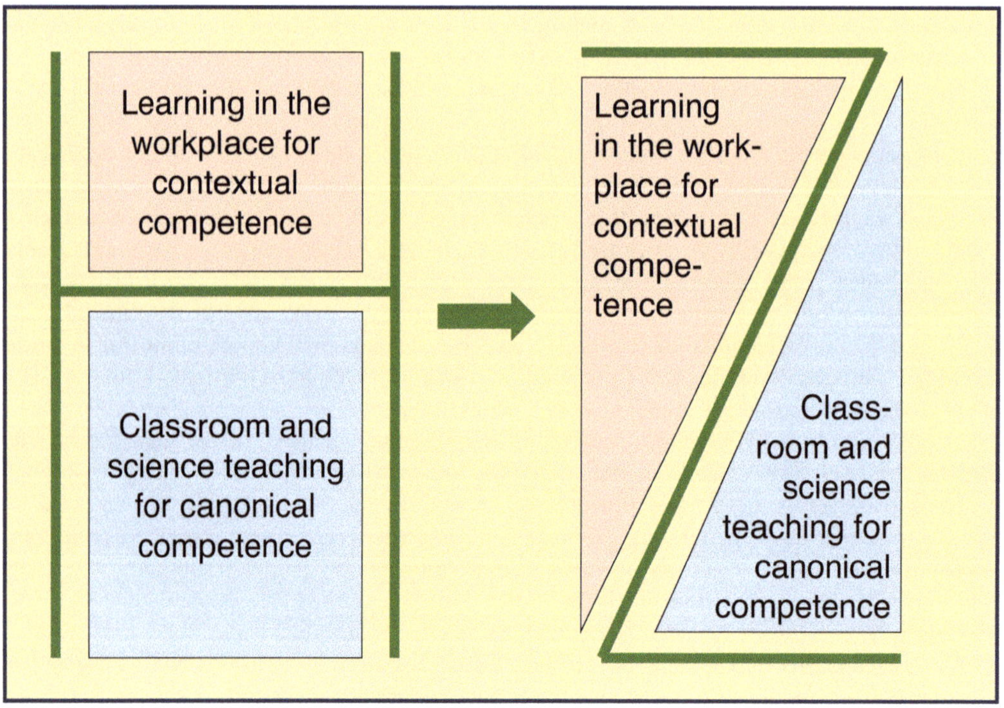

Figure 13.1: Modernization of health professions education toward vertically integrated or Z-shaped curricula with a focus on becoming a professional.

knowledge and skills in the workplace and contribute to patient care.[22,23] As trainees progress, the curriculum increases emphasis on the development of contextual competence in the workplace and supports their increasing capability and responsibility for patient care. At the same time, space is reserved to allow a return to the classroom even at advanced clinical stages to reinforce and reintegrate important foundational knowledge and skills.

Box 13.1: Curricular planning case study 1: adopting EPAs for pre-licensure trainees.

Overview

A pre-licensure education program would like to utilize EPAs to guide its curriculum and assessment efforts. The curriculum is divided into two stages: one that occurs primarily in the classroom using lectures and one that involves hands-on learning in the workplace. A committee is formed of education specialists and experts from the field who are recipients of the program's graduates. The committee reviews the program's goals and objectives along with typical job requirements from the field to determine what EPAs define the profession. As part of the EPA definitions, the committee includes a set of smaller EPAs that can be nested into the more complex core EPAs. They also determine for each EPA, where the skills and knowledge required to complete the EPA should be taught and which levels of entrustment are required to advance to the workplace stage of training and to graduate.

When the curriculum committee shares their proposed curricular plan, the faculty react with two very different responses. The faculty from the classroom stage note that they have been 'left out.' Several ask if their courses will be removed as they do not 'define the profession.' Some point out that they cannot use entrustment as an assessment tool if there are no opportunities to entrust. The faculty from the workplace stage are outraged that students will be expected to have supervision levels below required regulations. They cite safety concerns and legal ramifications.

Analysis

This case highlights problems that often occur when faculty from within different stages of training are not included in the EPA-based curriculum planning process. Key opportunities for faculty engagement have been missed and it will be much harder to gain buy-in. It is important to explain how the foundational science curriculum might map to core EPAs or more immediately to nested EPAs—and that the use of traditional assessment tools for knowledge and skills can and should still be utilized. Reviewing trainee qualities and behaviors that are important for entrustment and that can be assessed outside the workplace (e.g., agency, reliability, integrity, capability, and humility)[24] is another way to help classroom-based faculty connect to the overall educational mission. It is also critical to ensure that those who understand legal and program limitations related to trainee supervision are involved and help account for these limitations in the curriculum.[25]

This case also shows several best practices such as including stakeholders, who are 'recipients' of the program graduates, to ensure the EPAs are relevant to the profession. Working backward through stages of training to determine required levels of entrustment helps to ensure attention to developmental progression through the curriculum and to define advancement decisions. Additionally, nesting smaller EPAs into more complex core EPAs and mapping knowledge and skills to EPAs promote a cohesive curriculum.

Whether a program can create a 'Z-shaped' curriculum, there are key principles that are important to highlight when designing the curriculum. One is creating integrated content to support the application of knowledge to the care of patients. This can include the integration of different foundational sciences (e.g., anatomy, histology) into organs-based and problem-based curricula as well as the integration of foundational science learning and its application in the clinical context. The latter can be achieved by juxtaposing classroom, simulation, and workplace-based experiences. A second important principle is that of 'longitudinality.' Longitudinal supervisor–trainee relationships and experiences are important to support learning and enable valid entrustment decision. Some pre-licensure medical education programs have combined these two principles to create longitudinal integrated clerkships where trainees work in various specialty units throughout the year, learning, for instance, pediatrics at the same time as surgery with an assigned longitudinal supervisor in each specialty. A final principle is the engagement of all stakeholders including educators involved in the classroom-based curriculum, those representing recipients of the program graduates, and the trainees. See the case studies in Boxes 13.1 and 13.2 for examples of how these and other considerations discussed in this chapter can present challenges and potential solutions during curricular planning.

Box 13.2: Curricular planning case study 2: establishing programmatic assessment of EPAs for pre-licensure trainees.

Overview

A pre-licensure educational program implemented EPAs a few years ago. The program decided to use repeated low-stakes assessments of each EPA from a variety of faculty as the best approach for providing feedback to trainees and making advancement decisions during the workplace stage of training. The faculty approach the entrustment–supervision scale as a proficiency scale and are loath to 'rate' trainees at the lower end of the entrustment–supervision scale, and they continue to assess trainees only at the end of each rotation. Trainees complain about the paucity of assessments and feedback and are also surprised when, upon being reviewed for advancement decisions, they are told that they are 'not yet ready to move to the next stage' despite their 'passing' ratings.

Analysis

This situation highlights challenges in implementing an entrustment system in a pre-licensure program. Faculty and trainees may have difficulty transitioning from a proficiency rating and 'grades' mindset to that of entrustment–supervision. Faculty may rate trainees as being ready for more autonomy based on a history of using a higher part of a rating scale. Trainees in turn may interpret that as a 'passing' or high rating/grade and not a reflection of how much supervision they may still actually need to complete certain tasks.

This case demonstrates the importance of training both faculty and trainees on how entrustment–supervision scales function. Without a clear understanding of entrustment, supervision, and the goals of workplace-based assessments, faculty will have a difficult time pivoting from end-of-rotation evaluations to frequent low-stakes assessments and the interaction could become a checklist versus a process for entrustment. Similarly, trainees may remain focused merely on passing or receiving high ratings for clinical placements/rotations without understanding what is needed to achieve entrustment for an EPA or what it means to be ready to perform an EPA with distant or no supervision. This case also reinforces the importance of helping trainees seek feedback and build upon that feedback as part of their journey toward greater autonomy.

Conclusion

EPAs can be implemented in the pre-licensure stage of education, allowing trainees to contribute to patient care in a legitimate participatory role. Pre-licensure training lays a foundation of canonical competence, prepares trainees for entrustment, and reorients the trainee from student to emerging professional. The required knowledge, skills, and attitudes from EPA descriptions can help inform preworkplace-based curricula. Entrustment to perform specific EPAs informs the workplace-based curricula. The use of entrustment provides a means to explore and strengthen trainee qualities important for ongoing entrustment in later clinical stages of training and practice. Finally, an important step in building an EPA-based curriculum is the engagement of all stakeholders (e.g., classroom faculty, clinical administrators, trainees) and ensuring stakeholder understanding of the key principles and differences in an EPA-based curriculum.

Competing interests

The authors declare that they have no competing interests.

References

1. Chen HC, van den Broek WS, ten Cate O. The case for use of entrustable professional activities in undergraduate medical education. *Acad Med.* 2015;90(4):431–436. DOI: https://doi.org/10.1097/ACM.0000000000000586
2. Shorey S, Lau TC, Lau ST, Ang E. Entrustable professional activities in health care education: a scoping review. *Med Educ.* 2019;53(8):766–777. DOI: https://doi.org/10.1111/medu.13879
3. Bramley AL, McKenna L. Entrustable professional activities in entry-level health professional education: a scoping review. *Med Educ.* 2021;55(9):1011–1032. DOI: https://doi.org/10.1111/medu.14539
4. Francischetti I, Holzhausen Y, Peters H. Entrustable professional activities for junior Brazilian medical students in community medicine. *BMC Med Educ.* 2022;22(1):737. DOI: https://doi.org/10.1186/s12909-022-03762-4
5. Wijnen-Meijer M, van den Broek M, ten Cate O. Six routes to unsupervised clinical practice. *Acad Med.* 2021;96(3):475. DOI: https://doi.org/10.1097/ACM.0000000000003880
6. Forero DA, Majeed MH, Ruiz-Díaz P. Current trends and future perspectives for medical education in Colombia. *Med Teach.* 2020;42(1):17–23. DOI: https://doi.org/10.1080/0142159X.2019.1659944
7. Hamui-Sutton A, Vives-Varela T, Durán-Pérez VD, Gutiérrez-Barreto SE, Millán-Hernández M. Mapping an EPA-based comprehensive curricular proposal for UME. *MedEdPublish. (2016).* 2019;8:186. DOI: https://doi.org/10.15694/mep.2019.000186.1
8. Tielemans C, de Kleijn R, van der Schaaf M, van den Broek S, Westerveld T. The Westerveld framework for interprofessional feedback dialogues in health professions education. *Assess Eval High Edu.* 2023;48(2):241–257. DOI: https://doi.org/10.1080/02602938.2021.1967285
9. Hauer KE, ten Cate O, Boscardin C, Irby DM, Iobst W, O'Sullivan PS. Understanding trust as an essential element of trainee supervision and learning in the workplace. *Adv Health Sci Educ Theory Pract.* 2014;19(3):435–456. DOI: https://doi.org/10.1007/s10459-013-9474-4
10. ten Cate O, Chen HC, Hoff RG, Peters H, Bok H, van der Schaaf M. Curriculum development for the workplace using entrustable professional activities (EPAs): AMEE guide no. 99. *Med Teach.* 2015;37(11):983–1002. DOI: https://doi.org/10.3109/0142159X.2015.1060308
11. ten Cate O, Chen HC. The ingredients of a rich entrustment decision. *Med Teach.* 2020;42(12):1413–1420. DOI: https://doi.org/10.1080/0142159X.2020.1817348

12. Bray MJ, Bradley EB, Martindale JR, Gusic ME. Implementing systematic faculty development to support an EPA-based program of assessment: strategies, outcomes, and lessons learned. *Teach Learn Med.* 2021;33(4):434–444. DOI: https://doi.org/10.1080/10401334.2020.1857256
13. Harden RM. What is a spiral curriculum? *Med Teach.* 1999;21(2):141–143. DOI: https://doi.org/10.1080/01421599979752
14. ten Cate O, Khursigara-Slattery N, Cruess RL, Hamstra SJ, Steinert Y, Sternszus R. Medical competence as a multilayered construct. *Med Educ.* 2024;58(1):93–104. DOI: https://doi.org/10.1111/medu.15162
15. Merrill MD. Using the first principles of instruction to make instruction effective, efficient, and engaging. In: West RE, ed. *Foundations of Learning and Instructional Design Technology.* EdTech; 2017.
16. Pangaro L, ten Cate O. Frameworks for learner assessment in medicine: AMEE guide no. 78. *Med Teach.* 2013;35(6):e1197-e1210. DOI: https://doi.org/10.3109/0142159X.2013.788789
17. Jonker G, Booij E, Otte W, Vlijm C, ten Cate O, Hoff R. An elective EPA-based thematic final medical school year. An appreciative inquiry study among students, graduates and supervisors. *Adv Med Educ Pract.* 2018:9 837–845. DOI: https://doi.org/10.2147/AMEP.S176649
18. van der Vleuten CP, Schuwirth L, Driessen E, et al. A model for programmatic assessment fit for purpose. *Med Teach.* 2012;34(3):205–214. DOI: https://doi.org/10.3109/0142159X.2012.652239
19. Schuwirth LW, Van der Vleuten CP. Programmatic assessment: from assessment of learning to assessment for learning. *Med Teach.* 2011;33(6):478–485. DOI: https://doi.org/10.3109/0142159X.2011.565828
20. Epstein RM. Assessment in medical education. *N Engl J Med.* 2007;356(4):387–396. DOI: https://doi.org/10.1056/NEJMra054784
21. Wijnen-Meijer M, Van den Broek S, Koens F, ten Cate O. Vertical integration in medical education: the broader perspective. *BMC Med Educ.* 2020;20(1):509. DOI: https://doi.org/10.1186/s12909-020-02433-6
22. Wilson OW, Broman P, Tokolahi E, Andersen P, Brownie S. Learning outcomes from participation in student-run health clinics: a systematic review. *J Multidiscip Healthc.* 2023:143–157. DOI: https://doi.org/10.2147/JMDH.S385709
23. Chen HC, Sheu L, O'Sullivan P, ten Cate O, Teherani A. Legitimate workplace roles and activities for early learners. *Med Educ.* 2014;48(2):136–145. DOI: https://doi.org/10.1111/medu.12316
24. ten Cate O, Carraccio C, Damodaran A, et al. Entrustment decision-making: extending Miller's pyramid. *Acad Med.* 2021;96(2):199–204. DOI: https://doi.org/10.1097/ACM.0000000000003800
25. Zainuldin R, Tan HY. Development of entrustable professional activities for a physiotherapy undergraduate programme in Singapore. *Physiotherapy.* 2021;112:64–71. DOI: https://doi.org/10.1016/j.physio.2021.03.017

CHAPTER 14

Curriculum development for postgraduate training with entrustable professional activities

Marije P. Hennus, J. Damon Dagnone, Roberta I. Ladenheim, Daniel J. Schumacher, Mabel Yap, Olle ten Cate, H. Carrie Chen

Abstract

Entrustable professional activities (EPAs) are frequently implemented in training after licensing, in the postgraduate specialist stage of training. In this phase, trainees and supervisors must navigate the unique challenge of balancing patient care (service) and ongoing training (education). Opportunistic learning amid patient care represents a significant part of this stage of training. In this context, EPAs can play a pivotal role in scaffolding the service–education relationship and help anchor how best to operationalize workplace-based assessment. Specialty training can be highly variable across clinical settings and has many unpredictable elements. That may complicate training but it has also the benefit of building contextual agility and contextual competence.

This chapter aims to support readers and educators who are interested in building an EPA-based specialty training program. It highlights the key issues to be considered including (a) EPAs as organizational units for curriculum design, (b) things to think about in the creation of workplace curricula, (c) assessment considerations in an EPA-based postgraduate training program, (d) trainee experiences in postgraduate EPA-based curricula, (e) the role of interprofessional team members and patients in a postgraduate training program, and (f) challenges of EPA-based curricula in specialist training.

How to cite this book chapter:

Hennus MP, Dagnone JD, Schumacher DJ, Ladenheim RI, Yap M, ten Cate O, Chen HC. Curriculum development for postgraduate training with entrustable professional activities. In: ten Cate O, Burch VC, Chen HC, Chou FC, Hennus MP (Eds). *Entrustable Professional Activities and Entrustment Decision-Making in Health Professions Education*, Chapter 14, pp. 157–174. [2024] London: Ubiquity Press. DOI: https://doi.org/10.5334/bdc.n

This chapter uses cross-references to other chapters of the same book. For those who read this chapter as a standalone publication: all cross-references can be found at: https://doi.org/10.5334/bdc

Authors

- Marije P. Hennus, MD, PhD, MClinEd, University Medical Center Utrecht, Utrecht, the Netherlands. Correspondence: M.P.Hennus@umcutrecht.nl
- J. Damon Dagnone, MD, MSc, MMEd. Queens University, Kingston, Ontario, Canada, and Royal College of Physicians and Surgeons of Canada.
- Roberta I. Ladenheim, MD, MHPE, Universidad del Hospital Italiano de Buenos Aires, Argentina.
- Daniel J. Schumacher, MD, PhD. Cincinnati Children's Hospital Medical Center/University of Cincinnati College of Medicine, Cincinnati, Ohio, USA.
- Mabel Yap, MBBS, MSc, PhD. Ministry of Health Singapore, and National University Health System, Singapore.
- Olle ten Cate, PhD. University Medical Center Utrecht, the Netherlands, and University of California, San Francisco, California, USA.
- H. Carrie Chen, MD, PhD. Kaiser Permanente Bernard J. Tyson School of Medicine, Pasadena, California, USA.

Introduction

Entrustable professional activities (EPAs) are defined as units of professional practice that can be fully entrusted to a trainee as soon as they have demonstrated the necessary competence to execute an activity unsupervised. Initially conceived for postgraduate training, EPAs ground competency-based education (CBE), an outcomes-based approach to the design, implementation, and evaluation of education programs, in the essential activities required in clinical practice and define the transition from supervised to unsupervised practice.[1,2] Postgraduate training is also referred to as residency or fellowship training (medicine, dentistry, pharmacy, physical therapy, veterinary medicine) and often occurs post-licensure. In most health professions, licensure, or registration after completion of a degree-granting program, enables unsupervised practice without additional postgraduate training.

However, in medicine, many countries, especially in the Global North,[a] restrict practice for graduates with just a medical degree and require additional advanced training for general licensure and certification in a medical specialty for unsupervised work. Consequently, medical trainees entering postgraduate training have a license to practice, yet limited space to provide care to patients. They possess the core knowledge, skills, and attitudes (canonical competence), and have had some experience applying it in the clinical workplace (contextual competence), but they require direct or indirect supervision in performing health care tasks.[3] While expanding both canonical (that is, context-independent knowledge and skills) and contextual competence (that is, the ability to work in relevant contexts), postgraduate training provides a rich environment for the increasing development of personal practice approaches or styles (personalized competence).[3] Postgraduate training represents a phase in health professions education where trainees function as professionals with a license to practice, and thus with the right and duty to act, while also being expected to further build their competence.

Acknowledging these dual and sometimes competing roles of trainees in postgraduate training, as learners and service providers, is crucial. It necessitates a significant level of commitment and collaboration among stakeholders, including institutions, training programs, clinical supervisors, and trainees, and among patients willing to accept a trainee as their care provider. Programs and institutions need to be careful not to let service needs alone drive the curriculum of trainees (e.g., clinical duties, rotation schedules).[4] Clinical supervisors should recognize and seize opportunistic teaching moments during the busyness of daily professional duties. A supervisor in postgraduate training is often primarily a specialist practitioner who may not necessarily identify themselves as a teacher, lack defined roles in the training program, and lack training in how to supervise or teach trainees in the workplace.[5] Furthermore, they generally do not receive remuneration or time for teaching, which is expected to be squeezed into their busy clinical practice. Often their primary reason to work at teaching institutions is to perform high-level specialty practice or research, and the added expectations for supervising and teaching trainees may be experienced as a necessary burden. Recruitment of specialists is often based on service or research needs rather than teaching needs. This can affect the engagement and quality of teaching. While faculty development for clinician teachers in postgraduate education is strongly recommended, trainee agency is also important. Trainees need to actively seek out learning opportunities, request feedback, and shape the teaching encounters as necessary to meet their learning needs. Thus development in postgraduate learning settings is a dual enterprise.

In times of service stress and increased workplace needs or even during routine times, trainees' dual roles and the often-perceived tension between education and service may create a polarizing 'either/or' dynamic. This can pervade postgraduate training, both during combined teach-

[a] The nations of the world which are characterized by a high level of economic and industrial development and are typically located to the north of less industrialized nations: Oxford Dictionary.

ing and patient care moments and in the development of the curriculum. By defining essential tasks that align with both learning and clinical responsibilities, EPAs can to some extent alleviate this potential conflict of differing or competing priorities, by creating a 'both/and' phenomenon. EPAs help to frame trainee progression with increasing ability, responsibility, and autonomy in patient care with increasing contributions to clinical service, aligning the language of education with that of the workplace. Trainees, clinical supervisors, and educational leaders can use EPAs to define and sequence the required training experiences, thereby operationalizing desired educational outcomes with safe stepwise increases in service contributions. In essence, EPAs facilitate the 'marriage' of these seemingly opposing priorities, ensuring that trainees build contextual competence (upon expanding canonical competence) and start to develop personalized competence while delivering safe and high-quality patient care.

This chapter draws from established guidelines,[6] existing literature, and expert opinion to outline key challenges and considerations for curriculum planners in postgraduate training. It covers the use of EPAs as organizational units for curriculum design, including considerations for creating workplace curricula and assessments in postgraduate training. It discusses trainee experiences, the involvement of interprofessional team members and patients, and challenges of EPA-based specialist training programs.

EPAs as organizational units for curriculum design

Curricula for postgraduate training can be envisioned at three levels, the *macro, meso* and *micro* levels.[7] The highest, macro level, is a national curriculum. The meso level is the implementation of the national curriculum by institutions and programs, and the micro level is the curriculum established at the level of the trainee.

The macro curriculum at a national level

For many health professions, national specialty boards or accrediting bodies have prescribed expected graduation competencies, program duration, basic program structure (e.g., number of rotations, balance of inpatient/outpatient experiences), and general conditions for teaching, learning, and assessment. This may include expectations around roles of individual supervisors and assessors and procedures for advancement such as the use of competency committees (see Chapter 20 for more information). Boxes 14.1 to 14.5 provide examples of national EPA implementation projects in different countries with different strategies and at various stages (roughly early, mid-stage, and advanced) at the macro level in postgraduate training programs.

The meso-curriculum at a regional or institutional level

In most countries, accrediting bodies require institutions with significant numbers of residents (university medical centers or large nonuniversity teaching hospitals) to develop a local or regional curriculum, within the national core (macro) curriculum. This meso-level program should comply with local regulations and constraints, clinical structures, and available opportunities for rotations. Often pre-EPA curricula are or were defined by list of clinical experiences or rotations and goals/objectives, possibly within a competency framework.[8] Some national curricula now include a prominent role for EPAs, to link the competency expectations to activities in practice.[9–13] For those that do not, universities and programs can choose to interpret national curriculum guidelines into an EPA-based framework with locally defined EPAs and a locally developed EPA-based curriculum (see Chapter 9).

Box 14.1: Introducing EPAs in postgraduate education in Argentina (early).

In Argentina, EPAs were first integrated in undergraduate medical education, starting in 2017 at the Instituto Universitario Hospital Italiano de Buenos Aires. Subsequently, other universities adopted EPAs. The acceptance of EPAs within the academic community grew further over time, evidenced by increased participation in workshops and conferences, and thus with an emphasis on faculty development. This led to research projects with EPAs, along with the development of local guidelines. Next, an emerging faculty network across all of Latin America arose. By 2023, recognizing the effectiveness of EPAs for CBE, the National Ministry of Health began advocating for their incorporation into residency programs. This endorsement significantly accelerated the spread of the concept and heightened the interest among health care training stakeholders. Various stakeholders, including universities, health care institutions, and scientific societies, collaborated to establish consensus on the EPAs within different specialties in Argentina. The implementation of EPA concepts in postgraduate education, particularly in competence assessment, is still in an early stage. Achieving the implementation of EPA-based specialty training will require sustained efforts of faculty development, workplace-based assessment, the documentation of practice and learning experiences, conceptualizations of supervision and entrustment, and the establishment of clinical competency committees within training institutions. Argentina's experience underscores the usefulness of networking but also the need for sustained efforts to fully integrate EPA principles into health care education curricula.

Box 14.2: Introducing EPAs in postgraduate medical education in Singapore (mid-stage).

In Singapore, the introduction of EPAs into the postgraduate year 1 (PGY1) training curriculum in 2014 was a significant milestone. Successful pilots in selected health care professions from 2019 to 2020 paved the way for a nationwide initiative to integrate EPAs within all 50 postgraduate medical residency programs. This initiative, set to unfold over four academic years starting from July 2023, aims to achieve several goals: better defining postgraduate medical residency outcomes, enhancing existing curricula to meet training objectives, and tailoring assessments that are valid, reliable, and fit for purpose.

The integration of EPAs into the curriculum has led to the definition of key milestones within the training duration, outlining residents' expected levels of entrustment at specific time points. This clear definition of learning outcomes and trajectory encourages programs to intentionally structure rotations, case exposure, and didactic sessions to support residents in reaching these milestones. Residents progressing at different paces, whether faster or slower, now have opportunities for individualized learning experiences. This could include greater opportunities to perform meaningful tasks with more distant supervision or receive targeted remediation for specific competencies within the EPAs that require improvement. Assessment content areas, defined in exam blueprints, are also themed by EPAs, ensuring consistency between the learning and assessment processes. Additionally, workplace-based assessments are stipulated as sources of information within the EPA template. This prompts programs to design on-the-job experiences that facilitate the collection of these sources of information.[22]

Box 14.3: Introducing EPAs in postgraduate nursing education in the Netherlands (mid-stage).

In 2018, the Netherlands launched the CZO Flex Level project, named after the accrediting institution CZO, to reorganize postgraduate nursing training. In a nationally coordinated effort, all relevant training hospitals and education institutions in the country collaborated to redesign the postgraduate nursing education landscape, using EPAs to focus on more efficient training time, to enhance transfer across nursing specialties and to contribute to a better tuned continuum of initial education, postgraduate education, and continuing professional development. The preparatory project, involving 200 EPAs for 21 education programs, with input from large groups of health professionals, preceptors, educators, professional bodies, and trainees, was completed in 2022 and the new structure is being implemented from 2023. While data about the effect of the new structure on nursing competence, satisfaction, and career development are to be collected in the coming years, it has become clear that the project has generated enthusiasm and a strong wish to have health professions education contribute to solving major societal challenges in health care.[20]

Box 14.4: Introducing EPAs in postgraduate medical education in the Netherlands (advanced).

After experiences in some specialties, EPAs were nationally implemented for all of PGME in 2017–19.[31] The impetus for this process was a government plan to shorten the duration of all the postgraduate medical programs, in an attempt to reduce the national health budget, which includes residents' salaries. The medical community was resistant but offered to explore the possibility of flexibility (i.e., time-variability) in duration. While for some residents a cut in length might work, for others this would be irresponsible, and for still a few others there may be a justified need for increased length. To operationalize this flexibility the community turned to EPAs, and, with government support and financing, all specialty curricula were rewritten at national and regional levels. Absolute rules of fixed program lengths were replaced by recommended lengths and flexibility. Residents are entitled to part-time training (80% or 90% of a full-time schedule) in the event of family building, research pursuits or other reasons. In pediatrics, anesthesia, and ophthalmology, the majority of residents work part-time, with consequent lengthening of total duration.[28] Monitoring of resident development was based upon workplace-based observation and entrustment decisions, which eventually determine their readiness for unsupervised practice. The changes were threefold: (a) from closed to open curricula with core EPAs and space for electives, (b) individualization and personalization, and (c) a shift in focus from accountability to trust.[32]

The micro-curriculum at the individual level

CBE emphasizes mastering specific skills and knowledge rather than focusing solely on training duration, and promises increased flexibility and trainee-centeredness.[14] A critical component of CBE is therefore the tailoring of learning experiences to the individual,[15] ideally allowing individualized and time-variable progression and training completion.[16,17] This is an individualized curriculum at the micro level. EPA-based curricula are particularly well positioned to allow

Box 14.5: Introducing EPAs in postgraduate medical education in Canada (advanced).

The Royal College of Physicians and Surgeons of Canada (RCPSC) launched the Competence by Design (CBD) model beginning in 2017 for all specialty and subspecialty training programs in an effort to transform Canadian postgraduate medical training to a competency-based framework.[42] EPAs for each specialty were derived from facilitated specialty committee national workshops (in-person and virtual) across all 68 disciplines, whereby leaders across Canada were brought together to shape the future standards of their discipline on a national level. Within this new CBD model, EPAs for each specialty were created to be foundational building blocks across four discrete stages of postgraduate training: transition to discipline, foundations of discipline, core of discipline, and transition to practice. In so doing, resident advancement between these stages of training required successful completion of each sequential stage-specific set of EPAs within the current stage to be promoted to the next stage of training. Over the last seven years, nearly all 68 specialty disciplines have transitioned to the CBD model in Canada through a cohort-based multi-year implementation plan. All 68 have different EPAs to match their stage-specific needs within their disciplines and evolution of the national CBD model is under way. Program evaluation efforts and national forums are driving significant quality improvement processes at the national and institutional levels.[43] In particular, a national summit process outlines the needed action plan for the second iteration of the CBD framework.[44] Key issues for improvement across the 17 institutions in Canada include decreasing the significant assessment burden that occurred with initial CBD implementation, increased separation of assessment from in-the-moment feedback and coaching moments with frontline faculty, improvements in RCPSC communications and program evaluation of the project, and enhanced support for optimization of electronic platforms available across the country.

individualized, time-variable progression based on personal patterns and rates of achievement of entrustment for the program EPAs.[6] Typically, in postgraduate training programs, graduation expectations are set at the level of readiness for unsupervised practice.[18] A trainee may achieve a level of early entrustment for some EPAs and late entrustment for others. See Figure 14.1.

A sample curricular plan with anticipated progression for an average trainee can be shared with trainees at the start. Adaptations may then incorporate prior clinical experiences of the trainee. The individualized version of the blueprint can help set expectations and serve as a learning and development contract. As individual trainees progress, there may again be deviations from the anticipated schedule, based on individual strengths or challenges, clinical experiences encountered, and other external factors. Periodic review of trainee progression should allow for adjustments to the curricular plan—ideally increasing or decreasing specific clinical experiences in rotations as needed to create trainee-specific micro-level curricula enabling achievement of entrustment for each EPA.

Individualizing a trainee's curriculum can start even before the postgraduate training program commences. In many countries, the transition to advanced medical training does not occur immediately after completion of the medical degree program but after one or more years of general clinical experience.[19] Trainees may arrive with very different clinical strengths depending on their postdegree clinical practice. Programs can use an orientation phase to map out the new trainee's experience related to the program's EPAs and create a curricular plan individualized to that trainee.

Ideally, individualized curricula arise from a collaborative effort with trainees. The success of individualized pathways depends not only on program's opportunities but also on the trainee's

Graded supervision allows for
1 Observing the activity
2 Acting with direct, pro-active supervision present in the room
3 Acting with (re-active) supervision available within minutes
4 Acting unsupervised, i.e., under clinical oversight
5 Acting as the supervisor to a junior

Portfolio of: *trainee Jones*	PGY1		PGY2		PGY3		PGY4	
EPA a	1	2	2	2	3	4	4	5
EPA b	1	1	2	2	2	3	3	4
EPA c	2	2	3	4	5	5	5	5
EPA d	2	3	4	4	4	4	5	5

Figure 14.1: A simplified sample individualized EPA-based curriculum for a postgraduate trainee across postgraduate years (PGYs) 1 through 4.

engagement. Trainees must be active agents in identifying their own learning needs, seeking out learning experiences to advance their development, and requesting adjustments to their training path to maximize their learning. This is not a natural role that trainees assume, after a history of compliance with all undergraduate education rules and regulations. It is therefore important to offer an orientation of trainees to their role for setting their own expectations, showing agency and active engagement in reviewing and planning their individual micro-level curricula (see also Chapter 12). In postgraduate nursing training and in physician-assistant training in the Netherlands, variability in sets of EPAs, tailored to individual needs, is becoming common practice.[20,21]

Issues to consider in the creation of workplace curricula

The following subsections address common questions that emerge when building an EPA-based curriculum, assuming EPAs have already been defined for the relevant postgraduate training program (henceforth referred to as program EPAs).

Structuring and sequencing learning experiences

EPAs can help structure curricula and tailor clinical learning experiences. The first step is to identify the EPA framework. Is there a national framework that can be adopted? If not, an EPA framework should be created locally. Guidelines for this step can be found in Chapters 8, 9, and 11. EPA descriptions should not only include a specification of the EPA (what privileges will a qualification for this EPA in include?) but also the required knowledge, skills, attitudes, and experiences for entrustment with the EPA.

Next, the EPA framework must be mapped to existing clinical rotations, or optional rotations for elective program EPAs. For each rotation, an analysis should be made of the activities that actually happen in this context, of experiences necessary for trainees before entrustment can be considered, how specific knowledge and skills can be learned and practiced, and the level of the trainee upon entry to the rotation. Clinical experiences related to the EPA should preferably occur across a variety of settings. Entrustment with an EPA carries an expectation that the trainee has developed the agility to perform the EPA in multiple contexts. If needed, additional practice opportunities and opportunities across contexts may be sought. Simulation should be considered for rare but important clinical conditions or when clinical practice with real patients may not be possible (e.g., urgent life-threatening situations; complex procedures with high inherent patient risks). Simulated environments offer a controlled setting for safe skill acquisition and assessment of competence that complements the workplace curriculum (see also Chapter 15).

Sequencing clinical experiences in rotations can be guided by the aim to increase responsibilities thoughtfully. When are trainees first given opportunities to practice? Are they able to begin practice in simulated or highly supervised and scaffolded environments? Use of early small EPAs that nest under later and larger graduation EPAs may help with sequencing.[6] These smaller, nested EPAs can represent subcomponents of a later, larger EPA. For example, 'obtaining informed consent' and 'initiating a procedure' can be seen as subcomponents of the larger, end-of-program EPA 'Dialysis access.' They are smaller in scope or complexity (e.g., first only in stable patients) or limited to a specific context or patient population (e.g., first only in adult patients). As trainees progress, are they deliberately allowed to practice in contexts with less supervision and assume greater responsibility? Are opportunities offered to practice with minimal supervision prior to graduation and transitioning to unsupervised practice?

In the Canadian 'Competence By Design' (CBD) model, EPAs are defined for each of four phases of postgraduate medical training: transition to discipline, foundations of discipline, core of discipline, and transition to practice (Box 14.5). Still, rotations must be identified to determine where the necessary clinical experiences occur. For example, an end-of-program EPA 'Management of pain outside the operating room' for anesthesiologists can be separated into 'Management of pain for an emergency department patient' on the emergency department rotation and 'Management of pain for an intensive care patient' on an inpatient consult service rotation. Readiness to handle pain in both contexts is needed to allow for summative entrustment decision with the full EPA. Another approach to sequencing is to take case-complexity into account. To remain with the anesthesiology example, patients' preoperative condition and anesthesia risk can be categorized in American Society of Anesthesiology (ASA) I, II, III, and IV levels of increasing complexity, and junior residents can be more readily given greater autonomy to manage an ASA I patient in the operating room than an ASA III patient.

Sequencing decisions should be based on individual program needs and the structure of the program's rotations and curricular phases. A blueprint should preferably include expected levels of entrustment for each program EPA as trainees progress through the training program. For instance, expected levels of entrustment can be noted before graduation, before the end of each training phase, and before the end of each rotation, resulting in a two-dimensional map with EPAs, rotations, and expected levels of autonomy (similar to Figure 14.1 but representing program expectations rather than an individual trainee's progression). While the program blueprint expresses expectations, in practice individual trainees differ and deviations from the blueprint will always occur.

Curricular objectives that do not directly translate to EPAs

Training in the clinical setting naturally emphasizes clinical activities or EPAs as the description of those tasks and all expected competencies could be mapped to EPAs. However, one must acknowledge that a comprehensive curriculum includes more than training for clinical skills. The assertion that, if an objective is not reflected in a specific EPA, it is not important is not correct. Objectives such as attending to health inequities, considering climate change effects on patients, and interprofessional collaboration do not easily translate to EPAs.[23] The Royal Australasian College of Physicians and the Irish EPA-based Internship Curriculum provide a useful three-pillar framework, Do, Know, and Be, to structure postgraduate training (see also Chapters 2 and 8).[24,25] This emerged from the understanding that EPAs and entrustment, while focusing on performance of clinical tasks (*Do*), also require guidance on the essential underpinning knowledge (*Know*) and professional behaviors, values, and identity (*Be*) to ensure readiness of trainees for increased autonomy. In addition to detailing what graduates should be able to *Do* (EPAs) by the end of their training, this model also specifies what graduates should *Know* (including the ability to integrate knowledge into practice and commit to lifelong learning of evolving knowledge) to support the safe performance of EPAs. It also emphasizes how graduates should *Be* in developing their professional identity and professional behaviors (i.e., collaborator, role model, patient safety promoter), values (i.e., compassion, integrity, responsibility, etc.), and habits (i.e., reflection, lifelong learning).

Knowledge, skills, and professionalism are important *conditions* for entrustment. While *Know* and *Be* features can be attended to in EPA instructions and assessment, they often require their own, separate approaches, including lectures, online modules, regular progress testing (*Know*) or 360-degree feedback, learner reflections, and portfolios (*Be*). Four of the five trainee trustworthiness factors that enable supervisors to trust a trainee with critical health care activities (agency, reliability, integrity, and humility)[26] represent *Be* attributes and are weighed in entrustment decisions for EPAs. Calling out the *Be* expectations separately from the EPAs can help ensure the inclusion of curricula explicitly designed to support trainee development in these areas as well as assessments particularly suited to capturing these behaviors and habits.

Some components of knowledge and professional identity formation may not clearly link to EPAs. For example, knowledge of health care politics or advocacy for a healthier society can be EPA-independent and still represent important training objectives. Regardless of approach, the overall curriculum should explicitly develop and assess all competencies important to postgraduate practice, including those that cannot be easily captured in an EPA framework.

Postgraduate programs in small centers

Small postgraduate training programs based at single clinical institutions (e.g., hospital, clinic, medical center), may need to contend with limitations in service provision that can lead to interinstitutional training variation for the same specialty. For instance, a pediatric pharmacy program at a tertiary care hospital with transplant patients offers very different clinical experiences than one based at a rural community hospital with no transplant patients but other broad experiences. These limitations can conflict with the national macro-level curriculum and introduce undesirable variation in graduate outcomes at the institutional meso level. In cases of large variation in service provision, programs should consider interinstitutional partnerships to access essential experiences not available at the home training site(s) to improve standardization of training outcomes and ensure alignment with national curricular expectations.[27]

Dealing with the limitations of time-variability

Challenges arise when CBE principles, particularly those around time-variable progression or graduation of trainees, conflict with rules and regulations. While examples exist of time-variable options,[28] many programs cannot adapt training duration for individual trainees.[29] These programs, however, may create opportunities to qualify trainees who are ready early for more autonomy and only distant supervision, sometimes called 'sheltered independence' within the program.[30] This sustains trainee growth and ability to practice greater autonomy while still scaffolded by the training program. Some institutions have piloted the idea of *promotion in place*—where post-licensure trainees remain in the training program but are given greater autonomy and responsibilities comparable with those of a faculty member, and are allowed to function as a faculty member within the institution.[30] Another approach is to incorporate more elective time into the curriculum and offer additional selective or elective EPAs to allow exploration of specialized areas of interest. The framework of EPAs for a specialty may even include elective EPAs for trainees who advance quickly. This approach enriches the learning experience and allows trainees to develop customized portfolios of supplementary EPAs showcasing their unique fit for specific employment opportunities. For others, the elective space can be used to add individualized clinical experiences for targeted trainee-centered remediation to address specific areas for improvement for those progressing more slowly. This is implemented in pediatric specialty training at University Medical Center Utrecht, the Netherlands. Customization strategies create flexibility in less flexible systems, allowing continued trainee growth while also protecting against the graduation of trainees who may not yet be ready for unsupervised practice.

Assessment considerations in an EPA-based postgraduate training program

While this chapter is focused on curricula, some attention to assessment is warranted. We highlight two key considerations important for curricular design. For a more detailed discussion of assessment in EPA-based curricula, see Chapters 17–21.

The tension between frequent observations by different supervisors and the creation of a coherent longitudinal picture of the trainee

Creating a program of assessment that does not depend on a single examiner is central to modern workplace-based assessment, with or without EPAs. This is beneficial for increasing reliability and decreasing bias. In large programs, however, this programmatic assessment runs the risk of fragmentation if every observer is a new supervisor and there is no communication with others about the trainee of interest. As the purpose of assessment is not just *of* learning but also *for* learning,[33] the provision of frequent feedback and, ideally, longitudinal ongoing support for trainee development across their various clinical experiences requires adequate monitoring across time. While individual observation episodes may include feedback and learning conversations between trainees and individual supervisors, this feedback and learning is often limited to the observed episode and less likely to address longitudinal developmental patterns or needs. Here is where the educational team, often called a clinical competency committee (CCC), plays an important role. In several jurisdictions, CCCs are required bodies comprising at least three and often more members of the active teaching faculty. The CCC reviews the progress of all residents or fellows in the program and advises the program director in making official progression decisions or summative entrustment decisions.[34] Some CCCs meet monthly; others meet with a lower frequency. Adequate competency committees have the data to monitor development of all trainees in the program and their portfolio systems allow trainees to self-monitor progress, view aggregated feedback, and recognize their own performance patterns.[35,36]

Another approach to providing coherence is through coaching. Some programs are able to incorporate a coaching program into the structure of the curriculum that can help overcome the limitation of committees that cannot meet frequently.[37] Coaches can provide more frequent comprehensive feedback (i.e., based on all workplace-based and other assessment data received to that point) and guidance across clinical experiences in rotations to support longitudinal trainee development. While coaches can concentrate on specific skill development and performance improvement using EPAs as anchoring points, they can also encourage and track development in the *Know* and *Be* program expectations. Coaches can hold trainees accountable to the expectations around agency and engagement in their own learning plan; they can encourage trainees to seek out feedback and learning opportunities and foster trainee autonomy and accountability beyond workplace-based assessments.[38,39] They can also help trainees engage in deliberate practice[40] with setting learning targets, help interpret feedback to plan purposeful practice, and find rehearsal opportunities to improve performance. To realize their full potential, coaches should not be viewed by trainees as assessors but primarily as allies, facilitators of growth, and guides for creating their personal micro-level curricula. The Canadian CBD programs all employ coaches for the ongoing support and development of trainees.[41]

Data needed for summative entrustment decisions

A primary data source is the experiences with the performance of EPAs, reported after ad hoc entrustment decisions. However, the program of assessment should also collect data beyond EPA performance. Multisource (360-degree) feedback from peers, supervisors, interprofessional teammates, and potentially patients usually extends performance specific EPA assessments and is particularly useful to capture consistent professionalism behaviors and habits[45,46] (see Chapter 17 for more details). The combined results of these various assessments, including multisource feedback and knowledge tests, provide additional information on the *Know* and *Be* expectations not fully captured by the EPAs.

Valid summative entrustment decisions require sufficient sampling across a variety of contexts and among supervisors,[47] incorporation of both direct and indirect observation of clinical activities, and the use of both quantitative and qualitative data. These can be supplemented by artifacts from workplace activities (e.g., written notes and summaries, orthopedic cast), simulation activities and supplemented by data from the assessment in the *Know* and *Be* domains. Finally, trainee self-assessment of readiness for unsupervised practice for EPAs can provide additional insight. Portfolios and electronic dashboards[48,49] allow visualization and integration into a comprehensive picture of trainee progress; facilitate the tracking and sense-making of the multiple datapoints; support feedback, coaching, and summative decision-making; and enable the formulation of personalized learning plans and remediation strategies.[27]

Programs with a limited pool of supervisors submitting ad hoc entrustment decisions may have more difficulty achieving adequate sampling among supervisors and filling balanced competency committees. Care should be taken to maintain transparent procedures for arriving at decisions, to avoid the perception of unfairness, bias, and conflicts of interest.

Trainee experiences in postgraduate EPA-based curricula

Trainees are the center point of CBE, but few data exist regarding postgraduate trainees' perspectives on EPAs. A recent Canadian study revealed polarized views: some saw EPAs as valuable for professional growth, while others found them burdensome and disruptive to learning.[50] These perceptions were influenced by program administration, faculty assessors' engagement, and trainee behavior. The findings suggest that the trainee experience is influenced by the context and specifics for how EPA curricula are implemented. For the EPA system to function effectively, there must be a dynamic, interdependent relationship among all three CBE stakeholders (program administration, assessors and learners), with the system's value being only as strong as its weakest link.[50]

The role of interprofessional team members and patients in a postgraduate training program

In addition to the clinical teachers and supervisors, interprofessional team members and patients play critical roles in a postgraduate training program.

Interprofessional team members, as part of the clinical community of practice, collaborate with trainees to provide patient care. However, their relationships can sometimes be challenging. Team members' trust in the trainee can serve as an additional layer of gatekeeping for patient safety and access to learning opportunities. Depending on the trainee's role within the team, they might supervise an interprofessional team member (e.g., a resident supervising a physician assistant) while simultaneously learning from this—often more experienced—team member. Similarly, not only do interprofessional team members serve as colleagues but they can also be valuable assessors of the trainees.[45] Ideally these interprofessional team members feel part of the training program and these nuanced relationships with their shifting dynamics of supervision and learning need to be taken into consideration as part of the learning and assessment process.

Patients play a role in the educational process, being part of the patient–trainee–supervisor triad. Their trust in the trainee, in their supervisor, and in the training program can affect trainee access to learning opportunities. For instance, clinical supervisors may defer to patients' preferences and limit trainee performance of a procedure despite initial intention to entrust the trainee with the procedure.[51] Patients' involvement in the learning process can also offer unique perspectives on trainee competency and bedside manner, contributing valuable datapoints to a holistic assessment of trainee abilities.[52,53] Incorporating patient feedback into the EPA portfolio or in a multisource feedback procedure can be very valuable. While patient feedback contributes to practice-based learning, it requires careful navigation of conflicting roles and power dynamics in the treatment relationship.[54] Both patients and health care professionals need to embrace vulnerability and may require facilitation and guidance to use patient feedback effectively. Addressing power dynamics, and possibly shifting toward more collaborative relationships, is crucial for engaging patients in feedback conversations and leveraging their valuable perspectives.

Challenges of EPA-based curricula in specialist training

The wide introduction of EPAs in postgraduate education, with most reports highlighting their advantages,[55,56] does not mean that implementation has not faced challenges. First, Moore et al. recently reported how EPA frameworks are too often proposed with just EPA titles, with an inherent lack of clarity and risk of implementation problems.[57] Conversely, excessive detail and too much prescriptive granularity of activities can threaten the usefulness of EPAs.[58] New programs starting with long lists of newly defined EPAs often discover they need to lump them into broader units of practice to create a feasible program. The 45 rigorously defined Dutch anesthesiology EPAs[11] were reduced, in the first year of implementation, to 28 (larger) EPAs. That number appeared more feasible for serious entrustment decisions and a program of assessment. A balanced approach is needed to ensure that EPAs are specific enough to provide clear guidance for teaching and assessment but broad enough to be practical and flexible in real-world clinical settings. Hence, it is recommended that a complete set of EPAs for a training program should range from 20 to 30 EPAs, with no more than 10 per program year.[59] Next, time-variability, an inherent feature of CBE (with or without EPAs), brings significant practical hurdles,[29,60] as has been discussed above, while promising examples of time-variable postgraduate programs are emerging.[28,30] Finally, frequent observation and reports, features of programmatic assessment and applicable in EPA-based curricula, are often reported to be an unwelcome burden for clinical faculty as well as for trainees. The adoption of the Canadian CBD model unexpectedly increased trainee anxiety and their sense of assessment burden.[61] If EPAs become mere checkboxes that learners feel they must complete to 'pass,' EPAs can lose their original significance as units of practice for which one becomes qualified. Even if the administrative burden of workplace-based assessment for clinicians is actually less than they may perceive,[62] conditions must be created in which feedback, observation, and assessment minimally disrupt the clinical workflow; thoughtful implementation of automation with mobile devices may help.

Conclusion

Postgraduate training environments have specific challenges, primarily reflected in the need for trainees to care for patients while at the same time learning and working toward developing the competencies associated with unsupervised specialty practice. This process demands careful planning by education leaders, particularly given the complexity and opportunistic nature of the workplace learning environment. Using EPAs as a curricular framework, education leaders can begin to address tensions between education and service, implement CBE principles, and structure clinical learning experiences to support developmental progression of trainees toward unsupervised specialty practice.

Figure justification

Figure 14.1 was adapted from: ten Cate O. What entrustable professional activities add to a competency-based curriculum. *Acad Med.* 2014;89(4):691.

Competing interests

The authors declare that they have no competing interests.

References

1. ten Cate O. Entrustability of professional activities and competency-based training. *Med Educ.* 2005;39(12):1176–1177.
2. ten Cate O, Scheele F. Viewpoint: Competency-based postgraduate training: can we bridge the gap between theory and clinical practice? *Acad Med.* 2007;82(6):542–547. DOI: https://doi.org/10.1097/ACM.0b013e31805559c7
3. ten Cate O, Khursigara-Slattery N, Cruess RL, Hamstra SJ, Steinert Y, Sternszus R. Medical competence as a multilayered construct. *Med Educ.* 2024;58(1):93–104. DOI: https://doi.org/10.1111/medu.15162
4. Ngo E, Paterick ZR, Patel N, et al. Professional liability pertinent to graduate medical education: the intersection of medical education, patient care, and law. *J Med Pract Manage.* 2016;31(4):233–237.
5. Booij E, van Dam M, Jonker G, et al. An interprofessional faculty development program for workplace-based learning. 2024;13(1):266–273. DOI: https://doi.org/10.5334/pme.1242

6. ten Cate O, Chen HC, Hoff RG, Peters H, Bok H, Van Der Schaaf M. Curriculum development for the workplace using entrustable professional activities (EPAs): AMEE guide no. 99. *Med Teach.* 2015;37(11):983–1002. DOI: https://doi.org/10.3109/0142159X.2015.1060308
7. ten Cate O, Balmer DF, Caretta-Weyer H, Hatala R, Hennus MP, West DC. Entrustable professional activities and entrustment decision-making: a development and research agenda for the next decade. *Acad Med.* 2021;96(7):S96-S104. DOI: https://doi.org/10.1097/ACM.0000000000004106
8. Frank JR, Danoff D. The CanMEDS initiative: implementing an outcomes-based framework of physician competencies. *Med Teach.* 2007;29:642–647. DOI: https://doi.org/10.1080/01421590701746983
9. Hennus MP, Nusmeier A, Heesch GGMV, et al. Development of entrustable professional activities for paediatric intensive care fellows: a national modified Delphi study. *PLoS ONE.* Published online 2021:1–19. DOI: https://doi.org/10.1371/journal.pone.0248565
10. Amare EM, Siebeck M, Sendekie TY, Fischer MR, Berndt M. Development of an entrustable professional activities (EPA) framework to inform surgical residency training programs in Ethiopia: a three-round national Delphi method study. *J Surg Educ.* 2022;79(1):56–68. DOI: https://doi.org/10.1016/j.jsurg.2021.06.023
11. Wisman-Zwarter N, Van Der Schaaf M, ten Cate O, Jonker G, Van Klei WA, Hoff RG. Transforming the learning outcomes of anaesthesiology training into entrustable professional activities. *Eur J Anaesth.* 2016;33(8):559–567. DOI: https://doi.org/10.1097/EJA.0000000000000474
12. Hall AK, Oswald A, Frank JR, et al. Evaluating Competence by Design as a large system change initiative: readiness, fidelity, and outcomes. *Perspect Med Educ.* 13(1):95–107. DOI: https://doi.org/10.5334/pme.962
13. The American Board of Pediatrics. Entrustable professional activities for general pediatrics. Accessed May 31, 2024. https://www.abp.org/content/entrustable-professional-activities-general-pediatrics
14. Dagnone JD, Bandiera G, Harris K. Re-examining the value proposition for competency-based medical education. *Can Med Educ J.* 2021;12(3):155–158. DOI: https://doi.org/10.36834/cmej.68245
15. Van Melle E, Frank JR, Holmboe ES, et al. A core components framework for evaluating implementation of competency-based medical education programs. *Acad Med.* 2019;94(7):1002–1009. DOI: https://doi.org/10.1097/ACM.0000000000002743
16. Lucey CR, Thibault GE, ten Cate O. Competency-based, time-variable education in the health professions: crossroads. *Acad Med.* 2018;93(3S):S1-S5. DOI: https://doi.org/10.1097/ACM.0000000000002080
17. Schumacher DJ, Caretta-Weyer H, Busari J, et al. Competency-based time-variable training internationally: ensuring practical next steps in the wake of the COVID-19 pandemic. *Med Teach.* 2021;43(7):810–816. DOI: https://doi.org/10.1080/0142159X.2021.1925098
18. ten Cate O, Schwartz A, Chen HC. Assessing trainees and making entrustment decisions: on the nature and use of entrustment–supervision scales. *Acad Med.* 2020;95(11):1662–1669. DOI: https://doi.org/10.1097/acm.0000000000003427
19. O'Brien BC, Forrest K, Wijnen-Meijer M, ten Cate O. A global view of structures and trends in medical education. In: *Understanding Medical Education.* John Wiley & Sons, Ltd; 2018:7–22. DOI: https://doi.org/10.1002/9781119373780.ch2
20. Pool IA, van Zundert H, ten Cate O. Facilitating flexibility in postgraduate nursing education through entrustable professional activities to address nursing shortages and career prospects. *International Nursing Review.* Published online 2023, October 11. DOI: https://doi.org/10.1111/inr.12892

21. Wiersma F, Berkvens J, ten Cate O. Flexibility in individualized, competency-based workplace curricula with EPAs: analyzing four cohorts of physician assistants in training. *Med Teach.* 2017;39(5):535–539. DOI: https://doi.org/10.1080/0142159X.2017.1297526
22. Tan N, Chan YC, Tan K. Implementing neurology EPAs in Singapore using the consolidated framework for implementation research (1186). *Neurology.* 2020;94(15 Supplement):1186. DOI: https://doi.org/10.1212/WNL.94.15_supplement.1186
23. ten Cate O, Pool IA. The viability of interprofessional entrustable professional activities. *Adv Health Sci Educ.* 2019;25(5):1255–1262. DOI: https://doi.org/10.1007/s10459-019-09950-0
24. Boland J, Offiah G. Curriculum framework for the internship programme in Ireland. Published online October 2023. Accessed May 11, 2024. https://www.lenus.ie/handle/10147/638294
25. The Royal Australasian College of Physicians. Accessed June 2, 2024. https://www.racp.edu.au/trainees/basic-training/curricula-renewal/standards
26. ten Cate O, Chen HC. The ingredients of a rich entrustment decision. *Med Teach.* 2020;42(12):1413–1420. DOI: https://doi.org/10.1080/0142159X.2020.1817348
27. Royal College of Physicians and Surgeons of Canada. Competence by Design document suite – handbook and guidelines for review. Published online 2015. https://canmeds.royalcollege.ca/uploads/en/framework/CanMEDS%202015%20Framework_EN_Reduced.pdf
28. Hoff RG, Frenkel J, Imhof SM, ten Cate O. Flexibility in postgraduate medical training in the Netherlands. *Acad Med.* 2018;93(3S):S32. DOI: https://doi.org/10.1097/ACM.0000000000002078
29. Kogan JR, Whelan AJ, Gruppen LD, Lingard LA, Teunissen PW, ten Cate O. What regulatory requirements and existing structures must change if competency-based, time-variable training is introduced into the continuum of medical education in the United States? *Acad Med.* 2018;93(3S):S27-S31. DOI: https://doi.org/10.1097/ACM.0000000000002067
30. Goldhamer MEJ, Pusic MV, Nadel ES, Co JPT, Weinstein DF. Promotion in place: a model for competency-based, time-variable graduate medical education. *Acad Med.* 2024;99(5):518–523. DOI: https://doi.org/10.1097/ACM.0000000000005652
31. de Graaf J, Bolk M, Dijkstra A, van der Horst M, Hoff RG, ten Cate O. The implementation of entrustable professional activities in postgraduate medical education in the Netherlands: rationale, process, and current status. *Acad Med.* 2021;96(7):S29-S35. DOI: https://doi.org/10.1097/ACM.0000000000004110
32. de Heer MH, Driessen EW, Teunissen PW, Scheele F. Lessons learned spanning 17 years of experience with three consecutive nationwide competency based medical education training plans. *Front Med (Lausanne).* 2024;11:1339857. DOI: https://doi.org/10.3389/fmed.2024.1339857
33. Dannefer EF. Beyond assessment of learning toward assessment for learning: educating tomorrow's physicians. *Med Teach.* 2013;35(7):560–563. DOI: https://doi.org/10.3109/0142159X.2013.787141
34. Ekpenyong A, Padmore JS, Hauer KE. The purpose, structure, and process of clinical competency committees: guidance for members and program directors. *J Grad Med Educ.* 2021;13(2 Suppl):45–50. DOI: https://doi.org/10.4300/JGME-D-20-00841.1
35. Hauer KE, ten Cate O, Holmboe E, et al. Ensuring resident competence: a narrative review of the literature on group decision-making to inform the work of clinical competency committees. *J Grad Med Educ.* 2016;8(2):156–164. DOI: https://doi.org/10.4300/JGME-D-15-00144.1
36. Smit MP, de Hoog M, Brackel HJL, ten Cate O, Gemke RJBJ. A national process to enhance the validity of entrustment decisions for Dutch pediatric residents. *J Grad Med Educ.* 2019;11(4s):158–164. DOI: https://doi.org/10.4300/jgme-d-18-01006
37. Baenziger K, Chan M, Colman S. Coaching in postgraduate competency-based medical education: a qualitative exploration of three models. *Acad Psychiatr.* 2023;47(1):10–17. DOI: https://doi.org/10.1007/s40596-022-01628-x
38. Santiesteban L, Young E, Tiarks GC, et al. Defining advising, coaching, and mentoring for student development in medical education. *Cureus.* Published online July 27, 2022. DOI: https://doi.org/10.7759/cureus.27356

39. Wolff M, Deiorio NM, Miller Juve A, et al. Beyond advising and mentoring: competencies for coaching in medical education. *Med Teach*. 2021;43(10):1210–1213. DOI: https://doi.org/10.1080/0142159X.2021.1947479
40. Ericsson KA. Acquisition and maintenance of medical expertise: a perspective from the expert-performance approach with deliberate practice. *Acad Med*. 2015;90(11):1471–1486. DOI: https://doi.org/10.1097/ACM.0000000000000939
41. Richardson D, Landreville JM, Trier J, et al. Coaching in Competence by Design: a new model of coaching in the moment and coaching over time to support large scale implementation. *Perspect Med Educ*. 2024;13(1):33–43. DOI: https://doi.org/10.5334/pme.959
42. Frank JR, Karpinski J, Sherbino J, et al. Competence by Design: a transformational national model of time-variable competency-based postgraduate medical education. *Perspect Med Educ*. 13(1):201–223. DOI: https://doi.org/10.5334/pme.1096
43. Commitment to Action | Statement on enhanced flexibility for CBD program implementation. Accessed May 28, 2024. https://news.royalcollege.ca/en/newsroom/posts/commitment-to-action-statement-on-enhanced-flexibility-for-cbd-program-implementation.html
44. Microsoft Power BI. Accessed May 28, 2024. https://app.powerbi.com/view?r=eyJrIjoiNjc0ZmZlNTItMjgyNS00YTA2LWIzNDMtNjk2YWMyNjNlZDg1IiwidCI6ImM0OGUxZTJhLTljZjAtNGNkZC04MjIxLWRkZGM5MWRlMDgzNCJ9
45. van Keulen SG, de Raad T, Raymakers-Janssen P, ten Cate O, Hennus MP. Professional activities for pediatric intensive care fellows: a proof-of-concept study. *Teaching and Learning in Medicine*. Published online 2023. DOI: https://doi.org/10.1080/10401334.2023.2200760
46. Baines R, Regan de Bere S, Stevens S, et al. The impact of patient feedback on the medical performance of qualified doctors: a systematic review. *BMC Med Educ*. 2018;18:173. DOI: https://doi.org/10.1186/s12909-018-1277-0
47. Van Der Vleuten CPM, Schuwirth LWT. Assessing professional competence: from methods to programmes. *Med Educ*. 2005;39(3):309–317. DOI: https://doi.org/10.1111/j.1365–2929.2005.02094.x
48. Yilmaz Y, Carey R, Chan TM, et al. Developing a dashboard for faculty development in competency-based training programs: a design-based research project. *Can Med Educ J*. 2021;12(4):48–64. DOI: https://doi.org/10.36834/cmej.72067
49. McEllistrem B, Hennus MP, Fawns T, Hanley K. Exploring the Irish general practice training community's perceptions on how an entrustable professional activities dashboard implementation could facilitate general practice training in Ireland. Published online March 24, 2023:1–9. DOI: https://doi.org/10.1080/14739879.2023.2191340
50. Ahn E, LaDonna KA, Landreville JM, Mcheimech R, Cheung WJ. Only as strong as the weakest link: resident perspectives on entrustable professional activities and their impact on learning. *J Grad Med Educ*. 2023;15(6):676–684. DOI: https://doi.org/10.4300/JGME-D-23-00204.1
51. Tiyyagura G, Balmer D, Chaudoin L, et al. *The Greater Good: How Supervising Physicians Make Entrustment Decisions in the Pediatric Emergency Department*. Vol 14; 2014:597–602. DOI: https://doi.org/10.1016/j.acap.2014.06.001
52. Finnegan R, Flanagan O, Cantillon P, McGlacken-Byrne S. The hidden benefits of patient encounters. *Clin Teach*. 2023;20(1):e13544. DOI: https://doi.org/10.1111/tct.13544
53. Wykurz G, Kelly D. Developing the role of patients as teachers: literature review. *BMJ*. 2002;325(7368):818–821.
54. Sehlbach C, Bosveld MH, Romme S, Nijhuis MA, Govaerts MJB, Smeenk FWJM. Challenges in engaging patients in feedback conversations for health care professionals' workplace learning. *Med Educ*. Published online February 28, 2024. DOI: https://doi.org/10.1111/medu.15313
55. O'Dowd E, Lydon S, O'Connor P, Madden C, Byrne D. A systematic review of 7 years of research on entrustable professional activities in graduate medical education, 2011–2018. *Med Educ*. 2019;53(3):234–249. DOI: https://doi.org/10.1111/medu.13792
56. Liu L, Jiang Z, Qi X, et al. An update on current EPAs in graduate medical education: a scoping review. *Med Educ Online*. 26(1):1981198. DOI: https://doi.org/10.1080/10872981.2021.1981198

57. Moore SJ, Egerton T, Merolli M, Lees J, La Scala N, Parry SM. Inconsistently reporting post-licensure EPA specifications in different clinical professions hampers fidelity and practice translation: a scoping review. *BMC Med Educ.* 2023;23:372. DOI: https://doi.org/10.1186/s12909-023-04364-4
58. Van Loon KA, Driessen EW, Teunissen PW, Scheele F. Experiences with EPAs, potential benefits and pitfalls. *Med Teach.* 2014;36(8):698–702. DOI: https://doi.org/10.3109/0142159X.2014.909588
59. ten Cate O. An updated primer on entrustable professional activities (EPAs). *Revista Brasileira de Educação Médica.* 2019;43:712–720.
60. van Rossum TR, Scheele F, Sluiter HE, Paternotte E, Heyligers IC. Effects of implementing time-variable postgraduate training programmes on the organization of teaching hospital departments. *Med Teach.* 2018;40(10):1036–1041. DOI: https://doi.org/10.1080/0142159X.2017.1418850
61. Ott MC, Pack R, Cristancho S, Chin M, Van Koughnett JA, Ott M. 'The most crushing thing': understanding resident assessment burden in a competency-based curriculum. *J Grad Med Educ.* 2022;14(5):583–592. DOI: https://doi.org/10.4300/JGME-D-22-00050.1
62. Cheung K, Rogoza C, Chung AD, Kwan BYM. Analyzing the administrative burden of competency based medical education. *Can Assoc Radiol J.* 2022;73(2):299–304. DOI: https://doi.org/10.1177/08465371211038963

CHAPTER 15

The role of simulation in EPA-based curricula

Timo de Raad, Fremen Chihchen Chou,
Adrian P. Marty, Ryan Brydges

Abstract

Entrustable professional activities (EPAs) form the cornerstone of competency-based health professions education, focusing on the critical tasks trainees must master for their future unsupervised clinical practice. Recognizing the challenges in assessing EPAs, especially those caused by the rarity of some clinical events and the dynamic nature of health care settings, there is an increasing interest in utilizing simulation as a complementary approach. Using simulation modalities, educators can design controlled and relevant settings for learning and assessment, allowing students to apply theoretical knowledge, practical skills, and professional attitudes in a risk-free environment. This chapter delves into whether and how simulation can be integrated into EPA-based curricula to enhance training and preparation for performing EPAs, as well as to provide a controlled setting for assessing trainees' entrustment levels.

We explore the theoretical underpinnings for applying simulation in an EPA-based curriculum, highlighting its potential dual roles in bridging educational experiences with assessment activities, and relating both to real-world clinical practice. While we propose a model for the promising integration of simulation into EPA-based curriculum, we also note that the evidence supporting its efficacy remains preliminary. Further research must substantiate the role and value of simulation in an EPA-based training and assessment modality. Our model describes the possible application of EPAs that progresses from an

How to cite this book chapter:
de Raad T, Chou FC, Marty, AP, Brydges R. The roles of simulation in EPA-based curricula. In: ten Cate O, Burch VC, Chen HC, Chou FC, Hennus MP (Eds). *Entrustable Professional Activities and Entrustment Decision-Making in Health Professions Education*, Chapter 15, pp. 175–182. [2024] London: Ubiquity Press. DOI: https://doi.org/10.5334/bdc.o

This chapter uses cross-references to other chapters of the same book. For those who read this chapter as a standalone publication: all cross-references can be found at: https://doi.org/10.5334/bdc

individual's basic skill acquisition to their becoming capable of acting in complex, broader team-based clinical challenges. Incorporating simulation meaningfully into EPA-based curricula represents a transformative approach in preparing health care professionals for the challenges of clinical practice.

Authors

- Timo de Raad, PA-C, RN, MHPE. University Medical Center Utrecht, the Netherlands. Correspondence: T.deRaad@umcutrecht.nl
- Fremen Chihchen Chou, MD, PhD. China Medical University and China Medical University Hospital, Taichung, Taiwan.
- Adrian P. Marty, MD, MME. University Hospital Balgrist, University of Zurich, Zurich, Switzerland.
- Ryan Brydges, PhD. University of Toronto, Toronto, Canada.

Introduction

Entrustable professional activities (EPAs) undergird many models of competency-based health professions education.[1] EPAs are the tasks trainees must learn to perform effectively in all facets of their professional practice.[2] Most commonly, EPAs are assessed in the actual clinical workplace. However, multiple pressures, such as the low frequency of many EPA-indicated clinical events, have prompted scholars to seek ways to increase the opportunities to conduct EPA-related learning and assessments, including using simulation modalities.[2–5]

Simulation is a technique that creates a situation or environment to allow persons to experience a representation of a real [health care] event for practice, learning, evaluation, testing, or to gain understanding of systems or human actions.[6] Diverse uses, purposes, and technologies have led health care educators and leaders to use various simulation modalities (ranging from, e.g., manikins to simulated patients) for training, assessment, and quality improvement.[7] Simulation provides a controlled yet realistic environment where trainees construct understanding by applying the knowledge, skills, and attitudes essential for professional activities.

As EPA-based curricula become a foundational option across health care training programs and organizations, scholars have started investigating how and why simulation can function effectively in such curricula. Researchers in the EPA and simulation communities have, often separately (they tend to be different scholars), claimed that simulation can fulfill two purposes: functioning as (a) a preparatory setting for teaching EPA skills longitudinally throughout trainees' clinical training years[8,9] and (b) a technique for conducting assessments that inform high-stakes decisions on trainees' clinical competence.[2,4] In this chapter, we review the theoretical rationale and emerging evidence for the claims that simulation techniques can be effectively integrated into EPA-based curricula to provide: (a) tailored learning experiences for developing competencies that underpin EPAs, and (b) assessment data for making high-stakes decisions about trainees' performance outcomes.

EPA-based curricula may include an array of simulation learning settings, ranging from classroom-like activities in simulation centers to dynamic in situ scenarios in actual clinical contexts. We must consider the implications of using simulation across these diverse environments, including how and why this educational modality can effectively bridge the gap between educational experiences and real-world practices. We note that the theoretical rationale for linking EPAs and simulation currently outweighs the available evidence to evaluate the value of simulation's role in EPA-based curricula.[10] Thus, we aim to explore whether and how integrating EPAs and simulation-based training can enhance the quality and efficacy of health professions education.

Role of simulation in EPA-based curricula

We propose a central tenet that simulation should not be confined solely to the assessment of EPA performances; it may be equally or more potent as a learning modality. When designed well, simulation scenarios engage trainees, hone their skills, enhance their clinical reasoning, and build their confidence. In this way, simulation modalities become a key tool in educators' toolboxes as they design, implement, and evaluate EPA-based curricula. For example, in workplace settings, translational simulation (i.e., simulation scenarios that occur in the actual clinical setting) has become a refined use of simulation for evaluating whether individuals, teams, and the systems they work within require an educational intervention.[7] Likewise, in undergraduate and postgraduate settings, simulation has shown great potential as a modality for refining clinical competencies and preparing health care professionals for their future clinical practice.

The core components framework of competency-based medical education represents a potential blueprint for designing EPA-based curricula in health professions education.[11] Educators would begin by defining EPAs and then designing instructional activities and curricular sequences that support the required competencies for each EPA.[11] While classroom-based and workplace-based learning can fulfill many of the requirements of such a curriculum, simulation-based training can fill key gaps, enhancing the EPA-based curriculum with structured, comprehensive design and tailored learning experiences.

EPAs can be closely linked to simulation training activities: educators could use each EPA description written using the eight-item framework[12] as a 'mini curriculum' to inform their design of simulation scenarios. In particular, the framework's second item, 'specification and limitation,' and the fourth item, 'required knowledge, skills, attitudes and experiences' (KSAEs), both provide a foundational blueprint for designing simulation scenarios for EPA-based curricula. Specification, for instance, involves elaborating the EPA with chronological, bulleted subset tasks that could guide the designed components for the simulation scenarios. At the same time, KSAEs delineate the criteria for educators to cover during the debriefing, which typically follows simulation scenarios. In sum, we suggest that using EPAs to guide simulation design allows for tailored training programs aligned directly to identified needs in the curriculum blueprint. Involving experienced simulation educators would ensure that the complexity of scenarios is appropriately titrated to the perceived competence levels of trainees.

Role of simulation in assessing entrustment

Educators in health professions education set entrustment levels to determine when and how a trainee can be entrusted to subsequently perform clinical responsibilities unsupervised.[3] Simulation scenarios can conceivably be designed to align with each entrustment level, allowing educators to observe and assess trainees' performance in a controlled environment. Some authors suggest that if strong links between simulation-based and workplace-based assessments can be established, trainees' performance in EPA-related scenarios could complement or even replace high-stakes real-world assessments.[2,13]

To successfully assess entrustment levels on par with real-world practice, simulation-based assessment scenarios would have to be meticulously designed to have many features.[13,14] First, the designers would need to be clear about how the construct of interest (e.g., the competencies underlying a specific EPA) will be activated through the use of a simulation scenario (e.g., a manikin with actors role-playing colleagues). Second, the broad range of trainees (i.e., with different prior knowledge and varying levels of self-efficacy) must all be consistently stimulated to perform the EPA as expected. Third, those responsible for assessing the performance of the EPA must be trained to engage in a systematic and standardized observation of each trainee's performance. Fourth, the assessors must also be trained to translate their observations into a 'level of supervision' and, more importantly, to provide meaningful feedback according to previously established criteria. The extent to which simulation center staff and their clinical partners have the foundational skills and training to enact these features likely varies considerably across different health professions and health care organizations. Ultimately, significant and rigorous validation studies[14] would be needed to determine whether simulation could fulfill the role of complementing or even replacing real-world assessments. Many training programs are drawn to simulation for its potential to ease the assessment burden of EPAs in the workplace.[2,4,5,8,9] If the assessment of EPAs conducted in the simulation setting correlates highly with the assessment in the workplace, as with procedural/psychomotor skills,[13] then the many positive features of simulation—safe for patients, psychologically safe for trainees, effective for a range of clinical skills, highly controllable, highly flexible, and so on—become ever enticing.

Evaluating evidence: simulation's impact on EPA-based training and assessment

We reemphasize that conceptual papers severely outnumber empirical papers on integrating simulation into EPA-based curricula and assessments. That said, trends are emerging in how different medical education research teams have been reporting on using simulation modalities for EPA-based training and assessment.

Several groups have been using simulation-based activities as a 'capstone' method for training and for assessing entrustment readiness as learners (mostly medical students) approach the end of their training. For example, teams have investigated the use of simulation for assessing multiple EPA outcomes in medical students transitioning to residency.[15,16] Two other groups have extended this idea into a multiday formative and summative capstone course in medicine[17] and in pharmacy.[18] Hence, these researchers have identified simulation as a type of 'assurance,' checking to see that trainees have been adequately prepared for significant career transitions.

Researchers have also used simulation as a testbed for generating validity evidence for EPA-based assessments. Several studies have investigated whether simulation-based and workplace-based EPA assessments correlate quantitatively,[4,19,20] with the evidence showing moderate to no correlation for observable skills, like resuscitation. One explanation for these mixed findings may be found in an interview study, in which the same physician raters provided EPA ratings of polypectomy skills for the same trainees in the simulation-based vs. real-world endoscopy suite; notably, the raters reported defining and judging entrustment quite differently across the two settings.[2] Others have constrained assessment only to the simulation-based setting to understand how best to implement entrustment-supervision scales into existing processes like the Objective Structured Clinical Examination[21] or to examine the correlation between 'levels of supervision' and other relevant competency-based outcomes.[22] In all these studies, simulation appears to be viewed as most useful when researchers have identified EPAs that relate to directly observable skills, especially procedural skills and communication competencies.

The state of the evidence prompts us to advocate for a targeted research agenda that aims to establish the dual role of simulation in both EPA-based curricula and assessing EPAs. With these clear purposes as the foundation, researchers can build upon each other's work by conducting well-defined studies that contribute meaningfully to our collective knowledge advancement rather than conducting disparate studies that do not add to our foundational understanding. By examining the experiences and outcomes of institutions that have embraced simulation, researchers can provide educators with insights into the potential benefits and challenges of implementing simulation in their EPA-based curricula.[19]

Integrative model of simulation in EPA-based curricula

Based on the available literature, we have identified two major trends. First, reviews indicate that up to three times more studies focus on creating EPAs than on implementing EPA-based curricula.[23] Hence, our proposal that simulation can be used to implement EPA-based training and assessment has yet to be fully and systematically explored beyond theoretical proposals. Second, where empirical studies have been conducted on implementation, researchers tend to focus on the use of simulation for the assessment of EPAs rather than its use as a preparatory component to train for EPAs. Here, we challenge the simulation and EPA research communities to consider a provocative recommendation: that all trainees be required to experience every EPA and its related competencies, where those can be effectively delivered by educators using simulation, in a simulation-based setting before they are entrusted to perform the EPA on a patient.

Simulation-based education, as a modality for training and assessment, can involve scenarios that evolve from targeted, analytical tasks to holistic, real-world clinical scenarios, mirroring the

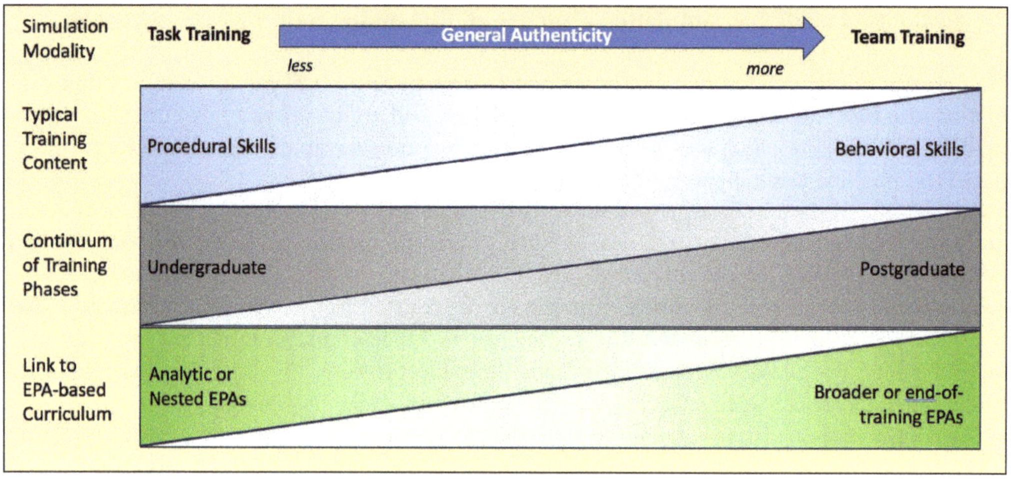

Figure 15.1: The role of simulation in an EPA-based curriculum.

progression of health care training from early learning to advanced practice.[24] In writing this chapter, we developed a preliminary model for educators to consider the pivotal role that simulation could play in developing trainees' competence in an EPA-based curriculum (Figure 15.1).

Early training—analytic and granular focus

In early training settings, simulation could be used to help trainees to independently hone granular tasks and essential procedural abilities. Educators might design part-task simulations with the aim of helping trainees to build core skills, like suturing or basic life support, in controlled settings. These activities correspond to analytic or nested EPAs (see Chapter 10), which focus on mastering specific components of broader professional activities.

Advanced training—holistic and end-of-training focus

As trainees progress from undergraduate to postgraduate programs, simulations would escalate in complexity, integrating technical and behavioral skills (e.g., communication, teamwork, decision-making). At advanced training stages, simulations could present comprehensive, realistic scenarios reflecting full-scale clinical encounters or complete patient care, resonating with holistic or end-of-training EPAs. Here, educators would examine how trainees perform when entrusted with complete professional tasks, simulating real-world practice and fusing procedural skills with the challenges of team-based health care.

Conclusion

Our preliminary model demonstrates how educators can formulate links between training content, trainees' progression, and the simulation purpose and modality best suited to the situation.[25] Our chapter raises and synthesizes key considerations for future directions of how to integrate simulation into EPA-based curricula as the landscapes of health professions education and simulation continue to evolve. We encourage researchers to use established frameworks—either those we have referenced or their own preferred ones—to systematically design, implement, and evaluate the impacts of using simulation modalities to support trainees' readiness for their future practice. Incorporating simulation into EPA-based curricula represents a transformative approach in health professions education.

Competing interests

The authors declare that they have no competing interests.

References

1. ten Cate O. Nuts and bolts of entrustable professional activities. *J Grad Med Educ.* 2013;5(1):157–158. DOI: https://doi.org/10.4300/JGME-D-12-00380.1
2. Jeyalingam T, Walsh CM, Tavares W, et al. Variable or fixed? Exploring entrustment decision-making in workplace- and simulation-based assessments. *Acad Med.* 2022;97(7):1057–1064. DOI: https://doi.org/10.1097/ACM.0000000000004661
3. ten Cate O, Chen HC, Hoff RG, Peters H, Bok H, van der Schaaf M. Curriculum development for the workplace using entrustable professional activities (EPAs): AMEE guide no. 99. *Med Teach.* 2015;37(11):983–1002. DOI: https://doi.org/10.3109/0142159X.2015.1060308
4. Weersink K, Hall AK, Rich J, Szulewski A, Dagnone JD. Simulation versus real-world performance: a direct comparison of emergency medicine resident resuscitation entrustment scoring. *Adv Simul.* 2019;4(1):9. DOI: https://doi.org/10.1186/s41077-019-0099-4
5. Dwyer T, Wadey V, Archibald D, et al. Cognitive and psychomotor entrustable professional activities: can simulators help assess competency in trainees? *Clin Orthop Relat Res.* 2016;474(4):926–934. DOI: https://doi.org/10.1007/s11999-015-4553-x
6. Lioce L, ed. *Healthcare Simulation Dictionary.* Agency for Healthcare Research and Quality; 2020. DOI: https://doi.org/10.23970/simulationv2
7. Nickson CP, Petrosoniak A, Barwick S, Brazil V. Translational simulation: from description to action. *Adv Simul.* 2021;6(1):6. DOI: https://doi.org/10.1186/s41077-021-00160-6
8. Herrigel DJ, Donovan C, Goodman E, et al. Simulation as a platform for development of entrustable professional activities: a modular, longitudinal approach. *Cureus.* Published online October 22, 2020. DOI: https://doi.org/10.7759/cureus.11098
9. Miller DT, Gibb W, Caretta-Weyer H, Ng K, Sebok-Syer SS, Gisondi MA. Filling the core EPA10 assessment void: a framework for individual assessment of core entrustable professional activity 10 competencies in medical students. *AEM Educ Train.* 2022;6(6). DOI: https://doi.org/10.1002/aet2.10787
10. Brydges R, Boyd VA, Tavares W, et al. Assumptions about competency-based medical education and the state of the underlying evidence: a critical narrative review. *Acad Med.* 2021;96(2):296–306. DOI: https://doi.org/10.1097/ACM.0000000000003781
11. Van Melle E, Frank JR, Holmboe ES, Dagnone D, Stockley D, Sherbino J. A core components framework for evaluating implementation of competency-based medical education programs. *Acad Med.* 2019;94(7):1002–1009. DOI: https://doi.org/10.1097/ACM.0000000000002743
12. ten Cate O, Taylor DR. The recommended description of an entrustable professional activity: AMEE guide no. 140. *Med Teach.* 2021;43(10):1106–1114. DOI: https://doi.org/10.1080/0142159X.2020.1838465
13. Brydges R, Hatala R, Zendejas B, Erwin PJ, Cook DA. Linking simulation-based educational assessments and patient-related outcomes: a systematic review and meta-analysis. *Acad Med.* 2015;90(2):246–256. DOI: https://doi.org/10.1097/ACM.0000000000000549

14. Cook DA, Hatala R. Validation of educational assessments: a primer for simulation and beyond. *Adv Simul.* 2016;1(1). DOI: https://doi.org/10.1186/s41077-016-0033-y
15. Brätz J, Bußenius L, Brätz I, Grahn H, Prediger S, Harendza S. Assessment of final-year medical students' entrustable professional activities after education on an interprofessional training ward: A case-control study. *Perspect Med Educ.* 2022;11(5):266–272. DOI: https://doi.org/10.1007/s40037-022-00720-0
16. Eliasz KL, Ark TK, Nick MW, Ng GM, Zabar S, Kalet AL. Capturing entrustment: using an end-of-training simulated workplace to assess the entrustment of near-graduating medical students from multiple perspectives. *Med Sci Educ.* 2018;28(4):739–747. DOI: https://doi.org/10.1007/s40670-018-0628-0
17. Salzman DH, McGaghie WC, Caprio T, et al. Use of a simulation-based capstone course to teach and assess entrustable professional activities to graduating medical students. *Med Sci Educ.* 2016;26(3):453–456. DOI: https://doi.org/10.1007/s40670-016-0267-2
18. Croft H, Gilligan C, Rasiah R, Levett-Jones T, Schneider J. Development and inclusion of an entrustable professional activity (EPA) scale in a simulation-based medicine dispensing assessment. *Curr Pharm Teach Learn.* 2020;12(2):203–212. DOI: https://doi.org/10.1016/j.cptl.2019.11.015
19. Keating S, McLeod-Sordjan R, Lemp M, Willenbrock D, Fried AM, Cassara M. Evaluating entrustable professional activities in a nurse practitioner readiness for practice simulation. *J Nurse Pract.* 2021;17(5):611–614. DOI: https://doi.org/10.1016/j.nurpra.2021.01.003
20. Prudhomme N, O'Brien M, McConnell MM, Dudek N, Cheung WJ. Relationship between ratings of performance in the simulated and workplace environments among emergency medicine residents. *CJEM.* 2020;22(6):811–818. DOI: https://doi.org/10.1017/cem.2020.388
21. Holzhausen Y, Maaz A, März M, Sehy V, Peters H. Exploring the introduction of entrustment rating scales in an existing objective structured clinical examination. *BMC Med Educ.* 2019;19(1). DOI: https://doi.org/10.1186/s12909-019-1736-2
22. Fincke F, Prediger S, Schick K, et al. Entrustable professional activities and facets of competence in a simulated workplace-based assessment for advanced medical students. *Med Teach.* 2020;42(9):1019–1026. DOI: https://doi.org/10.1080/0142159X.2020.1779204
23. O'Dowd E, Lydon S, O'Connor P, Madden C, Byrne D. A systematic review of 7 years of research on entrustable professional activities in graduate medical education, 2011–2018. *Med Educ.* 2019;53(3):234–249. DOI: https://doi.org/10.1111/medu.13792
24. Rotthoff T, Kadmon M, Harendza S. It does not have to be either or! Assessing competence in medicine should be a continuum between an analytic and a holistic approach. *Adv Health Sci Educ.* 2021;26(5):1659–1673. DOI: https://doi.org/10.1007/s10459-021-10043-0
25. Petrosoniak A, Brydges R, Nemoy L, Campbell DM. Adapting form to function: can simulation serve our healthcare system and educational needs? *Adv Simul.* 2018;3(1). DOI: https://doi.org/10.1186/s41077-018-0067-4

CHAPTER 16

Entrustable professional activities and transitions across the continuum of training and practice

Olle ten Cate, David A. Turner, Martin V. Pusic, Daniel J. Schumacher

Abstract

Transitions of trainees in the health professions to new contexts, to new training stages, and to unsupervised health care practice are critical learning periods where entrustable professional activities (EPAs) can play a pivotal role. For entrustment decisions, the critical questions are: are trainees prepared for a next phase, often with more autonomy, and are graduates prepared for the requirements of practice, often unsupervised?

This chapter addresses EPA-related issues from the perspective of these transitions and how they apply to the entire continuum of education and practice. Supervision plays a key role, both before transitions and after.

Authors

- Olle ten Cate, PhD. University Medical Center Utrecht, Utrecht, the Netherlands and University of California, San Francisco, USA. Correspondence: t.j.tencate@umcutrecht.nl
- David A. Turner, MD. American Board of Pediatrics, Chapel Hill, North Carolina, and Duke University Medical Center, Durham, North Carolina, USA.
- Martin V. Pusic, MD, PhD. Harvard University, Boston, Massachusetts, USA.
- Daniel J. Schumacher, MD, PhD, Cincinnati Children's Hospital Medical Center/University of Cincinnati College of Medicine, Cincinnati, Ohio.

How to cite this book chapter:

ten Cate O, Turner DA, Pusic MV, Schumacher DJ. Entrustable professional activities and transitions across the continuum of training and practice. In: ten Cate O, Burch VC, Chen HC, Chou FC, Hennus MP. (Eds). *Entrustable Professional Activities and Entrustment Decision-Making in Health Professions Education*, Chapter 16, pp. 183–193. [2024] London: Ubiquity Press. DOI: https://doi.org/10.5334/bdc.p

Introduction

Transitions are ubiquitous in health professional training—from classrooms to the clinical workplace, from one clinical environment to another, from supervised to unsupervised practice, from one institution to another, from prelicensure to licensed practitioner, and, in general, from training to practice. Entrustment with entrustable professional activities (EPAs) can reflect a transition on a granular level, as entrustment decisions bring trainees into situations where they have a greater responsibility and autonomy to act. EPAs have been defined as units of professional practice that trainees must be prepared to perform without supervision after a period of training. Originally proposed for postgraduate medical training,[1] EPAs were soon embraced by undergraduate programs. Accounts of proposals or uses of EPAs have now been published in all health professions. Given that EPAs define a profession, they are also suitable for individuals in practice after training, for instance to recognize when they have gaps in their abilities or when new activities are added to the profession that they did not encounter before completing training.

Entrustment with health care tasks does not occur only at the end or after completion of training. Even if formal regulation of the permission to practice health care is linked to credentialing, licensing, or board certification, supervised execution of health care tasks happens from the moment a trainee starts their first clinical rotation and a preceptor assigns and supervises professional tasks.[2] Even after completion of all training, a specialist may encounter new areas of work not experienced before. How practicing physicians acquire new knowledge and skills varies and may be different for unfamiliar surgical[3] and medical[4] tasks, but the assumption of responsibility for new professional activities is relevant across the continuum of education and practice. In other words, EPAs do not necessarily represent an educational construct; in fact, 'units of practice' constitute professional work, not educational exercises.

Figure 16.1 shows the transitions with the continuum from an international perspective, acknowledging the great variety of stages in training and practice worldwide. Each of these stages

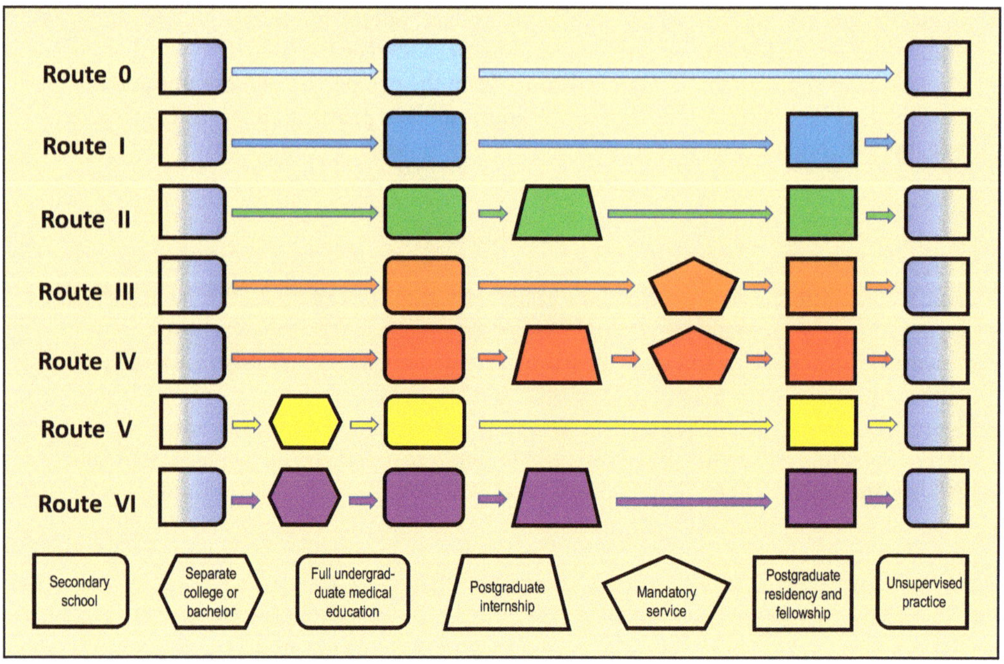

Figure 16.1: Transitions within the medical continuum worldwide. Adapted from Wijnen-Meijer et al. (2021).[5]

Box 16.1: A theoretical note: developing situation awareness after transitions.

Passing the threshold for summative entrustment with a health care task (an EPA) is a significant transition moment. Following Dreyfus's skill development model (novice–advanced beginner–competent–proficient–expert), this is when a trainee would be 'competent.'[10,11] Passing this threshold, that is, becoming allowed to work unsupervised, either within training or after training, is only the beginning of a trajectory toward proficiency and expertise. In an excellent overview, US Air Force industrial engineer Endsley (2018) explains the crucial role of developing situation awareness (SA) and how this occurs in three stages toward expertise: *perception* of relevant situational cues, *comprehension* of the dynamics in the environment, and *projection*, i.e., forecasting of relevant future happenings, illustrating this with examples from team sports, aviation, and medicine.[12] The mastery of an EPA at the threshold moment of readiness for unsupervised execution does not yet imply the automation of task execution that is needed for a high case load and robust execution under variable circumstances, because full SA has not been reached. A lower case load with ample time for each case is needed initially after a transition, also to avoid overload, feelings of moral injury (able, but not having enough time to do the job well), and burnout.[13]

may employ EPAs, while intermittent service periods can benefit from qualifications for EPAs. For each stage, the preceding phase should prepare trainees to work at a designated level of supervision.

Assuming clinical responsibility of professional work is a critical transition point. Transitions, from classroom to clinical phases of education and from education to practice, have always caused concerns.[6] Moving from possessing knowledge to executing clinical responsibilities is especially stressful. The weeks and months after such transitions have been called 'critically intensive learning periods.'[7] While preparation for such transitions can often be optimized, they are unavoidable difficult phases of professional growth that pose immense opportunities to learn to become resilient.[8] The first time a trainee passes the threshold of competence and is initially entrusted with unsupervised task execution, performance can be high-quality, but is not routinized and may take time.[9] After that transition, the development of situation awareness helps to speed up task execution and allows the increase of caseloads (Box 16.1).

In this chapter, we address critical issues related to EPAs and the continuum of education and practice, including its transitions. While competency-based education (CBE) has dominated the language of health professions *education*, competency-based *practice* throughout a clinical career is really its eventual purpose.[14]

Preparing early trainees for first EPAs

EPAs can be envisioned for early trainees but, as they reflect contributions to patient care activities for which one can (and must) become qualified, classroom education can never fully prepare trainees for EPA entrustment. Examples of legitimate EPAs for early trainees, however, can be found. For instance, some programs require medical students to become an emergency medical technician in the first year[15] or offer work in a supervised but student-run clinic for underserved populations (patient triage, history and physical examinations, patient education, and laboratory and immunization procedures).[2] These can also be offered as electives leading to formalized health care activities that require qualification and permission.

As early trainees (and their patients) are highly vulnerable, adequate training and supervision and clear regulations are of utmost importance. If well secured, however, such experiences are highly valuable. They provide an orientation to the profession to strengthen (or redirect) convictions of career choice. In addition, they provide a relevant context for the effort needed for foundational, canonical knowledge acquisition. This vertical curricular integration combines the *knowing, doing,* and *being* from the outset of professional training and identity formation, and is likely to prepare trainees for transition to more responsibilities.[16]

True entrustment with contributions to care in undergraduate education

Prelicensure trainees are often restricted in their autonomy to contribute to patient care. While that is needed and justified for the sake of patient (and trainee) safety, strong restrictions will cause more significant transition gaps after graduation compared to a more gradual preparation of trainees for responsibility. In international comparisons, the freedom of senior, but prelicensure, trainees differs vastly. In some jurisdictions, senior prelicensure trainees may not do much more than a physical and history, fully checked by a licensed attending, while in other settings prelicensure trainees can bear a significant weight of primary patient care with limited and indirect supervision. In terms of the Chen-adapted entrustment–supervision scale,[17] these variations before graduation range from 3a (all findings double-checked) for only limited tasks to 4a (remote supervision, reachable by phone) for quite significant tasks, including uncomplicated child delivery, as an example. Heavy responsibilities prepare learners well, but patient safety requires clear regulation of supervision. This dichotomy is where summative entrustment decisions, after adequate assessment of trainees, are critical to convince collaborators and the public that significant responsibilities are justified.

Entrustable professional activities and the transition to residency

EPAs define a circumscriptive profession. For EPAs for medical school, this is the entire profession of medicine, but in a general sense. EPAs achieved in medical school must prepare pluripotent (not pluricompetent) students for a diverse range of fields, from psychiatry to neurosurgery. Thus, EPAs at the transition from medical school to residency deserve special consideration. The Association of American Medical Colleges (AAMC) in the US navigated this issue by defining the EPAs they believed any practicing physician should potentially need to perform, regardless of specialty,[18,19] with the additional expectation that these would fit with subsequent EPAs for various specialties. The AAMC developed a set of 13 Core EPAs for Entering Residency (AAMC Core EPAs), such as developing differential diagnoses, ordering and interpreting common tests, documenting clinical encounters, and contributing to a culture of safety and improvement.[19]

The first specialty in the US attempting to align undergraduate and postgraduate EPAs was pediatrics. As part of a time-variable pilot (Education in Pediatrics Across the Continuum, or EPAC), pediatric educators mapped their general pediatrics EPAs[20] to the AAMC Core EPAs and transitioned medical students in this small pilot to pediatric residency early, based on their individual readiness.[21,22] Next, they aligned the general pediatrics EPAs to EPAs for each pediatric subspecialty for individuals who complete fellowship training. This includes EPAs common to general pediatrics and every subspecialty, such as 'Leading a team' and 'Serving as a consultant for other healthcare workers providing care to children.'[23]

Entrustment decisions and the transition to new training contexts

As trainees progress through the training continuum, there are both formative and summative considerations regarding an individual's readiness to execute a given EPA. The focus on EPAs can effectively improve feedback and progression along a developmental trajectory,[24–26] but summative entrustment decisions regarding readiness to practice EPAs in new contexts are important. Some programs award a 'statement of awarded responsibility' (STAR) when readiness for unsupervised practice has been demonstrated for an activity, a common practice among all Dutch postgraduate medical and nursing programs that serves as an informal mini-certification.[1,27] Testifying to this readiness may serve just to complete a training stage, such as in Canada's Competence-by-Design (CBD) model,[28] or to proceed to greater autonomy and responsibility in patient care. The CBD model requires learners to achieve mastery of a set of EPAs before progressing to their next context, which is devoted to other EPAs. A risk of this model is that trainees feel they need to 'chase' ratings for EPAs, not to allow for practicing with more autonomy but to tick off a program requirement.[29]

EPA qualifications also serve an important role in transitioning into completely new training environments, like the transition from undergraduate medical education (UME) to graduate medical education (GME). As noted above, in the US, the AAMC Core EPAs were developed and piloted in UME, and data suggest that there is an association between perceived readiness to perform these EPAs with transition to GME training.[30] Data also demonstrate that readiness to execute these AAMC Core EPAs may be lacking at the time of transition.[31,32] These data can be used to identify gaps that exist between UME and GME training, which serves as further evidence for the need to think about CBE and assessment as a genuine continuum to mitigate the abrupt transitions that are a part of many medical education systems.[14,18,33]

Transportability of summative entrustment decisions

Before formal licensing and specialty certification, summative decisions for EPAs at level 4 of supervision (basically, 'allowed to practice unsupervised, with oversight only') serve to qualify senior trainees to exercise responsibilities that are compatible with a posttransition phase. These summative decisions or STARs can be translated to digital badges[34] and should be acknowledged by members of the health care team. However, trainees can transition to a new context, for instance to a different, affiliated hospital during training. The question then arises as to the extent to which STARs uphold in this new context. Should new supervisors accept the trainee's STAR status and can they be allowed to work autonomously during night shifts? The recommendation is twofold: to basically accept the status in the new context, but also to incorporate an orientation phase, including sufficient observation to confirm the STAR status. For new environments, the recommendation thus is: 'trust, but verify.'

In nursing, where transition programs are widely used to support graduates in a practice environment,[35] a Dutch nationwide EPA model was recently created for postgraduate training to provide more flexibility to address both career development and the needs of health care[36] by using the concept of transdisciplinary EPAs.[37]

EPAs and transitions from training to full practice

Entering the first phase of full responsibility in practice following training is a critically important step.[38,39] Readiness to execute EPAs can serve as the basis for the decision to enter practice, and they provide an opportunity to clearly define the entrance requirements needed for practice in a profession or specialty.[40] However, in the siloed medical education systems that exist in many contexts, there may be inconsistency regarding how prepared a graduate needs to be at the time of transition into practice. Using the example of pediatrics in the US, EPAs were developed to define the activities expected of pediatricians and pediatric subspecialists, and, as these have been investigated over the last few years, data demonstrate substantial variability in graduates' preparedness to execute these activities at the conclusion of training. In general pediatrics, less than 80%

Box 16.2: Transition-to-practice models that focus on oversight of junior attendings.

- 'Promotion-in-place' is a US pilot program that allows residents to graduate in a time-variable fashion into a fully certified independent role within the residency institution, the advantage being that close supervision and support remains available during the early independent period.[44]
- Several US procedural specialty boards require the newly graduated surgeon to collect detailed information on a full, consecutive case series that is then reviewed at the time of their oral board examination, providing a window into the match between the individual's readiness for entrustment in a specific practice context.
- Comprehensive cardiac sonography was recently defined in 24 very specific EPAs, 10 of which were rated as core for postgraduate training, seven as requiring supervision after postgraduate training, and eight as requiring additional focused training and supervision for certified cardiologists.[45]

of graduating residents in one study demonstrated readiness for unsupervised practice for 6 of the 17 general pediatric EPAs[41] and, in the pediatric subspecialties, program directors suggested that unsupervised practice should not be the minimum expectation at the time of graduation for most EPAs.[42,43]

Considering transitions, it may not be realistic to list unsupervised practice as the strict minimum expectation for transitioning to full certification as a health professional. Rather than viewing the ongoing need for some supervision as deficiencies of individual trainees, or a deficiency in a training program, we suggest that this represents an ongoing, dynamic entrustment interface that must be negotiated not only at the time of certification and transition to practice but in an ongoing fashion throughout a practitioner's career. This recognizes both individual variability and contextual variability. Box 16.2 provides some examples.

Consider veterinary training and the readiness to manage emergency care for domestic animals. The variety of medical conditions, in the variety of potential animals, cannot all be taught and confirmed in undergraduate veterinary education. For every recent vet there will be deficiencies (and continued postgraduate residency is not the norm in veterinary medicine). Veterinary graduates are qualified but not *fully* competent.[46]

The notion of 'readiness for practice' is not absolute. The newly graduated practitioner *must* ensure further skill development, requiring the availability of a more experienced backup practitioner and special practice sessions.[46] In addition, the adaptation to the context may regard very different new skills. Clinical competency committees, qualifying trainees for the completion of training, should therefore reliably evaluate the trainee's *ability to recognize* the need for support and guidance. The designation 'not yet ready to be entrusted' is a signal to the learner (and the system) that extra support will be needed. To return to the realm of emergency veterinary practice, Figure 16.2 shows a recent Dutch project to negotiate on Day 1 after the transition to this new environment, how much supervision will be needed and for how long.[47] Similar approaches may be developed in transition phases for other health professions.

Once further into practice, a role for EPAs can be envisioned in the ongoing maintenance and updating of skills for practitioners. An important competency 'edge' for every practitioner involves adjusting to changing circumstances over a career. At the person level, 'disuse atrophy' may lead to de facto loss of readiness for critical activities, with implications for both continuing education and for ongoing certification.[48] EPAs can clarify where the edges are. At the context level,

EPA Checklist for new employees in emergency veterinary care

Essential EPAs in emergency veterinary care		For this EPA I estimate I require this level of supervision*					I strive to be ready for unsupervised practice after X months					
Initial treatment of a dog or cat with...		1	2	3	4	5	0	1	2	3	4	5
1	trauma, bleeding(en), wound(s)											
2	cardiorespiratory arrest (needing CPR)											
3	epilepsy											
4	dilated stomach/volvulus (excl. surgical intervention)											
5	dysuria / stranguria / pollakiuria											
6	intoxication											
7	dyspnea											
8	luxatio bulbi											
9	acute glaucoma											
10	acute blindness											
11	perforated cornea											
12	dystocia (including caesarean section)											
13	pyometra (including hysterectomy)											
14	dental urgency											
15	acute heart failure (myocardial, pericardial, arrhythmia)											
16	diarrhea, vomiting and/or abdominal pain											
17	anemia											
18	acute paresis/paralysis											
19	foreign body in nose/oropharynx, larynx, trachea, esophagus											
20	heatstroke											
21	allergic reaction											
22	diabetic ketoacidosis/hyperglycaemia											
23	determining indication and performing euthanasia											

***Level of supervision**

1. Ready to be present but not enacting the EPA
2. Ready to practice this EPA with supervisor physically present
3. Ready to practice this EPA with indirect (on-call) supervision
4. Ready for unsupervised practice
5. Ready to provide supervision to junior learners

Name: ...	Date: ...	Discussed with supervisor: ...

Figure 16.2: Example of a self-evaluation tool to negotiate supervision needs after transition.

practice is likely to keep changing rapidly over the course of a practitioner's career. New EPAs can arise with others being sunsetted, as practice evolves. For example, six collaborating emergency medicine organizations maintain a practice model, termed the 'Model of the Clinical Practice of Emergency Medicine' and made up of three main 'dimensions'—patient acuity, physician tasks, and physician competencies[49]—with the tasks dimension aligning with the EPA framework. This collaborative model, with the emergency medicine community coming together to ensure ongoing relevance of the guiding elements of a profession, ensures that inclusive cocreated frameworks strike the right balance between protecting the public and respecting individual practitioner autonomy. Another example is from physician assistant training, where EPAs are being added to the individual's portfolio after training.[50]

A next step could be to define for individual specialists what the core activities are, for all in their specialty must be ready to perform at any time (defining the common ground of the specialty), and what one's individual, dynamic portfolio of additional EPAs[14] shows they are ready to perform at a specific moment.

EPAs are usually associated with a single program, in either postgraduate or undergraduate education. In this chapter we have argued how EPAs can play a pivotal role across the educational continuum, and particularly around moments of transition. The role of supervision, a key variable in guarding the safety and quality of care, and simultaneously fostering the development of learners, cannot be stressed enough in this process.

Figure justifications

Figure 16.1 was adapted from Wijnen-Meijer et al. (2021).[5] Figure 16.2 was taken from ten Cate & Favier, 2022.[47]

Competing interests

The authors declare that they have no competing interests.

References

1. ten Cate O, Scheele F. Competency-based postgraduate training: can we bridge the gap between theory and clinical practice? *Acad Med.* 2007;82(6):542–547. DOI: https://doi.org/10.1097/ACM.0b013e31805559c7
2. Chen HC, Sheu L, O'Sullivan P, ten Cate O, Teherani A. Legitimate workplace roles and activities for early learners. *Med Educ.* 2014;48(2):136–145. DOI: https://doi.org/10.1111/medu.12316
3. Jaffe TA, Hasday SJ, Knol M, et al. Strategies for new skill acquisition by practicing surgeons. *J Surg Educ.* 2018;75(4):928–934. DOI: https://doi.org/10.1016/j.jsurg.2017.09.016
4. Grossman SN, Han SC, Balcer LJ, et al. Rapid implementation of virtual neurology in response to the COVID-19 pandemic. *Neurology.* 2020;94(24):1077–1087. DOI: https://doi.org/10.1212/WNL.0000000000009677
5. Wijnen-Meijer M, van den Broek M, ten Cate O. Six routes to unsupervised clinical practice. *Acad Med.* 2021;96(3):475. DOI: https://doi.org/10.1097/ACM.0000000000003880
6. Becker HS, Geer B, Huges EC, Strauss AL. *Boys in White. Student Culture in Medical School.* University of Chicago Press; 1961.
7. Kilminster S, Zukas M, Quinton N, Roberts T. Preparedness is not enough: understanding transitions as critically intensive learning periods. *Med Educ.* 2011;45(10):1006–1015. DOI: https://doi.org/10.1111/j.1365-2923.2011.04048.x
8. Rosenbaum L. Being well while doing well – distinguishing necessary from unnecessary discomfort in training. *N Engl J Med.* 2024;390(6):568–572. DOI: https://doi.org/10.1056/NEJMms2308228
9. Balziano S, Heyman E, Prat D. Patellar fracture surgery performed autonomously by residents, yields similar short-term outcomes to surgery performed by fellowship-trained surgeons. *J Surg Educ.* April 26, 2024. DOI: https://doi.org/10.1016/j.jsurg.2024.03.002
10. Dreyfus HL, Dreyfus SE. *Mind over Machine.* Free Press; 1986.
11. ten Cate O, Chen HC, Hoff RG, Peters H, Bok H, van der Schaaf M. Curriculum development for the workplace using entrustable professional activities (EPAs): AMEE Guide No. 99. *Med Teach.* 2015;37(11):983–1002. DOI: https://doi.org/10.3109/0142159X.2015.1060308

12. Endsley MR. Expertise and situation awareness. In: Ericsson KA, Hoffman RR, Kozbelt A, Williams AM, eds. *The Cambridge Handbook of Expertise and Expert Performance*. Cambridge University Press; 2018:714–742. DOI: https://doi.org/10.1017/9781316480748.037
13. Injured, not sidelined: NOS episode 2.10. *N Engl J Med*. 2024;390(15):e37. DOI: https://doi.org/10.1056/NEJMp2400700
14. ten Cate O, Carraccio C. Envisioning a true continuum of competency-based medical education, training, and practice. *Acad Med*. 2019;94(9):1283–1288. DOI: https://doi.org/10.1097/ACM.0000000000002687
15. Brenner J, Bird J, Ginzburg SB, et al. Trusting early learners with critical professional activities through emergency medical technician certification. *Med Teach*. 2018;40(6):561–568. DOI: https://doi.org/10.1080/0142159X.2018.1444745
16. Wijnen-Meijer M, ten Cate O, van der Schaaf M, Burgers C, Borleffs J, Harendza S. Vertically integrated medical education and the readiness for practice of graduates. *BMC Med Educ*. 2015;15:229. DOI: https://doi.org/10.1186/s12909-015-0514-z
17. Chen HC, van den Broek WES, ten Cate O. The case for use of entrustable professional activities in undergraduate medical education. *Acad Med*. 2015;90(4):431–436. DOI: https://doi.org/10.1097/ACM.0000000000000586
18. Carraccio C, Englander R, Gilhooly J, et al. Building a framework of entrustable professional activities, supported by competencies and milestones, to bridge the educational continuum. *Acad Med*. 2017;92(3):324–330. DOI: https://doi.org/10.1097/ACM.0000000000001141
19. Englander R, Flynn T, Call S, et al. Toward defining the foundation of the MD degree: core entrustable professional activities for entering residency. *Acad Med*. 2016;91(10):1352–1358. DOI: https://doi.org/10.1097/ACM.0000000000001204
20. Andrews JS, Bale JF, Soep JB, et al. Education in Pediatrics Across the Continuum (EPAC): first steps toward realizing the dream of competency-based education. *Acad Med*. 2018;93(3):414–420. DOI: https://doi.org/10.1097/ACM.0000000000002020
21. Murray KE, Lane JL, Carraccio C, et al. Crossing the gap: using competency-based assessment to determine whether learners are ready for the undergraduate-to-graduate transition. *Acad Med*. 2019;94(3):338–345. DOI: https://doi.org/10.1097/ACM.0000000000002535
22. Geraghty JR, Ocampo RG, Liang S, et al. Medical students' views on implementing the core EPAs: recommendations from student leaders at the core EPAs pilot institutions. *Acad Med*. 2021;96(2):193–198. DOI: https://doi.org/10.1097/ACM.0000000000003793
23. Mink RB, Schwartz A, Herman BE, et al. Validity of level of supervision scales for assessing pediatric fellows on the common pediatric subspecialty entrustable professional activities. *Acad Med*. 2018;93(2):283–291. DOI: https://doi.org/10.1097/ACM.0000000000001820
24. Bremer AE, Ruczynski LIA, Bot P, Fluit CRMG, van de Pol MHJ. A qualitative study on how entrustable professional activities support medical students in their transitions across clerkships. *Perspect Med Educ*. 2023;12(1):187–197. DOI: https://doi.org/10.5334/pme.825
25. Arnstead N, Campisi P, Takahashi SG, et al. Feedback frequency in competence by design: A quality improvement initiative. *J Grad Med Educ*. 2020;12(1):46–50. DOI: https://doi.org/10.4300/JGME-D-19-00358.1
26. Berger S, Stalmeijer RE, Marty AP, Berendonk C. Exploring the impact of entrustable professional activities on feedback culture: a qualitative study of anesthesiology residents and attendings. *Acad Med*. 2023;98(7):836–843. DOI: https://doi.org/10.1097/ACM.0000000000005188
27. Sigurdsson V, ten Cate O. Do summative entrustment decisions actually lead to entrustment? *Clin Teach*. October 10, 2023:e13668. DOI: https://doi.org/10.1111/tct.13668
28. Hall AK, Oswald A, Frank JR, et al. Evaluating competence by design as a large system change initiative: readiness, fidelity, and outcomes. *Perspect Med Educ*. 2024;13(1):95–107. DOI: https://doi.org/10.5334/pme.962

29. Ott MC, Pack R, Cristancho S, Chin M, Van Koughnett JA, Ott M. 'The most crushing thing': understanding resident assessment burden in a competency-based curriculum. *J Grad Med Educ.* 2022;14(5):583–592. DOI: https://doi.org/10.4300/JGME-D-22-00050.1
30. Obeso V, Grbic D, Emery M, et al. Core entrustable professional activities (EPAs) and the transition from medical school to residency: the postgraduate year one resident perspective. *Med Sci Educ.* 2021;31(6):1813–1822. DOI: https://doi.org/10.1007/s40670-021-01370-3
31. Lindeman BM, Sacks BC, Lipsett PA. Graduating students' and surgery program directors' views of the Association of American Medical Colleges core entrustable professional activities for entering residency: where are the gaps? *J Surg Educ.* 2015;72(6):e184–92. DOI: https://doi.org/10.1016/j.jsurg.2015.07.005
32. Angus SV, Vu TR, Willett LL, Call S, Halvorsen AJ, Chaudhry S. Internal medicine residency program directors' views of the core entrustable professional activities for entering residency: an opportunity to enhance communication of competency along the continuum. *Acad Med.* 2017;92(6):785–791. DOI: https://doi.org/10.1097/ACM.0000000000001419
33. Aschenbrener CA, Ast C, Kirch DG. Graduate medical education: its role in achieving a true medical education continuum. *Acad Med.* 2015;90(9):1203–1209. DOI: https://doi.org/10.1097/ACM.0000000000000829
34. Mehta NB, Hull AL, Young JB, Stoller JK. Just imagine: new paradigms for medical education. *Acad Med.* 2013;88(10):1418–1423. DOI: https://doi.org/10.1097/ACM.0b013e3182a36a07
35. Alshawush K, Hallett N, Bradbury-Jones C. The impact of transition programmes on workplace bullying, violence, stress and resilience for students and new graduate nurses: a scoping review. *J Clin Nurs.* 2022;31(17–18):2398–2417. DOI: https://doi.org/10.1111/jocn.16124
36. Pool IA, van Zundert H, ten Cate O. Facilitating flexibility in postgraduate nursing education through entrustable professional activities to address nursing shortages and career prospects. *Int Nurs Rev.* October 11, 2023. DOI: https://doi.org/10.1111/inr.12892
37. Pool I, Hofstra S, van der Horst M, ten Cate O. Transdisciplinary entrustable professional activities. *Med Teach.* 2023;45(9):1019–1024. DOI: https://doi.org/10.1080/0142159X.2023.2170778
38. Teunissen PW, Westerman M. Junior doctors caught in the clash: the transition from learning to working explored. *Med Educ.* 2011;45(10):968–970. DOI: https://doi.org/10.1111/j.1365-2923.2011.04052.x
39. Hampton KB, Smeltzer SC, Ross JG. Evaluating the transition from nursing student to practicing nurse: an integrative review. *J Prof Nurs.* 2020;36(6):551–559. DOI: https://doi.org/10.1016/j.profnurs.2020.08.002
40. Taylor D, Park YS, Smith C, Cate OT, Tekian A. Constructing approaches to entrustable professional activity development that deliver valid descriptions of professional practice. *Teach Learn Med.* 2021;33(1):89–97. DOI: https://doi.org/10.1080/10401334.2020.1784740
41. Schumacher DJ, West DC, Schwartz A, et al. Longitudinal assessment of resident performance using entrustable professional activities. *JAMA Netw Open.* 2020;3(1):e1919316. DOI: https://doi.org/10.1001/jamanetworkopen.2019.19316
42. Turner DA, Schwartz A, Carraccio C, et al. Continued supervision for the common pediatric subspecialty entrustable professional activities may be needed following fellowship graduation. *Acad Med.* 2021;96(7S):S22-S28. DOI: https://doi.org/10.1097/ACM.0000000000004091
43. Weiss PG, Schwartz A, Carraccio CL, et al. Achieving entrustable professional activities during fellowship. *Pediatrics.* 2021;148(5). DOI: https://doi.org/10.1542/peds.2021-050196
44. Goldhamer MEJ, Pusic MV, Nadel ES, Co JPT, Weinstein DF. Promotion in place: a model for competency-based, time-variable graduate medical education. *Acad Med.* January 29, 2024. DOI: https://doi.org/10.1097/ACM.0000000000005652
45. Perry R, Forshaw A, Childs J, Chester D, Edwards C. Cultivating competency in cardiac sonography: aligning entrustable professional activities with industry expectations. *Heart Lung Circ.* March 7, 2024. DOI: https://doi.org/10.1016/j.hlc.2024.01.027

46. Duijn C, Bok H, ten Cate O, Kremer W. Qualified but not yet fully competent: perceptions of recent veterinary graduates on their day-one skills. *Vet Rec*. 2020;186(7):216. DOI: https://doi.org/10.1136/vr.105329
47. ten Cate O, Favier RP. Approaching training-practice gaps after the transition: a practice proposal for supervision after training. *Front Med (Lausanne)*. 2022;9:881274. DOI: https://doi.org/10.3389/fmed.2022.881274
48. Pusic MV, Kessler D, Szyld D, Kalet A, Pecaric M, Boutis K. Experience curves as an organizing framework for deliberate practice in emergency medicine learning. *Acad Emerg Med*. 2012;19(12):1476–1480. DOI: https://doi.org/10.1111/acem.12043
49. Beeson MS, Bhat R, Broder JS, et al. The 2022 model of the clinical practice of emergency medicine. *J Emerg Med*. 2023;64(6):659–695. DOI: https://doi.org/10.1016/j.jemermed.2023.02.016
50. de Raad T, Wiersma F, Kuilman L, ten Cate O. The fate of entrustable professional activities after graduation: a survey study among graduated physician assistants. *J Contin Educ Health Prof*. 2023;43(1):28–33. DOI: https://doi.org/10.1097/CEH.0000000000000467

SECTION D

Assessment

CHAPTER 17

Workplace-based assessment to support entrustment decision-making: four sources of information

Olle ten Cate, Gersten Jonker, Yoon Soo Park, Eric S. Holmboe, Vanessa C. Burch

Abstract

A program of assessment that enables summative decisions about the trainee's readiness, such as a clinical competency committee, requires a synthesis of various sources of information and sufficient data points. Besides information about knowledge and skills, assessed outside the workplace (written examinations and standardized skills tests), workplace-based assessment can be categorized into four sources of information about a trainee: direct observation, conversation, longitudinal observation, and evaluation of 'products' of patient care. Direct observation of a trainee happens during a natural patient care activity in an authentic clinical setting, usually 10 to 20 minutes, followed by a few minutes of focused feedback. Conversations are a five- to 20-minute one-on-one discussion with a trainee to probe knowledge, understanding, reasoning, and/or decision-making. Longitudinal observation or monitoring checks the natural, unplanned observation of a trainee over time by collaborators and others (including patients) who have natural encounters with the trainee, often in the form of multisource feedback. Product evaluation pertains to the assessment of trainees through their output of patient care that does not require their direct presence during the assessment.

How to cite this book chapter:

ten Cate O, Jonker G, Park YS, Holmboe ES, Burch VC. Workplace-based assessment to support entrustment decision-making: four sources of information. In: ten Cate O, Burch VC, Chen HC, Chou FC, Hennus MP. (Eds). *Entrustable Professional Activities and Entrustment Decision-Making in Health Professions Education*, Chapter 17, pp. 197–211. [2024] London: Ubiquity Press. DOI: https://doi.org/10.5334/bdc.q

This chapter uses cross-references to other chapters of the same book. For those who read this chapter as a standalone publication: all cross-references can be found at: https://doi.org/10.5334/bdc

All four sources of information are discussed with examples and literature references. We end with notes on documentation of information, and feedback processes as an intrinsic component of workplace-based assessment.

Authors

- Olle ten Cate, PhD. University Medical Center Utrecht, Utrecht, the Netherlands and University of California, San Francisco, USA. Correspondence: t.j.tencate@umcutrecht.nl
- Gersten Jonker, MD, PhD. Department of Anesthesiology, University Medical Center Utrecht, Utrecht, the Netherlands.
- Yoon Soo Park, PhD. Department of Medical Education, University of Illinois College of Medicine, Illinois, USA.
- Eric Holmboe, MD. Intealth, Philadelphia, Pennsylvania, USA.
- Vanessa C. Burch, MD, PhD. Colleges of Medicine of South Africa, South Africa.

Workplace-based assessment to support feedback and summative entrustment decisions

In 1990, George Miller, a senior scholar in medical education, presented a famous model of assessment, arguing that significant advances had been made across his lifetime to increase the psychometric quality of the assessment of knowledge, applied knowledge and reasoning, and integrated knowledge and skills in a standardized environment.

However, the 'does' level in the pyramid that was named after him was left for a necessary future advance in medical education.[1] Workplace-based assessment reflects the assessment at this fourth level of the pyramid but it was not well developed at the time.

Since Miller's publication, workplace-based assessment (WBA) has been developed in many ways[2,3] to include tools, forms, procedures, and approaches. Assessment of trainees in the health professions, to determine their readiness to practice, has evolved from limited static moments of high-stakes assessment into a more continuous and developmental interaction with trainees to support learning, combined with evaluating their readiness for practice requiring varying levels of supervision and support.[4] Readiness for practice is increasingly translated to entrustment: the decision to transfer patient care responsibilities to a trainee who has shown to possess the required competencies.

Entrustment decisions require solid information about the trainee. In the clinical workplace, a multitude of sources of information is available to inform their development and their readiness for practice.

WBA is assessment in the variable context of patient care. While trainees have acquired generalized, context-independent knowledge and skill (this can be called a canonical layer of competence), working in practice requires the ability to apply generalized knowledge and skills in circumstances that vary. This 'contextual' layer of competence must be evaluated to justify summative entrustment decisions. Students must meet standards of contextual performance derived from observations in actual practice before permission to practice should be granted. In contrast with assessment under standardized conditions, WBA requires case-by-case judgments by individuals, because the conditions in the workplace (patient cases, assessors' experience and expertise, team composition, time of day, and day of week) cannot be easily standardized. Assessors are

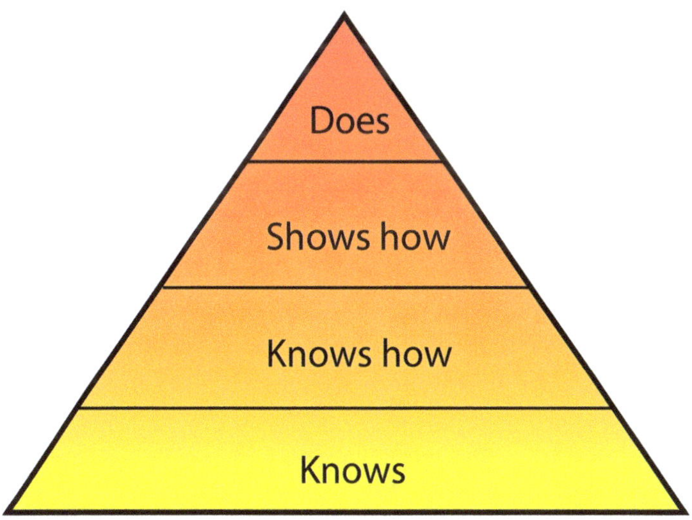

Figure 17.1: Miller's pyramid.

often clinician-preceptors who happen to be available in the workplace but they can also include others, such as interprofessional personnel. Traditional psychometric criteria that work well with standardized assessment (e.g., written tests) are seldom met in workplace-based assessment.[5,6] A different approach is required, including aggregation of data from multiple sources.[7] Crossley et al. have argued that good, intuitive, questions when assessing trainees will lead to more reliable answers.[8] 'Would you entrust this learner with care for the next patient?' is a more intuitive question than 'Please rate trainee for professionalism on a nine-point scale.' The concept of entrustment decisions is essentially new as a way of assessing trainees, although it has been informally practiced for as long as anyone can remember. Entrustment for unsupervised future practice may be conceptualized as a fifth level in Miller's pyramid, beyond observing how well a trainee has 'done' in the past so far.[9]

While the assessment of knowledge and reasoning, as well as standardized skills assessments, are very important in health professions education, the focus in this chapter is on assessment in the workplace, to support decisions of entrustment with tasks in health care.

EPAs and entrustment decision-making within workplace-based assessment

Assessment usually concerns a conclusion regarding work done and thus draws a *retrospective* summative conclusion. A *prospective* view implies an estimation of readiness for future practice, which requires more than retrospection of completed exams and assignments. A trainee, for example, with high scores on exams, and often doing well while observed in the clinical workplace, but who is not inclined to ask for help if needed, or does not collaborate well, may be less trustworthy for future tasks than someone who maybe scored less well on knowledge exams but who knows when to ask for help and how to mobilize resources when needed to bring a clinical problem to a satisfactory end,[10] or 'knows what to do when you don't know what to do.'[a]

Permission to practice patient care can be fully unsupervised, but in education it usually refers to permission under a specified level of supervision. Translated to a commonly used entrustment–supervision (ES) scale,[12] *observation only* (level 1) permits no trainee contribution to care, *direct supervision* (level 2) signifies a supervisor being present to observe and take over the activity if needed, and *indirect supervision* (level 3) means that a supervisor is not present but on site and available to assist if needed or if so requested. Off-site supervision (level 4), e.g., by phone, relies heavily on a trainee's readiness to work with virtually no supervision, and their willingness to seek help if really needed.

Ad hoc entrustment decisions are those that occur 'on the fly' in the clinical moment ('now you go ahead with this patient; call me if you need me'). This reflects individual supervisor decisions, in contrast to *summative* entrustment decisions, which have the nature of a formalized qualification, supported by a team decision.

Entrustable professional activities (EPAs), being units of practice to be entrusted to trainees once they demonstrate the required competence, can be regarded as tasks (or bundles of tasks) that can be well observed, overseen, and monitored. A summative entrustment decision should be made only when a trainee has demonstrated readiness for more autonomy. That requires thoughtful decision-making, based on various data sources, by a team of knowledgeable educators, often called a (clinical) *competency committee* or entrustment committee.[10]

---

[a] Derived from a child-pedagogy book[11] and cited in Dr. Ian Bates's 2017 keynote talk at a Dutch HPE conference.

Multiple sources of information in the workplace are available to estimate competence and add to the grounding of trust.[13] Clearly, a valid, holistic picture of the trainee cannot be based on a single observation. Following the premise of *programmatic assessment*,[14] many and varied observations together must build an adequate picture of the trainee's readiness to practice. This includes not just knowledge and skills but also professional attributes like humility, agency, integrity, and reliability.[15]

In a program that is serious about a stepwise increase in the progressive autonomy and responsibility of trainees, clinical education should include formalized moments of summative entrustment for EPAs. EPAs can be narrow or broad tasks, depending on what the activity includes, but an educational program should organize their EPAs such that summative entrustment decisions to qualify trainees for unsupervised practice (level 4; in undergraduate medical education for indirect supervision: level 3) are made not more than a few times per year, reflecting significant steps toward more autonomy. Early in education, EPAs are usually small in scope (e.g., taking general neurological histories; placing IUDs; removing a small benign lump); later they can be broad (e.g., running the internal medicine ward day service; running the Friday anesthesia night shift).

Four sources of assessment information to support summative entrustment decisions

The emphasis in WBA is on contextual competence. The presumption is that trainees possess a foundation of canonical knowledge and skills; they are assessed with the purpose of entrustment with clinical tasks. To arrive at summative entrustment decisions, a clinical competency committee must rely on data from various sources. These sources can be categorized into four groups: direct observations, conversations, longitudinal observations, and evaluations of 'products' of the trainee's care provision.[16,17] In a *program of assessment*, sources of information must be identified that align best with a particular EPA and inform a summative entrustment decision. The recommendation is to draw from all four sources of information.

1. Direct observation

A direct, focused observation of a trainee during a natural patient care activity in an authentic clinical setting usually takes 10 to 20 minutes, followed by a few minutes of rating and feedback. Trainee and supervisor should have a shared understanding of its purpose, i.e., both to assess and to support the trainee with performance feedback. The most common types of direct observation focus on a clinical encounter or a procedure.

Forms and scales. Traditional rating forms have been criticized because they do not align well with the thinking of a clinical assessor.[8] Numerical scales (e.g., 1–9, or unsatisfactory–satisfactory–superior; or below–meets–exceeds expectations) are increasingly replaced by ES scales, either retrospective ('how much guidance was needed?')[28,29] or prospective ('based on my observations so far, I recommend that this trainee is ready for supervision level [X] for this EPA').[12] Ample space for narrative, descriptive assessment data is also increasingly recommended, albeit that more research is needed to optimize its quality and use.[30,31]

How many observations? There is no simple answer, as this depends on the task, the trainee, and their stage of training or development. Complex tasks may require much practice under direct supervision; simple, low-risk tasks require less. An advanced or skillful trainee may

Table 17.1: Four sources of workplace information to support summative entrustment decisions.

	Defined	Examples and references
Direct observation	Focused observation of a trainee during a natural patient care activity in an authentic clinical setting, usually 10–20 minutes, followed by a few minutes of focused feedback	Among the dozens of tools[18] and guidelines,[19] observation of history and physical examination in clinical encounters using mini-CEX and observation of procedural skills using DOPS are frequently used.[3] ES scales are used to support entrustment decisions made[12]
Conversation	A five- to 20-minute one-on-one discussion with a trainee to probe knowledge, understanding, reasoning and/or decision-making	Case-based discussions (CBDs) and chart-stimulated recall (CSR)[2,3,20] focus on knowledge and reasoning, and performed actions; entrustment-based discussions (EBD)[21] focus on anticipated action and risk assessment. Brief teaching conversations[22] such as SNAPPS* and OMP* and pre- and debriefings of encounters contribute to trainee evaluation
Longitudinal observation	The natural, unplanned observation of a trainee over time by collaborators and others (including patients) who have natural encounters with the trainee	Multisource feedback procedures[23] are typically longitudinal. Automated procedures can be done.[24,25] The Mini-PAT is a well-known MSF form[2] and the A RICH framework[15] may inform narrative comments
Product evaluation	Assessment of trainees through their outputs of patient care that do not require their direct presence during the assessment	Examples are entries into health records (discharge letters), physical products (dentistry, plastic surgery, orthopedics, etc.), patient experiences, clinimetrics, complication rates, and readmissions[26,27]
* See text		

require less than a beginner, and patient availability and clinical workload[32] can be a limiting factor for observations.

Important, however, is that only requiring a fixed number of observations neglects the importance of individual differences. There is nothing wrong with a threshold number ('at least X'), as long as 'completing the number' is not used to conclude that the trainee is competent.[33] It is more important to consider the number of *recent satisfactory* performances, preferably under different circumstances. Up to eight satisfactory observations have been suggested for undergraduate medical EPAs as thresholds for entrustment,[34] but for some EPAs fewer may be enough. Obviously, older observations, when a trainee is still inexperienced, should not weigh as much as recent ones. Sampling should reflect a thoughtful representation, adequate for the entrustment decision, but that does not mean that every trainee should be observed as much; underperforming trainees, for instance, generally require more observations.

Who initiates the observations? In many programs, it is the trainee who initiates direct observations by inviting clinicians to observe and report. There is benefit of trainee ownership and control of their curriculum and development, which alleviates staff of the burden of planning observations.[35] A downside is that trainee-initiated observations are not always a random 'snapshot' or adequate sample of practice and may stimulate trainees to document their best performances, including requests for hindsight documentation when an activity was done well in the presence

Box 17.1: Direct observation.

A clinical encounter with a patient. This can include history taking, physical examination of the patient, a conversation with the patient about a clinical decision, asking for informed consent, breaking bad news, etc. Observations are documented on a structured form. This invites the observer to evaluate interviewing skills, physical examination skills, humanistic qualities, clinical judgment, counseling skills, organization/efficiency, and an overall score, plus free comments.

A procedure involving a patient, requiring technical skill. Procedures can range from inserting an IV, vaccination, venous or arterial blood withdrawal, various punctures, a surgical procedure, administering a cognitive screening test, etc. Usually it is not only technical skill that is evaluated but also the interaction.

of a clinician. That is not always problematic, but it can create an imbalanced picture. Showing one's 'best practices' is not a problem in itself, as long as it does not mask critical deficiencies. In contrast, supervisor-selected convenient observation moments can contribute to bias, including leniency bias.[36] Cocreation of individualized WBA among trainees and multiple supervisors is recommended to arrive at a balanced selection of observations.

Faculty and trainee experiences with direct observation. Direct observation requires faculty effort that cannot be spent on efficient patient care. Resistance against implementing direct observation is frequently heard,[37] but establishing an observation-based training culture does not necessarily imply a huge time commitment.[38] Trainees may feel awkward or uncomfortable asking attending faculty to observe them.[39,40] Also, when trainees experience every observation as a critical, high-stakes assessment moment, rather than a welcomed, low-stakes learning moment,[41] a culture change is needed, to reframe a teaching hospital as more than just a health care institution. When formative assessment and feedback become routine, and not just incidental, observation can be experienced as a natural component of the training culture, rather than a continuous examination.

2. Conversation

Case-based discussions (CBDs) with trainees—if focused on a trainee's case that has been documented in a health record, also called chart-stimulated recall (CSR)—is a well-established method to capture trainee knowledge and understanding needed to perform patient care. Unlike standardized reasoning tests, these conversations generally relate to cases in the local context, often the trainee's own patients, and test what some authors call situated cognition,[42] rather than decontextualized cognition. CBDs and CSR particularly focus on what a trainee's reasoning and rationales are (or were) as related to the case. These conversations are 10 to 20 minutes including feedback and documentation. The procedures are well described elsewhere.[2,3,20]

Some conversational approaches have been designed as individual teaching moments rather than assessments, but they do add to a preceptor's picture of the trainee. Well known are SNAPPS (Summarize history and findings–Narrow the differential–Analyze–Probe the Preceptor about uncertainties–Select issues for further study), which is trainee-driven, and the One-Minute Preceptor (Get a commitment–Probe for underlying reasoning–Teach a general rule–Reinforce what was done well–Correct mistakes), which is more supervisor-driven.[43]

One approach that is particularly suitable for entrustment decision-making is the 'entrustment-based discussion.'[21] This 10- to 20-minute conversation has a focus on risk assessment when anticipating an entrustment decision, either directly after an EPA has been performed or before an upcoming activity (supporting ad hoc entrustment). Box 17.2 explains the procedure.

Box 17.2: Four steps in the entrustment-based discussion.[21]

1. **Explain the activity**

What are procedural steps? Have you done this before? What are critical parts?

2. **Why is/was that needed?**

Relevant anatomy/physiology, indications, rationale in this patient's management

3. **What are/were associated risks?**

What are consequences of inadequate performance, what could happen?

4. **What would you do if…?**

Give scenario (unusual or uncooperative patient, different history and physical findings, different test results, comorbidity) and probe for actions.

All these encounters are meant to be brief, regular, and formative, rather than long, infrequent, and merely assessment-focused. Long oral exams, such as a 'long case' (an hour or more with a patient and a subsequent interrogation) at the end of rotations are no longer considered adequate WBA methods.[44]

3. Longitudinal observation

Not all important behaviors, relevant for summative entrustment decisions, can be captured in brief direct observations and discussions. During direct observation, the trainee is usually aware of being observed and may not behave completely naturally[45]; longitudinal observation does not happen in an arranged setting and is better suited to capture qualities of professionalism, relevant to entrustment decisions (arriving at meetings on time, doing what was promised, setting priorities, communicating adequately interprofessionally, etc.). Longitudinal observation is the natural, unplanned observation of a trainee over time by collaborators or others (including patients) who have natural encounters with the trainee. Features that are suitable for longitudinal observation include the behavioral characteristics that are important for entrustment. These were recently summarized and grouped into five categories as the 'A RICH' entrustment decision (Box 17.3).[15]

Box 17.3: Trainee features relevant for *A RICH* entrustment decision.[15]

Agency:	Self-confident, proactive toward work, team, safety, and own development
Reliability:	Conscientious; predictable; accountable; responsible
Integrity:	Truthful; having good, benevolent, intentions; being patient-centered
Capability:	Having focused knowledge and skills, experience, adaptive expertise
Humility:	Observing personal limits; willing to ask help; receptive to feedback

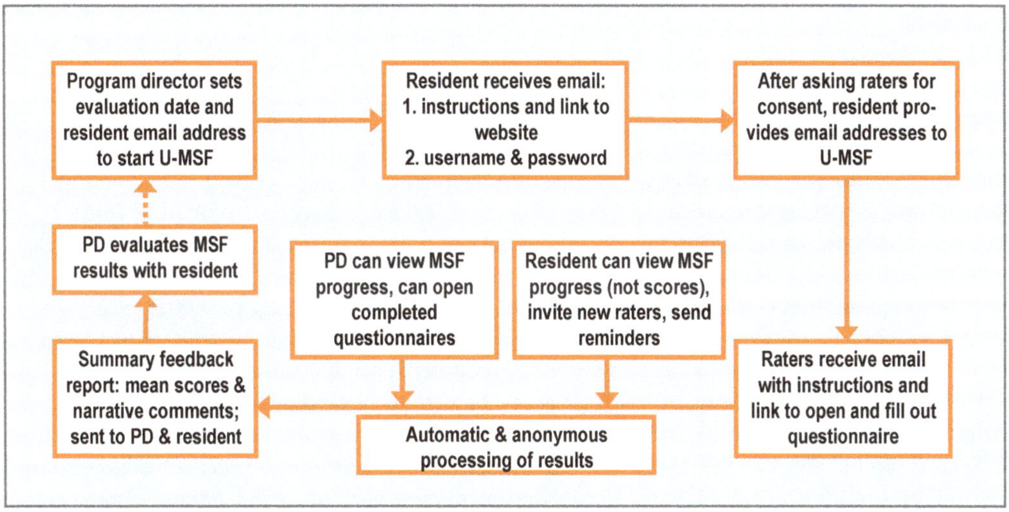

Figure 17.2: Example of an automated MSF procedure.

Opinions of supervisors and others may accumulate over time to build a picture of a trainee in colleagues with whom the trainee works. Such informal opinions are not sufficiently grounded for important decision-making; more formalized, structured approaches are needed. One such procedure is multisource feedback (MSF) or 360-degree evaluation, in which clinical staff members, peers and other trainees, interprofessional colleagues, and patients and their families may be included. For longitudinal observation, assessors must be asked in advance to observe over a period of time (a week, a weekend shift, a rotation). While MSF may require quite some logistical effort,[46] web-based methods can alleviate most of the administrative burden. Figure 17.2 shows a MSF procedure that has been successfully applied in many residency programs in the Netherlands as a fully automated procedure with little administrative effort.[24,25]

Trainees in this example select their own observers (six medical colleagues, six nonmedical colleagues, and 10 patients), who then respond to a brief email survey, combining a rating scale with adequate space for narrative comments. The automated, anonymous reports (two to three pages), generated by the system, have proved to be highly useful, in particular the narrative component.[24,25] Another regularly used example of an MSF form is the mini-Peer Assessment Tool (mini-PAT).[2] While the A RICH components are less suitable for rating scales, they may inform MSF raters' frame of reference for narrative comments, over longitudinal periods of time. The trainee's reflection on an MFS report is important, and can be supported by a coach or mentor.[25]

Longitudinal monitoring provides critical information for clinical competency committees. MSF reports can show trends, if various sources point in a similar direction. This analysis should inform CCCs; even less structured longitudinal information can be useful but needs to be corroborated by views from different observers, akin to quality journalism that relies on multiple independent sources.

4. Product evaluation

One of the quality features of entrustable professionals activities is that the EPA is 'measurable in its outcome,' enabling a judgment of 'well done' or not 'well done.'[47,48] This looks at the result or product of an activity. By product evaluation we mean the assessment of trainees through their output of patient care, while not requiring their direct presence during the assessment. Those familiar with Kirkpatrick's four hierarchical levels of educational effectiveness (satisfaction → learning → behavior change → results)[49] will agree that most WBA focuses on 'learning' (as established in tests and performances) and on some behavior change but less on 'results,' i.e., on effective health care provided. In other sectors of society, professional services and their providers are frequently evaluated by products (artifacts such as reports, designs, manufactured and engineered products), but in health care product evaluation happens less frequently. The effect of learning, training, and competence on patient care, including benefits to patients, is not easy to demonstrate or measure but it is worth pursuing.[50] Products of individuals in health care can include entries in an electronic health record, discharge summaries, physical products from procedures performed, quality improvement and patient safety (QIPS) measures, patient experiences, clinimetrics,[26] portfolio-logged patient encounters, and other, specialty-specific products. Research output, reports created by a trainee, and presentations can sometimes be included, even if less linked to clinical care.

Some procedural professions and specialties yield clear products (dentistry, e.g., a crown; plastic surgery, e.g., a facial reconstruction; orthopedic surgery, e.g., fractured bone reconstruction, as evidenced by imaging). While these may still reflect team efforts, the product is visible. In non-procedural specialties, such as in psychiatry, the suicidal status must be documented, and written patient handovers, coherence of patient records, and therapeutical adherence can be measured.

While surgical complication rates and patient readmissions are other outcome measures, they may be even less easily directly linked to individual effort, while some examples, for instance in obstetric care, do exist.[51] Some scholars argue that in health care the quality or competence of teams is more important than those of individuals,[52] but teams do not graduate from programs and are not licensed to practice. To link individual competence to the products in health care, it has been suggested that contribution analysis may be used to determine each individual's contribution to the team outcome.[53,54] Resident-sensitive or trainee-attributable quality measures are being explored, developed, and researched for WBA linked to EPAs[27,55]; more research and development needs to be done before these measures can be used for product evaluation.

Summative entrustment decision-making in clinical competency committees can include, besides observations and discussions, an assessment of products of care, but that means these should be made visible to the assessors. As with other elements of WBA, this requires a two-stage procedure: formative evaluation with feedback to trainees and documentation in a portfolio, and weighing of these for summative decisions by the decision-making team.

Documentation

WBAs conducted in daily clinical practice must be documented to enable data aggregation, and support validity and transparency in summative entrustment decision-making. The ambition of programmatic assessment, combined with the constraints of a clinical environment, is high-quality, efficient documentation. Electronic portfolios and mobile apps[56] now facilitate realization of these ambitions through dashboards that systematically synthesize multiple sources of information. Technology should cause minimal disruption to clinical workflow, not only to minimize additional effort but also to maintain the authenticity of the workplace context. Oral feedback can be recorded, transcribed, sent to portfolios,[57] and aggregated with scores to produce insightful visual displays for program directors and competency committees. Rating forms must include carefully designed questions and items,[8] to optimize the response process by observers without requiring instruction that is too detailed. Other chapters discuss the use of rating scales (Chapter 19) and technology support (Chapter 20) for WBA more deeply. Narrative information is becoming more prominent in WBA, both for feedback conversations and for documentation to support summative decisions by the educational team.[58] New advances in learning analytics and AI are likely to optimize conclusions and decisions about trainees and programs in the near future.[53–55]

Feedback

Assessment, evaluation, feedback, and teaching in the workplace cannot be disentangled. Recommendations to separate coaching and mentoring from assessment to improve objectivity[59] are debatable, simply because a preceptor or tutor has more relevant knowledge about a trainee's readiness for entrustment than does an independent assessor, who may not know the trainee well enough. Role conflicts between assessing versus coaching are better resolved by: (a) regarding direct observation as low stakes and formative; (b) requiring feedback conversations to be more than providing comments and support improvement as an inherent component of observation; (c) leaving high-stakes decision-making regarding progress and summative entrustment to an educational team; (d) involving trainees in the assessment process as much as possible through feedback conversations; and (e) cocreation of developmental paths. Assessment in the clinical workplace is largely meant to support learning[60–62] as a continuous endeavor, and only use distinct moments for making summative decisions.

Faculty development

Skills increase with training and deliberate practice.[63] That is true for clinical skills as well as skills for observation and assessment of trainees. Experts easily forget how much clinical practice experience is needed to gain expertise;[b] this holds similarly to observation and assessment. Faculty development for observing and evaluating trainees must be supplemented with regular, deliberate assessment practice.

Assessment is not only done by clinical supervisors but also by peers (e.g., residents evaluating medical students) and others in the clinical environment, such as for multisource feedback. While the recommendation is to create procedures that are simple and self-explanatory, instruction and training are also needed for high-quality observation and feedback,[19] including so-called 'frame-of-reference' training, where the educational team shares norms and criteria to build the quality of their judgments. Chapter 23 provides more information on faculty development.

Conclusion

WBA with the purpose to support summative entrustment decision-making needs to draw on various sources of information available in the clinical workplace. The collection of this information should happen as an integral component of daily clinical business and belongs to the culture of any clinical setting that is responsible for educating health professionals. Four sources of information (direct observation, longitudinal observation, conversations, and evaluation of care produced by trainees) all have their place in a program of assessment, one of the important components of competency-based education.[65]

Figure justifications

Figure 17.1 is derived from Miller (1990).[1]

---

[b] As an example, machine learning studies reveal that up to 100,000 annotated specimens in nephropathology may be needed before an algorithm has learned to recognize a glomerulus;[64] senior pathologists may forget how many they saw to become an expert.

Competing interests

The authors declare that they have no competing interests.

References

1. Miller GE. The assessment of clinical skills/competence/performance. *Acad Med.* 1990;65(9 Suppl):S63-S67. DOI: https://doi.org/10.1097/00001888-199009000-00045
2. Norcini J, Burch V. Workplace-based assessment as an educational tool: AMEE guide no. 31. *Med Teach.* 2007;29(9):855–871. DOI: https://doi.org/10.1080/01421590701775453
3. Norcini JJ, Zaidi Z. Workplace-based assessment. In: Swanwick T, Forrest K, O'Brien B, eds. *Understanding Medical Education.* 3rd ed. Wiley; 2018:319–334.
4. Holmboe ES, Yamazaki K, Hamstra SJ. The evolution of assessment: thinking longitudinally and developmentally. *Acad Med.* 2020;95(11S):S7-S9. DOI: https://doi.org/10.1097/ACM.0000000000003649
5. Govaerts MJB, van der Vleuten CPM, Schuwirth LWT, Muijtjens AMM. Broadening perspectives on clinical performance assessment: rethinking the nature of in-training assessment. *Adv Health Sci Educ Theory Pract.* 2007;12(2):239–260. DOI: https://doi.org/10.1007/s10459-006-9043-1
6. Ryan MS, Gielissen KA, Shin D, et al. How well do workplace-based assessments support summative entrustment decisions? A multi-institutional generalisability study. *Med Educ.* January 2, 2024. DOI: https://doi.org/10.1111/medu.15291
7. Moonen-van Loon JMW, Overeem K, Donkers HHLM, van der Vleuten CPM, Driessen EW. Composite reliability of a workplace-based assessment toolbox for postgraduate medical education. *Adv Health Sci Educ Theory Pract.* 2013;18(5):1087–1102. DOI: https://doi.org/10.1007/s10459-013-9450-z
8. Crossley J, Johnson G, Booth J, Wade W. Good questions, good answers: construct alignment improves the performance of workplace-based assessment scales. *Med Educ.* 2011;45(6):560–569. DOI: https://doi.org/10.1111/j.1365-2923.2010.03913.x
9. ten Cate O, Carraccio C, Damodaran A, et al. Entrustment decision-making: extending Miller's pyramid. *Acad Med.* 2021;96(2):199–204. DOI: https://doi.org/10.1097/ACM.0000000000003800
10. Schumacher DJ, Michelson C, Winn AS, Turner DA, Martini A, Kinnear B. A realist synthesis of prospective entrustment decision-making by entrustment or clinical competency committees. *Med Educ.* December 13, 2023. DOI: https://doi.org/10.1111/medu.15296
11. van Manen M. *Pedagogical Tact - Knowing What to Do When You Don't Know What to Do.* Routledge; 2016. DOI: https://doi.org/10.4324/9781315422855
12. ten Cate O, Schwartz A, Chen HC. Assessing trainees and making entrustment decisions: on the nature and use of entrustment-supervision scales. *Acad Med.* 2020;95(11):1662–1669. DOI: https://doi.org/10.1097/ACM.0000000000003427
13. ten Cate O, Hart D, Ankel F, et al. Entrustment decision-making in clinical training. *Acad Med.* 2016;91(2):191–198. DOI: https://doi.org/10.1097/ACM.0000000000001044
14. Hauer KE, O'Sullivan PS, Fitzhenry K, Boscardin C. Translating theory into practice: implementing a program of assessment. *Acad Med.* 2018;93(3):444–450. DOI: https://doi.org/10.1097/ACM.0000000000001995
15. ten Cate O, Chen HC. The ingredients of a rich entrustment decision. *Med Teach.* 2020;42(12):1413–1420. DOI: https://doi.org/10.1080/0142159X.2020.1817348
16. ten Cate O, Chen HC, Hoff RG, Peters H, Bok H, van der Schaaf M. Curriculum development for the workplace using entrustable professional activities (EPAs): AMEE guide no. 99. *Med Teach.* 2015;37(11):983–1002. DOI: https://doi.org/10.3109/0142159X.2015.1060308

17. McBride ME, Adler MD, McGaghie WC. Workplace-based assessment. In: Yudkowsky R, Park YS, Downing SM, eds. *Assessment in Health Professions Education*. 2nd ed. Routledge; 2020:160–172.
18. Kogan JR, Holmboe ES, Hauer KE. Tools for direct observation and assessment of clinical skills of medical trainees - a systematic review. *JAMA*. 2009;302(12):1316–1326.
19. Kogan JR, Hatala R, Hauer KE, Holmboe E. Guidelines: the do's, don'ts and don't knows of direct observation of clinical skills in medical education. *Perspect Med Educ*. 2017;6(5):286–305. DOI: https://doi.org/10.1007/s40037-017-0376-7
20. Holmboe ES, Durning SJ, eds. *Assessment of Clinical Competence*. 3rd ed. Elsevier; 2025.
21. ten Cate O, Hoff RG. From case-based to entrustment-based discussions. *Clin Teach*. 2017;14(6):385–389. DOI: https://doi.org/10.1111/tct.12710
22. Irby DM, Wilkerson L. Teaching when time is limited. *BMJ*. 2008;336(7640):384–387. DOI: https://doi.org/10.1136/bmj.39456.727199.AD
23. Lockyer J. Multisource feedback in the assessment of physician competencies. *J Contin Educ Health Prof*. 2003;23(1):4–12. DOI: https://doi.org/10.1002/chp.1340230103
24. Alofs L, Huiskes J, Heineman MJ, et al. User reception of a simple online multisource feedback tool for residents. *Perspect Med Educ*. 2015;4(2):57–65. DOI: https://doi.org/10.1007/s40037-015-0173-0
25. Buis CAM, Eckenhausen MAW, ten Cate O. Processing multisource feedback during residency under the guidance of a non-medical coach. *Int J Med Educ*. 2018;9:48–54. DOI: https://doi.org/10.5116/ijme.5a7f.169d
26. Fava GA, Tomba E, Sonino N. Clinimetrics: the science of clinical measurements. *Int J Clin Pract*. 2012;66(1):11–15. DOI: https://doi.org/10.1111/j.1742-1241.2011.02825.x
27. Schumacher DJ, Holmboe ES, van der Vleuten C, Busari JO, Carraccio C. Developing resident-sensitive quality measures: a model from pediatric emergency medicine. *Acad Med*. 2018;93(7):1071–1078. DOI: https://doi.org/10.1097/ACM.0000000000002093
28. Gofton WT, Dudek NL, Wood TJ, Balaa F, Hamstra SJ. The Ottawa Surgical Competency Operating Room Evaluation (O-SCORE): a tool to assess surgical competence. *Acad Med*. 2012;87(10):1401–1407. DOI: https://doi.org/10.1097/ACM.0b013e3182677805
29. Zwischenberger JB, Hatchett SP, Rahman NA, Chadha P, Sebok-Syer SS, George BC. Implementing workplace-based assessments at scale: The SIMPL approach. *Ann Surg Open*. 2023;4(4):e353. DOI: https://doi.org/10.1097/AS9.0000000000000353
30. Holmboe ES, Osman NY, Murphy CM, Kogan JR. The urgency of now: rethinking and improving assessment practices in medical education programs. *Acad Med*. 2023;98(8S):S37-s49. DOI: https://doi.org/10.1097/ACM.0000000000005251
31. Burch V. The changing landscape of workplace-based assessment. *Journal of Applied Testing Technology*. 2019;20(S2):37–59.
32. Park YS, Hicks PJ, Carraccio C, Margolis M, Schwartz A, PMAC Module 2 Study Group. Does incorporating a measure of clinical workload improve workplace-based assessment scores? Insights for measurement precision and longitudinal score growth from ten pediatrics residency programs. *Acad Med*. 2018;93(11S):S21-S29. DOI: https://doi.org/10.1097/ACM.0000000000002381
33. ten Cate O. The false dichotomy of quality and quantity in the discourse around assessment in competency-based education. *Adv Health Sci Educ Theory Pract*. 2015;20(3):835–838. DOI: https://doi.org/10.1007/s10459-014-9527-3
34. Harvey A, Paget M, McLaughlin K, et al. How much is enough? Proposing achievement thresholds for core EPAs of graduating medical students in Canada. *Med Teach*. 2023;45(9):1054–1060. DOI: https://doi.org/10.1080/0142159X.2023.2215910
35. Holleran C, Konrad J, Norton B, Burlis T, Ambler S. Use of learner-driven, formative, ad-hoc, prospective assessment of competence in physical therapist clinical education in the United States: a prospective cohort study. *J Educ Eval Health Prof*. 2023;20:36. DOI: https://doi.org/10.3352/jeehp.2023.20.36

36. Albanese MA. Challenges in using rater judgements in medical education. *J Eval Clin Pract.* 2000;6(3):305–319. DOI: https://doi.org/10.1046/j.1365-2753.2000.00253.x
37. Ras T, Stander Jenkins L, Lazarus C, et al. 'We just don't have the resources': supervisor perspectives on introducing workplace-based assessments into medical specialist training in South Africa. *BMC Med Educ.* 2023;23(1):832. DOI: https://doi.org/10.1186/s12909-023-04840-x
38. Cheung K, Rogoza C, Chung AD, Kwan BYM. Analyzing the administrative burden of competency based medical education. *Can Assoc Radiol J.* 2022;73(2):299–304. DOI: https://doi.org/10.1177/08465371211038963
39. Ott MC, Pack R, Cristancho S, Chin M, Van Koughnett JA, Ott M. 'The most crushing thing': understanding resident assessment burden in a competency-based curriculum. *J Grad Med Educ.* 2022;14(5):583–592. DOI: https://doi.org/10.4300/JGME-D-22-00050.1
40. Ahn E, LaDonna KA, Landreville JM, Mcheimech R, Cheung WJ. Only as strong as the weakest link: resident perspectives on entrustable professional activities and their impact on learning. *J Grad Med Educ.* 2023;15(6):676–684. DOI: https://doi.org/10.4300/JGME-D-23-00204.1
41. Schut S, Maggio LA, Heeneman S, van Tartwijk J, van der Vleuten C, Driessen E. Where the rubber meets the road - an integrative review of programmatic assessment in health care professions education. *Perspect Med Educ.* 2021;10(1):6–13. DOI: https://doi.org/10.1007/s40037-020-00625-w
42. Rencic J, Schuwirth LWT, Gruppen LD, Durning SJ. A situated cognition model for clinical reasoning performance assessment: a narrative review. *Diagnosis (Berl).* 2020;7(3):227–240. DOI: https://doi.org/10.1515/dx-2019–0106
43. Pascoe JM, Nixon J, Lang VJ. Maximizing teaching on the wards: review and application of the One-Minute Preceptor and SNAPPS models. *J Hosp Med.* 2015;10(2):125–130. DOI: https://doi.org/10.1002/jhm.2302
44. Boursicot K, Roberts TE, Burdick WP. Structured assessment of clinical skills. In: Swanwick T, Forrest K, O'Brien BC, eds. *Understanding Medical Education.* 3rd ed. John Wiley & Sons Inc; 2019:335–346.
45. LaDonna KA, Hatala R, Lingard L, Voyer S, Watling C. Staging a performance: learners' perceptions about direct observation during residency. *Med Educ.* 2017;51(5):498–510. DOI: https://doi.org/10.1111/medu.13232
46. Lockyer J. Multisource feedback. In: Holmboe ES, Durning SJ, Hawkins RE, eds. *Evaluation of Clinical Competence.* 2nd ed. Elsevier; 2018:204–214.
47. ten Cate O. Entrustability of professional activities and competency-based training. *Med Educ.* 2005;39(12):1176–1177. DOI: https://doi.org/10.1111/j.1365-2929.2005.02341.x
48. Taylor DR, Park YS, Egan R, et al. EQual, a novel rubric to evaluate entrustable professional activities for quality and structure. *Acad Med.* 2017;92(11S Association of American Medical Colleges Learn Serve Lead: Proceedings of the 56th Annual Research in Medical Education Sessions):S110-S117. DOI: https://doi.org/10.1097/ACM.0000000000001908
49. Kirkpatrick DL, Kirkpatrick JD. *Evaluating Training Programs: The Four Levels.* 3rd ed. Berrett-Koehler Publishers, Inc; 2006.
50. Yardley S, Dornan T. Kirkpatrick's levels and education 'evidence.' *Med Educ.* 2012;46(1):97–106. DOI: https://doi.org/10.1111/j.1365-2923.2011.04076.x
51. Epstein AJ, Nicholson S, Asch DA. The production of and market for new physicians' skill. *American Journal of Health Economics.* 2016;2(1):41–65. DOI: https://doi.org/10.1162/AJHE_a_00033
52. Lingard LA. Rethinking competence in the context of teamwork. In: Hodges BD, Lingard L, eds. *The Question of Competence: Reconsidering Medical Education in the Twenty-First Century.* Cornell University Press; 2012.

53. ten Cate O, Carrie Chen H. The parts, the sum and the whole - evaluating students in teams. *Med Teach.* 2016;38(7):639–641. DOI: https://doi.org/10.3109/0142159X.2016.1170794
54. Schumacher DJ, Dornoff E, Carraccio C, et al. The power of contribution and attribution in assessing educational outcomes for individuals, teams, and programs. *Acad Med.* 2020;95(7):1014–1019. DOI: https://doi.org/10.1097/ACM.0000000000003121
55. Schumacher DJ, Kinnear B, Burk-Rafel J, Santen SA, Bullock JL. The next era of assessment: can ensuring high-quality, equitable patient care be the defining characteristic? *Acad Med.* December 18, 2023. DOI: https://doi.org/10.1097/ACM.0000000000005603
56. Marty AP, Linsenmeyer M, George B, Young JQ, Breckwoldt J, ten Cate O. Mobile technologies to support workplace-based assessment for entrustment decisions: guidelines for programs and educators: AMEE guide no. 154. *Med Teach.* 2023;45(11):1203–1213. DOI: https://doi.org/10.1080/0142159X.2023.2168527
57. Young JQ, McClure M. Fast, easy, and good: assessing entrustable professional activities in psychiatry residents with a mobile app. *Acad Med.* 2020;95(10):1546–1549. DOI: https://doi.org/10.1097/ACM.0000000000003390
58. Cook DA, Kuper A, Hatala R, Ginsburg S. When assessment data are words: validity evidence for qualitative educational assessments. *Acad Med.* 2016;91(10):1359–1369. DOI: https://doi.org/10.1097/ACM.0000000000001175
59. Cavalcanti RB, Detsky AS. The education and training of future physicians - why coaches can't be judges. *JAMA.* 2011;306(9):993–994.
60. Schuwirth LWT, Van der Vleuten CPM. Programmatic assessment: from assessment of learning to assessment for learning. *Med Teach.* 2011;33(6):478–485. DOI: https://doi.org/10.3109/0142159X.2011.565828
61. Wiliam D. What is assessment for learning? *Studies in Educational Evaluation.* 2011;37(1): 3–14. DOI: https://doi.org/10.1016/j.stueduc.2011.03.001
62. Castanelli D. Sociocultural learning theory and assessment for learning. *Med Educ.* 2023;57(5):382–384. DOI: https://doi.org/10.1111/medu.15028
63. Ericsson KA, Krampe RT, Tesch-Römer C. The role of deliberate practice in the acquisition of expert performance. *Psychol Rev.* 1993;100(3):363–406. DOI: https://doi.org/10.1037/0033-295X.100.3.363
64. Fogo AB, Kronbichler A, Bajema IM. AI's threat to the medical profession. *JAMA.* 2024;331(6):471–472. DOI: https://doi.org/10.1001/jama.2024.0018
65. Van Melle E, Frank JR, Holmboe ES, et al. A core components framework for evaluating implementation of competency-based medical education programs. *Acad Med.* 2019;94(7):1002–1009. DOI: https://doi.org/10.1097/ACM.0000000000002743

CHAPTER 18

Entrustment with health care tasks: balancing trainee autonomy, supervision, and patient safety

Gersten Jonker, Jennifer M. Klasen, Marije P. Hennus, Jacqueline de Graaf, Daniel J. Schumacher, Olle ten Cate

Abstract

For entrustment with unsupervised practice, an ultimate goal of health care education, modulating trainee autonomy during training is necessary and critical. Trainees benefit from experiencing autonomy during clinical training, but patient safety necessitates restrictions. Balancing these two must be modulated by titrating supervision to an adequate intensity. The patient, trainee, and supervisor constitute a triad in the workplace that revolves around safe and effective provision of health care tasks and effective education. In forming an 'educational alliance' with the trainee, the supervisor adjusts their role, based on the trainee's needs and desires, variations in practice, patient safety considerations, and the trainee's developmental stage. Programs that capitalize on entrustable professional activities and entrustment decision-making have a deliberate focus on the conditions for entrustment of trainees with health care tasks.

Entrustment decisions about trainee autonomy happen in daily clinical practice in teaching hospitals as ad hoc decisions, sometimes implicit and unarticulated, but often deliberate and negotiated in sound educational trainee–supervisor alliances.

Summative entrustment decisions, made by a team and grounded in adequate assessment data, are meant to formally privilege the trainee for future task execution with increased autonomy, within the restrictions by rules and regulations.

A solid summative entrustment decision process allows for defensible adjustments in responsibility and accountability, and backs supervisors in applying appropriate supervision levels. Entrustment with tasks after established readiness for autonomous performance is educationally advantageous and could have a positive impact on patient safety.

How to cite this book chapter:
Jonker G, Klasen J, Hennus MP, de Graaf J, Schumacher DJ, ten Cate O. Entrustment with health care tasks: balancing trainee autonomy, supervision, and patient safety. In: ten Cate O, Burch VC, Chen HC, Chou FC, Hennus MP (Eds). *Entrustable Professional Activities and Entrustment Decision-Making in Health Professions Education*, Chapter 18, pp. 213–223. [2024] London: Ubiquity Press. DOI: https://doi.org/10.5334/bdc.r

Authors

- Gersten Jonker, MD, PhD. University Medical Center Utrecht, Utrecht, the Netherlands.
- Jennifer M. Klasen, MD, PhD, MME. St. Claraspital and University Hospital Basel, Basel, Switzerland.
- Marije P. Hennus, MD, PhD, MSc Clin Ed. University Medical Center Utrecht, Utrecht, the Netherlands.
- Jacqueline de Graaf, MD, PhD. Radboud University Medical Center, Nijmegen, the Netherlands.
- Daniel J. Schumacher, MD, PhD, MEd. Cincinnati Children's Hospital Medical Center/ University of Cincinnati College of Medicine, Cincinnati, Ohio, USA.
- Olle ten Cate, PhD. University Medical Center Utrecht, Utrecht, the Netherlands and University of California, San Francisco, USA.

Introduction

The postgraduate medical education reform movement in the 1990s was in part born out of major concerns about patient safety. The 1984 death of 18-year-old Libby Zion, daughter of a well-known New York prosecutor and journalist, resulted from unsupervised care by overworked junior residents in a busy lengthy shift. This led to regulations aimed at ensuring adequate supervision and capping resident duty hours, first in New York and, in 2003, nationally in the USA.[1,2] In the wake of this incident and with the Institute of Medicine's *To Err Is Human* and other reports,[3,4] the question of what postgraduate trainees were actually allowed to do became prominent, constraining trainee autonomy and making attending specialists much more active. This North American trend affected medical training elsewhere but has been most prominent in Canada and the USA.

Following these changes, some studies showed that patient safety and trainee well-being indeed improved, but education did not.[5] In fact, graduating residents seemed less prepared for unsupervised work, paradoxically jeopardizing patient safety after training.[6,7] Even the US Accreditation Council for Graduate Medical Education (ACGME), which determines rules for duty hours and program execution, now signals that the decrease in autonomy and the 'seniorization' of resident tasks is becoming worrisome.[8] There are many examples across several specialties[8] of tasks that can easily be envisioned as entrustable professional activities (EPAs, even if not called by that name) and where evidently entrustment is lacking. However, recent studies in surgery suggest that the decrease in resident autonomy across decades has not improved patient outcomes.[9–11] Trainees who do not experience a sufficient sense of responsibility and autonomy before completion of training will face challenges after training in bearing responsibility in unsupervised practice. A proper balance, or sweet spot, must be achieved, to secure both patient safety and educational value, including an experience of graded autonomy in patient care.

EPAs, defined as units of professional practice to be entrusted to trainees,[12] provide a way to organize autonomy in a curriculum with the aim to unite patient safety and educational needs in order to reestablish the right balance.

Supervision is key in this balance and can be defined as '[t]he provision of guidance and support in learning and working effectively in health care by observing and directing the execution of tasks or activities to ensure that they are done correctly and safely, from a position of being in charge.'[13]

This chapter explores the link between trainee autonomy, entrustment of health care tasks, and patient safety. The chapter elaborates on the triad of patient, trainee, and supervisor, on types of entrustment decisions, and on barriers and enablers of entrustment in the workplace.

The authors are aware of the gaps between potential benefits and current evidence, or between ideals and current practice. This chapter aims to provide guidelines for safe health care task entrustment.

The patient, trainee, and supervisor triad

In balancing safety and autonomy, three actors assume a role: the patient, the trainee, and the supervisor. The dynamics of their intricate and triadic interplay revolve around the axis of safety of health care tasks. The patient, assuming the key role, is not just the focus of health care intervention but is also vital in trainee learning and development. The trainee, in turn, is challenged to embrace autonomy and cultivate a sense of responsibility while often working at the edge of their competence. The supervisor takes the role of the navigator of the scenario, uniting patient safety and trainee learning. While navigating, the supervisor must balance roles of teacher, assessor, and patient guardian, while not micromanaging clinical teaching situations at the same time.[14]

During clinical work, the supervisor titrates trainee guidance and support by choosing and switching between observing and (re)directing. The supervisor incorporates teaching opportunities into routine patient encounters, pausing throughout exchanges to provide brief explanations, clarify concepts, or explore evidence-based treatments. By grabbing these teachable moments, skilled supervisors maximize learning opportunities within patient care, transforming it into an integrated process that actively secures that training *contributes* to patient safety, rather than compromising it.[15]

The supervisor continuously adapts the degree of trainee autonomy, drawing upon experience and intuition (i.e., their gut feeling about readiness of a trainee to take over) in permitting autonomy versus deciding to 'step in.'[15,16] In granting autonomy, the supervisor acknowledges an acceptable variability in practice and even allows for mistakes, while constantly judging the boundaries that guarantee patient safety.[15]

Trainee development and graded autonomy are often depicted as linear or curvilinear. On average, this may be true; however, for individual trainees learning curves are much more haphazard.[16] Pushed by a myriad of interacting variables influenced by supervisors, trainees, and patients within the complexity of workplace learning, development and autonomy cannot evolve linearly. Building on earlier work defining five factors that contribute to decisions on how much trust is granted, and thus how much autonomy is allowed (trainee, supervisor, context, relationship and task),[17,18] we propose to add 'patient' as a separate factor (Table 18.1). Although the patient is often regarded as a component of the task,[18] in daily ad hoc entrustment decisions, patient variables weigh in (clinical characteristics, complexity, acuity, and patient preference), irrespective of the particular task.

The nonlinearity of development adds depth to the understanding how learning occurs in unpredictable, changing contexts.[15] Amid these complexities, the educational alliance of trainee and supervisor emerges as a linchpin, binding the triad together. It represents a collaborative effort where trust is not only in the clinical abilities of the trainee but also in the shared commitment to quality care and patient safety. The educational alliance fosters an environment where the trainee can learn, make mistakes, and grow,[20] while the supervisor navigates the fine line between guidance and autonomy while guarding patient safety.

Entrustment: ad hoc and summative decisions

The Oxford English Dictionary[21] defines entrustment as assigning the responsibility for something valued or important to someone. In health professions education, especially in competence-based education operationalized with EPAs, entrustment refers to granting autonomy to trainees to perform health care tasks without direct supervisory involvement, implying a degree of risk for patient safety. Entrustment can be ad hoc, conferred by a supervisor and specific to the moment, or summative, implying a more permanent and comprehensive decision.[22]

Ad hoc entrustment

Ad hoc decisions of entrustment, such as leaving an anesthesiology resident alone in the operating room,[23] can be deliberate, but are often implicit and unarticulated, made in the moment. Every day, clinical supervisors consider when and whether to allow a trainee to perform a particular task on their own. Conversely, trainees face tasks at the edge of their competence and consider whether to perform it autonomously or ask for supervisor guidance and support. In all these decisions, the safety of the patient is of high importance.

Table 18.1: Factors influencing degree of ad hoc trainee autonomy allowed in performing health care tasks.

Factor	Examples
Trainee	Learning need, agency, reliability, integrity, capability, humility[19]
Supervisor	Clinical ability, clinical experience, supervisory expertise, propensity to trust, identification of learning opportunity
Supervisor–trainee relationship	Degree of acquaintance, like-mindedness, prior collaborative experience, interpretation and negotiation of applied supervision
Patient	Clinical characteristics, complexity, acuity, preference, socioeconomic status, language, etc.
Task (patient independent)	General difficulty of the task, general risks of the task
Context	Abilities of team members, opportunity to intervene quickly, need for hands/staffing, time of the day, institutional culture of delegating work to trainees

In a productive educational alliance, trainee and supervisor negotiate the appropriate level of supervision and autonomy for a particular task. Intentional ad hoc entrustment decisions are part of a deliberate educational approach[24] belonging to the core components of CBME (i.e., tailored learning experiences and sequenced progression).[25] Typically, a supervisor making an ad hoc entrustment decision relies on a combination of the estimated trustworthiness of the trainee, the perceived risk of the situation, the urgency of the task, patient characteristics, and the appropriateness of the assigned task for the trainee at that specific moment (see Table 18.1).[26] Typically, an ad hoc entrustment decision is a situational, short-term prospective decision for a single occasion.

After an ad hoc entrustment decision, the situation may be evaluated by trainee and supervisor in a feedback conversation. From a patient perspective, ad hoc decisions may be high-stakes, but from the perspective of trainee progression they are low-stakes and formative; their evaluation is one data point in the trainee's portfolio. Even in low-stakes assessments, using an entrustment–supervision scale[27] forces supervisors to determine the appropriate supervision level for future occurrences of similar ad hoc entrustment situations. This prospective thinking incorporates risk estimations for future performance and thus takes patient safety into account. Ad hoc entrustments do not imply precedents but do, in aggregate, inform a summative entrustment decision. Multiple low-stakes assessments of multiple occasions by multiple assessors with multiple assessment tools collectively paint a fuller picture of trainee performance. As such, assessments of ad hoc entrustment decisions contribute to summative entrustment decisions endorsing readiness for unsupervised practice.

Summative entrustment

In contrast with ad hoc entrustment, a summative entrustment decision is not made by a single supervisor. In a program that provides significant curricular ownership to trainees, they should know when they are ready for a next step and should proactively request formalized, summative entrustment for a unit of professional practice. Such decisions are deliberately made by a program director with their clinical competency committee and are grounded in thorough evaluation of sufficiency and relevance of assessment data points, including evaluations of ad hoc entrustment decisions collected from various assessors over time.[26] A summative entrustment decision is designed to result in the certification and privileging of the trainee for future task execution with a specified level of supervision.[26] The decision results in tangible adjustments to the official permissions granted to a trainee at a specific level of supervision. The supervisory team should be compelled to enact the decrease in supervisor involvement.

In contrast with ad hoc decisions, when all factors of Table 18.1 weigh in, summative entrustment decisions focus largely on trainee factors.[25] Decision-makers can use five key groups of trainee features, succinctly captured by the mnemonic 'A RICH': agency (proactivity toward work, team, safety, personal development), reliability (conscientious, predictable, accountable, responsible), integrity (truthful, benevolent, patient-centered), capability (task-specific knowledge, skills, experience, situational awareness), and humility (recognizes limits, asks for help, receptive to feedback).[19]

A summative entrustment decision goes beyond assessing current performance of an EPA. It extrapolates to cover the spectrum of EPA manifestations, also under unfamiliar conditions, and implies trust in the trainee's future performance. When a trainee is entrusted with an EPA without supervision, the entrustment not only extends beyond the moment of the decision but also has implications well beyond graduation into practice.[28] Entrustment decisions are not merely an attestation of achievement of competence, nor of the end-of-training, but a high-stakes statement of trust in the trainee to provide safe and high-quality care within the scope of the EPA.

Formalizing summative entrustment

Being summatively entrusted with an EPA in patient care should be translated into language in a way that both the trainee and their environment are clear about the trainee's privileges. Statement of awarded responsibility (STAR) has been proposed as term[29] for this qualification or authorization. To allow for time-variable progression in a time-fixed model, the recently introduced concept of promotion-in-place (PiP) seems promising.[30] PiP provides residents who are deemed competent early with a status of 'sheltered independence' while still in training. While PiP regards the readiness for the full breadth of a specialty, STARs are a similar approach for smaller units, i.e., EPAs.[22]

Barriers to and enablers of entrustment during education

The educational philosophy of EPAs and entrustment decisions implies relevant consequences for the entitlement to practice patient care when the readiness for a decrease in supervision is established. This should translate to progressive responsibilities in patient care and a gradual decrease in supervision.

Supervision is crucial and supervisors have dual obligations: to provide learning opportunities and to guard patient safety. From a position of being in charge, the supervisor has the power and obligation to grant and restrict a trainee's autonomy and vary the level of supervision based on their judgments and preferences.

The restriction of responsibility arises further from various regulations, issued by several authorities that set limitations to patient care practice by trainees. In the tensions between educational wishes and regulatory restrictions, the following parties exercise their formal duties (Table 18.2; similar examples can be found in nursing and other health professions with restricted privileges).

Table 18.2: Institutions that have the power to restrict trainee autonomy.

Authority	Role and power	Examples
The law	The law gives patients the option to sue care providers in case of substandard care	The medical license prohibits medical practice by unqualified individuals
Medical boards	Medical and specialty boards certify and can withdraw certification, which de facto affects the possibility to practice	A supervising physician is found to be intoxicated while working clinically with medical students and residents, and the medical board for their jurisdiction suspends their medical license
Hospitals, clinics, and medical centers	Clinical employers issue privileges for all health care professional employees and can restrict or terminate employment if these agreements are breached	A supervising surgeon is repeatedly not in the operating room or even able to be found while surgical residents are operating on patients, leading their medical privileges to be limited before being revoked if compliance with hospital rules for supervising trainees is not met
Insurance companies	Insurance companies set conditions for reimbursement of costs, and usually exclude trainees as independent care providers	A rural hospital employing an emergency medicine resident (licensed, but not yet board-certified) who moonlights in emergency medicine to supplement salary is unable to charge professional fees for moonlighting work, nor is the resident
Accreditors of hospitals and educational programs	Accreditors set standards. Breaches of these may lead to loss of accreditation status of a hospital or educational program	The US ACGME, and the 'Joint Commission' accredit graduate medical education and hospitals respectively; Box 18.1 shows the JC standard for supervision of trainees

The ACGME in the USA distinguishes in its common program requirements—in contrast to the five general levels of supervision used throughout this book—three levels of supervision they deem most germane to postgraduate training: direct (supervisor present with trainee and patient), indirect (supervisor not present but quickly available), and oversight (supervisor available to review after care is delivered).[31] The trainee's individual level of training and patient complexity and acuity must factor into decisions regarding the level of supervision provided, ensuring that the supervision is appropriate for each patient.

The supervisor is pivotal in the process, having the final responsibility and liability as long as a trainee has not received an unrestricted license, a training certificate,[c] or a specialty certification. This makes entrustment decisions significant. In a process where valid summative entrustment decisions are made by a team, grounded in sufficient data and deliberation, a supervisor should feel backed to lean on that process. When adverse events happen after a summative entrustment decision for a particular EPA has been made (e.g., 'the resident may now run the Wednesday-morning clinic'), the supervisor in charge of the care for particular patients may still be liable but should be able to adequately defend the basis for the trust in the trainee, and the adverse event may reflect a happening that could have occurred with any attending professional. However, the fact that a medical malpractice lawsuit may attempt to place responsibility on the attending

---

[c] In the USA, residents in accredited programs are licensed to practice through a *training certificate*. This permits them to practice under supervision until fully licensed. Residents can seek a full license before the end of residency, depending on personal or institutional priorities (https://www.ama-assn.org).

Box 18.1: Case example from the Joint Commission's Standards for accredited hospitals (2012).[32]

Standard MPE.4: 'The [health care] organization understands and provides the required frequency and intensity of medical supervision for each type and level of medical student and resident trainee.'

The required level of supervision is consistent with the level of training and level of competence of the medical student and resident trainee. Competence cannot be assumed and must be demonstrated early in the training program. A medical school student understands if supervision is provided by a resident or by the patient's primary physician or by a medical school faculty member. [Trainees] understand if the supervision includes daily signing of all notes and orders, or signing of the care plan and progress notes every other day or making a separate entry in the patient's record. There must be evidence of that supervision and uniform expectations for the mentoring/supervision process. Measurable elements of MPE.4 include (amongst others):

- Organization policy identifies the required level of supervision for each level of trainee.
- The level to be provided is based on the demonstrated competence of the trainee.
- Each trainee understands the level, frequency, and documentation of their supervision.
- The organization provides the required level of supervision for each trainee.
- Patient care records are reviewed for compliance with the requirements and frequency.

supervisory physician rather than the trainee who is deemed ready for less supervision can lead supervisors to provide more supervision than is needed. This can rob trainees of opportunities to care for patients with less supervision during training.

The regulations of accreditors (e.g., Box 18.1) align well with the levels of supervision used with entrustment decisions for EPAs. While supervisors have individual responsibilities and liabilities are based on various regulations, the space they have to exercise their education responsibility to offer trainees appropriate opportunities in patient care should be backed by the educational team or competency committee and the culture at the department or health care unit.

Conclusion

An entrustment decision in health professions education is a decision to trust a trainee to perform a health care task without direct supervisory presence.[33] This gives the patient a prominent position. The stakes of ad hoc entrustment decisions may be low with regard to trainee progress, yet they are high because of potential implications for patient safety.

The trainees attending to Libby Zion, discussed above, were not positioned to bear the responsibility for her care. In the context of a busy night shift, they were entrusted with her care with deficient supervision. One can—and, we would contend, should—argue that the supervisors were more to blame than the trainees. In a strong educational alliance, ad hoc entrustment decisions are explicit and intentional, taking risks for patient safety into account. Supervisors should weigh and accept practice variations and serve as guardrails, supporting trainees whenever needed and serving as a stopgap for mishaps whenever they can. The decision can be evaluated in a formative, prospective workplace assessment.

In contrast, a deliberate and defensible summative entrustment decision is made by the supervisory team, after establishing readiness, supported by valid assessment data. It is not primarily a decision that considers learner progress but entails an estimation of future performance and risk in a spectrum of circumstances. It is a high-stakes statement of trust in the trainee to provide safe and high-quality care within the scope of the EPA. These decisions should lead to formal changes in autonomy, responsibility, and accountability, even if a supervisor retains final responsibility. After a valid summative entrustment decision, adverse events can still happen, even among experts, and this does not necessarily imply a deficient decision. However, entrusting and transferring tasks only after established readiness for autonomous performance has a positive impact on patient safety.

Competing interests

The authors declare that they have no competing interests.

References

1. Leape LL. The girl who died twice: every patient's nightmare: the Libby Zion case and the hidden hazards of hospitals. *JAMA*. 1996;275(13):1031. DOI: https://doi.org/10.1001/jama.1996.03530370069035
2. Bell BM. Supervision, not regulation of hours, is the key to improving the quality of patient care. *JAMA*. 1993;269(3):403–404.
3. Institute of Medicine (US) Committee on Quality of Health Care in America. *To Err Is Human: Building a Safer Health System*. (Kohn LT, Corrigan JM, Donaldson MS, eds.). National Academies Press (US); 2000. DOI: https://doi.org/10.17226/9728
4. *Independent Inquiry into Care Provided by Mid Staffordshire NHS Foundation Trust: January 2005–March 2009*. The Stationery Office; 2010:815.
5. Fletcher KE, Reed DA, Arora VM. Patient safety, resident education and resident well-being following implementation of the 2003 ACGME duty hour rules. *J Gen Intern Med*. 2011;26(8):907–919. DOI: https://doi.org/10.1007/s11606-011-1657-1
6. Mattar SG, Alseidi AA, Jones DB, et al. General surgery residency inadequately prepares trainees for fellowship: results of a survey of fellowship program directors. *Ann Surg*. 2013;258(3):440–449. DOI: https://doi.org/10.1097/SLA.0b013e3182a191ca
7. Halpern SD, Detsky AS. Graded autonomy in medical education—managing things that go bump in the night. *N Engl J Med*. 2014;370(12):1086–1089. DOI: https://doi.org/10.1056/NEJMp1315408
8. Dacey RG, Nasca TJ. Seniorization of tasks in the academic medical center: a worrisome trend. *J Am Coll Surg*. 2019;228(3):299–302. DOI: https://doi.org/10.1016/j.jamcollsurg.2018.11.009
9. Oliver JB, McFarlane JL, Kunac A, Anjaria DJ. Declining resident surgical autonomy and improving surgical outcomes: correlation does not equal causality. *J Surg Educ*. 2023;80(3):434–441. DOI: https://doi.org/10.1016/j.jsurg.2022.10.009
10. Tonelli CM, Cohn T, Abdelsattar Z, Luchette FA, Baker MS. Association of resident independence with short-term clinical outcome in core general surgery procedures. *JAMA Surg*. 2023;158(3):302–309. DOI: https://doi.org/10.1001/jamasurg.2022.6971
11. Kunac A, Oliver JB, McFarlane JL, Anjaria DJ. General surgical resident operative autonomy vs patient outcomes: are we compromising training without net benefit to hospitals or patients? *J Surg Educ*. 2021;78(6):e174-e182. DOI: https://doi.org/10.1016/j.jsurg.2021.09.017

12. ten Cate O, Taylor DR. The recommended description of an entrustable professional activity: AMEE guide no. 140. *Med Teach.* 2021;43(10):1106–1114. DOI: https://doi.org/10.1080/0142159X.2020.1838465
13. ten Cate O. Supervision and entrustment in clinical training: protecting patients, protecting trainees. *WebM&M Case Studies https://psnet.ahrq.gov/webmm/case/461.* November 9, 2018:1.
14. Chan TM. The helicoptering attending: diagnosis & management of supervisory micromanagement. https://icenet.blog/2021/12/23/. December 23, 2021:1.
15. Klasen J. *Allowing Failure as an Unspoken Pedagogy in Residency Training.* PhD Thesis. Maastricht University; 2024.
16. Pusic MV, Boutis K, Hatala R, Cook DA. Learning curves in health professions education. *Acad Med.* 2015;90(8):1034–1042. DOI: https://doi.org/10.1097/ACM.0000000000000681
17. Dijksterhuis MG, Voorhuis M, Teunissen PW, et al. Assessment of competence and progressive independence in postgraduate clinical training. *Med Educ.* 2009;43(12):1156–1165. DOI: https://doi.org/10.1111/j.1365-2923.2009.03509.x
18. Hauer KE, ten Cate O, Boscardin C, Irby DM, Iobst W, O'Sullivan PS. Understanding trust as an essential element of trainee supervision and learning in the workplace. *Adv Health Sci Educ Theory Pract.* 2014;19(3):435–456. DOI: https://doi.org/10.1007/s10459-013-9474-4
19. ten Cate O, Chen HC. The ingredients of a rich entrustment decision. *Med Teach.* 2020;42(12):1413–1420. DOI: https://doi.org/10.1080/0142159X.2020.1817348
20. Telio S, Ajjawi R, Regehr G. The 'educational alliance' as a framework for reconceptualizing feedback in medical education. *Acad Med.* 2015;90(5):609–614. DOI: https://doi.org/10.1097/ACM.0000000000000560
21. Hughes AM. Oxford English Dictionary. *Isis.* 2008;99(3):586. DOI: https://doi.org/10.1086/593289
22. Sigurdsson V, ten Cate O. Do summative entrustment decisions actually lead to entrustment? *Clin Teach.* October 10, 2023:e13668. DOI: https://doi.org/10.1111/tct.13668
23. Weller JM, Misur M, Nicolson S, et al. Can I leave the theatre? A key to more reliable workplace-based assessment. *Br J Anaesth.* 2014;112(6):1083–1091. DOI: https://doi.org/10.1093/bja/aeu052
24. Conroy M, McCallister J, Gustin J. Entrustment decision-making in the intensive care unit: it's about more than the learner. *ATS Scholar.* October 11, 2023. DOI: https://doi.org/10.34197/ats-scholar.2023-0060OC
25. Van Melle E, Frank JR, Holmboe ES, et al. A core components framework for evaluating implementation of competency-based medical education programs. *Acad Med.* 2019;94(7):1002–1009. DOI: https://doi.org/10.1097/ACM.0000000000002743
26. ten Cate O, Hart D, Ankel F, et al. Entrustment decision-making in clinical training. *Acad Med.* 2016;91(2):191–198. DOI: https://doi.org/10.1097/ACM.0000000000001044
27. ten Cate O, Schwartz A, Chen HC. Assessing trainees and making entrustment decisions: on the nature and use of entrustment–supervision scales. *Acad Med.* 2020;95(11):1662–1669. DOI: https://doi.org/10.1097/ACM.0000000000003427
28. Touchie C, Kinnear B, Schumacher D, et al. On the validity of summative entrustment decisions. *Med Teach.* 2021;43(7):780–787. DOI: https://doi.org/10.1080/0142159X.2021.1925642
29. ten Cate O, Scheele F. Competency-based postgraduate training: can we bridge the gap between theory and clinical practice? *Acad Med.* 2007;82(6):542–547. DOI: https://doi.org/10.1097/ACM.0b013e31805559c7
30. Goldhamer MEJ, Pusic MV, Nadel ES, Co JPT, Weinstein DF. Promotion in place: a model for competency-based, time-variable graduate medical education. *Acad Med.* 2024;99(5):518–523. DOI: https://doi.org/10.1097/ACM.0000000000005652
31. NN. *Common Program Requirements (Residency).* Accreditation Council for Graduate Medical Education; 2023.

32. NN. Standards for academic medical center hospitals: medical education programs, clinical research programs. In: *Accreditation Standards Hospitals*. 4th ed. Joint Commission International; 2012:Suppl 1–24.
33. ten Cate O. Entrustment decisions: bringing the patient into the assessment equation. *Acad Med*. 2017;92(6):736–738. DOI: https://doi.org/10.1097/ACM.0000000000001623

CHAPTER 19

Scales, numbers, and words to support entrustment decisions about trainees

Vanessa C. Burch, Jacqueline de Graaf, Jennie B. Jarrett, Severin Pinilla, Alan Schwartz, Olle ten Cate

Abstract

This chapter focuses on reporting trainee performance in workplace-based assessment programs. Tools that translate observations into assessment documentation typically include several components of observed activities, or competencies, and rating scales with multiple gradations of proficiency. Over the past two decades, introduction of the concept of entrustment and entrustable professional activities has led educators to create scales that focus on the amount of supervision, support, or help trainees need to complete a workplace-based activity. More recently, entrustment–supervision (ES) scales have shifted the focus to reporting readiness for future activities, using specified levels of supervision to be recommended for trainees. This chapter describes the use of these scales for ad hoc and summative entrustment decision-making, including adaptations for profession-specific or context-specific circumstances and variable levels of trainee proficiency.

Scales for entrustment and supervision are more holistic than those for reporting observed behavior, and include both specific and general trainee features. Expert supervisor judgment includes an inherent subjective element, because experts show legitimate differences, but unwanted bias must be excluded. Narrative feedback comments can supplement and explain scale scores providing a holistic picture, guided by tools such as the 'A RICH' framework. Entrustment decisions are crucial in an EPA-based curriculum, and ES

How to cite this book chapter:

Burch VC, de Graaf J, Jarrett JB, Pinilla S, Schwartz A, ten Cate O. Scales, numbers, and words to support entrustment decisions about trainees. In: ten Cate O, Burch VC, Chen HC, Chou FC, Hennus MP. (Eds). *Entrustable Professional Activities and Entrustment Decision-Making in Health Professions Education*, Chapter 19, pp. 225–235. [2024] London: Ubiquity Press. DOI: https://doi.org/10.5334/bdc.s

This chapter uses cross-references to other chapters of the same book. For those who read this chapter as a standalone publication: all cross-references can be found at: https://doi.org/10.5334/bdc

scale values must be embedded in a program of assessment in which feedback conversations with trainees remain essential.

Authors

- Vanessa C. Burch, MD, PhD. Colleges of Medicine of South Africa, Cape Town, South Africa. Correspondence: vanessa.burch@cmsa.co.za
- Jacqueline de Graaf, MD, PhD. Radboud University Medical Center, Nijmegen, the Netherlands.
- Jennie B. Jarrett, PharmD, MMedEd, PhD. University of Illinois Chicago College of Pharmacy, Chicago, Illinois, USA.
- Severin Pinilla, MD, MEd, PhD. University Hospital of Old Age Psychiatry and Psychotherapy, Bern, Switzerland.
- Alan Schwartz, PhD, JD. University of Illinois Chicago, Chicago, Illinois, USA.
- Olle ten Cate, PhD. University Medical Center Utrecht, Utrecht, the Netherlands and University of California, San Francisco, USA.

Introduction

Reporting on the performance of trainees within a program of workplace-based assessment requires tools that translate observations into assessment documentation. This chapter explores the evolving conversation about such documentation, specifically the concept of entrustment with a focus on determining future supervision likely to be required by a trainee or licensed professional, rather than just reporting on currently observed competencies. The chapter also addresses the quantity of workplace-based observations needed, the role of narrative comments in holistic assessment decision-making, and the need to accommodate inherent expert observer subjectivity while remaining cognizant of unwanted bias. Finally, the chapter reflects on feedback that advances trainee autonomy in the workplace.

Traditional workplace-based assessment scales

Many paper forms and, more recently, digital forms have been proposed to document the performance of trainees in the workplace. These include, among many, the mini-CEX, direct observation of procedural skills (DOPS), and case-based discussion.[1] Common scales to assess performance often include three or four general values (below expectations–meets expectations–above expectations; or poor–marginal–good–excellent). Other examples use nine or 10 scale values with a cut-off between five and six for fail and pass. Scales can focus on a single dimension (how did the trainee do in general?) or pertain to several dimensions (history, physical examination, knowledge and reasoning, communication, professional conduct, or other) or combine a series of skills with an overall judgment. Rating forms often include ancillary information (names of ratee and rater, specialty, program year, setting, case complexity) and space for narrative feedback. The core purpose is to record the observed performance and report on trainee performance using the scale provided. As a record of observed performance, this is a retrospective report.

A common concern with these traditional performance assessment scales is eloquently illustrated by Crossley when he says:

> *[M]y judgement about the performance of my trainee, based on my interpretation of his performance, with a particular patient or client, with a particular problem, in a particular context today, is always highly meaningful, [but does] this judgement have anything to say about my judgement with the same trainee in a completely different context, or anyone's judgement about the same trainee in any context?*[2]

As Crossley contends, maybe we are asking the wrong questions to expect a reliable answer[3] and we should instead ask 'is this trainee ready for more autonomy?'[4]

Entrustment–supervision scales

Over the past two decades, introduction of the concept of entrustment and EPAs has led educators to create scales focusing on the amount of supervision, support, or help needed to complete an activity in the workplace. Entrustment–supervision (ES) scales differ from traditional scales in their focus on (a) entrustment with tasks and (b) level of supervision or support required.[5,6] ES scales reflect a shift in focus from the pursuit of 'objective proficiency ratings,' using predominantly numerical scales with brief anchoring statements, to decision-making about the level of supervision trainees require to safely complete workplace-based activities. From the perspective of clinical training, autonomy can be described in terms of a required level of supervision. The most generic entrustment–supervision scale includes five levels: (1) observe only, (2) act under direct supervision, (3) act under indirect supervision, (4) act unsupervised, and (5) act as a supervisor. The literature provides many variations of ES scales.[5]

ES scales can be retrospective or prospective. While supervision is factored into both scales, the first regards the supervision or help provided during an activity, and is not particularly focused on entrustment regarding a future activity. In contrast, prospective ES scales focus on readiness to trust future performance at a specified level of supervision.[5] They ask supervisors to estimate readiness using a scale based on autonomy. These scales, and variations thereof, frame the judgment to include an estimation of readiness and risks associated with entrustment. Paired with narrative feedback, ES scales can highlight specific actions or gaps that are relevant when considering entrustment. Prospective ES scales are a good preparation for summative entrustment decisions, which should be based on multiple evaluations of observations and case-based discussions. Table 19.1 shows published examples of retrospective and prospective ES scales.

Prospective ES scales, which focus on *decisions* of entrustment, also differ from proficiency scales by their ordinal nature. Entrustment decisions reflect discrete steps toward granted autonomy and are not a continuous scale of ability. Note that, when entrustment decisions about increased trainee autonomy do not lead to the actual granting of increased autonomy ('To what extent *would* I trust the trainee with Task X,' in theory only),[10] they are better called 'entrustment determinations.'[11] Entrustment determinations are problematic in that they run the risk of reducing ordinal ES scales to continuous proficiency scales of trustworthiness, and just add more scales to the existing ones. True entrustment scales with concrete consequences cannot be continuous, because the decision to entrust a trainee with a task is a discrete act.

Working with prospective ES scales is not easy, either for clinicians[12] or for members of a clinical competency committee (CCC)[13] because it requires a deeper understanding of trainees than is needed when just documenting an observation.[14] However, entrustment decisions should not be avoided just because they are difficult to make. To ask a supervisor about the readiness of a trainee for less supervision involves weighing benefits and risks,[15] which requires thoughtful consideration. Preparing trainees for a qualification or license to practice (for an EPA or a full profession respectively) is a key role of educators and programs, and it is exactly what such entrustment decisions entail. It may be easy to give a score for observed proficiency but hard yet important to estimate the consequences of entrustment for patient care.

Critical in ES scale use is the distinction between ad hoc and summative decisions of entrustment. Ad hoc judgments and decisions, made and evaluated by individual supervisors for

Table 19.1: Examples of retrospective and prospective entrustment–supervision scales.

	Explanation	Examples used with direct observation
Retrospective entrustment–supervision scale (examples are the O-SCORE[7] or OCAT[8] scale)	This scale uses supervision levels to indicate how much support was provided in an observed performance	1. I had to do it 2. I had to talk them through 3. I had to prompt them from time to time 4. I needed to be there just in case 5. I did not need to be there
Prospective entrustment–supervision scale	This scale uses supervision levels to indicate how much supervision the trainee should receive in future performances of a similar activity[9]	Based on this observation, my judgment is that this trainee, for this activity, is: 1. not yet ready for direct supervision 2. ready for direct, proactive supervision 3. ready for indirect, reactive supervision 4. ready to perform without supervision 5. ready to supervise junior trainees

specific patient care encounters in the workplace, lead to reports and scale use, as the examples in Table 19.1 show. Summative decisions are made by a team—often a CCC in postgraduate medical education or entrustment committee in undergraduate education—building on a variety of information sources, and are true decisions for qualification and privileging.[9] Following principles of programmatic assessment, summative entrustment decisions must be based on multiple data points. Permission to practice health care and execute specified EPAs under indirect supervision is an example that could apply to senior medical students, aligning well with the autonomy of a medical license.

Context-specificity of entrustment–supervision scales

Various ES scales and, more generally, levels of supervision, can deviate from the common, original framework of five levels (Table 19.2, column 1). Depending on the context, specifications or adaptations of this generic framework are useful. A modified, expanded scale created by Chen et al.[16] for undergraduate medical education is frequently used (Table 19.2, column 2). This expanded scale is useful for reporting on trainees' progress in the early stages of training. Similarly, the scale created by Jarrett et al. (Table 19.2, column 3) utilizes the expanded model further modified for pharmacy trainees, by noting the physical location of the supervisor to quickly orient them to the use of the scale in relation to the performance of the trainee.[17] Expansion allows faculty to better

Table 19.2: Generic and expanded entrustment–supervision scales.

Generic ES scale	Expanded scales	
	Chen-modified ES scale[16]	**Jarrett-modified ES scale[17]**
1. Not allowed to practice the EPA	1a. Not allowed to observe 1b. Allowed to observe	1a. Would not trust, not allowed to observe 1b. Trust to thoughtfully observe, has foundational knowledge
2. Allowed to practice under direct, proactive supervision (supervisor in the room)	2a. As co-activity with supervisor 2b. With supervisor in room ready to step in as needed	2a. Trust to perform task with the supervisor, requiring direction, guidance and help 2b. Trust to perform task with the supervisor present and ready to step in and is new in performing the task alone
3. Allowed to practice under indirect, reactive supervision (supervisor not in the room)	3a. With supervisor immediately available; all findings/decisions double-checked 3b. With supervisor immediately available; key findings/decisions double-checked 3c. With supervisor distantly available; findings/decisions reviewed on request	3a. Trust to perform task with supervisor nearby and all findings are immediately checked 3b. Trust to perform task with supervisor nearby and key findings are immediately checked 3c. Trust to perform task with supervisor remote, but on demand and work is audited soon after completion
4. Allowed to practice unsupervised	4a. With supervisor not around but available by phone 4b. With supervisor not available by phone	4. Trust to perform task independently and unsupervised
5. Allowed to act as supervisor for more junior trainees		5. Trust to perform task independently as well as supervise and teach others

represent their opinion about supervision needs in the future and provides ample opportunity to document progress of junior trainees. Since graduates of several health professions become licensed to enter full unsupervised clinical practice upon graduation, with no further postgraduate training requirements, this expanded scale example accurately describes assessment of the work completed.

Many discipline-specific retrospective ES scales are in use internationally. Examples include the 'Zwisch scale,' used with the mobile app SIMPL in surgical education—the scale has four values: 'show and tell,' 'active help,' 'passive help,' and 'supervision only.'[18] It is somewhat similar to the O-SCORE scale, developed for postgraduate surgery training in Canada,[7] which uses the values one to five as depicted in the upper right cell of Table 19.1. An ES scale used in one anesthesia program frames supervision as the duration a supervisor can leave the operating theater (for coffee, for lunch, etc.).[19] A triple-tool scale in pathology using procedures, situations, or reporting[20] and a retrospective ES scale under consideration in internal medicine uses the supervisor's expectation as a benchmark ('to ensure safe care I (1) had to step in much more than expected, (2) stepped in a little more than expected, (3) provided usual supervision, (4) could step back a little more than usual, (5) stepped back much more than usual').[a] Stepping in ('hands-on') and out ('hands-off') also depends on the context, the trainee, and the tasks expected to be performed in a given role.[21]

In other words, clinical specialties need to adapt ES scales depending on the nature of the work and expectations of the workplace. For example, level 2 entrustment (supervisor present during the activity) is infrequently reported for junior internal medicine residents, while this level predominates in surgical specialties, where even senior trainees spend many hours under direct supervision in the operating room,[22] and may be characterized by different steps, such as permission to do part of an operation ('Open entry to the abdomen' and 'Fascial and abdominal closure') as early EPAs, nested later within full surgery EPAs, or to act with a supervisor present but unscrubbed, which could be characterized as a new level 2c (supervisor present to instruct, but not able to step in immediately). It is recommended that, for each specialty and profession, a logical scale of supervision and entrustment be established to reflect a stepwise, deliberate increase in autonomy based on relevant, documented observations. This requires a shared mental model of ES scales by both supervisors and trainees.

Making trustworthy entrustment decisions

Since the 20th century, education in the health professions has pursued objectivity over subjectivity in assessment.[23] Assessment outside the workplace, including standardized testing of canonical (i.e., non-disputed) knowledge and skills, should meet traditional reliability criteria. Workplace-based assessment, however, which focuses on the application of knowledge and skills in patient- and context-specific practice, often cannot meet the criteria established for 'high-stakes' standardized tests, in particular reliability criteria proposed in classical test theory. As a result, no single instrument will meet the goals of workplace-based assessment—to accurately identify areas for trainee development, work collaboratively with trainees through self-reflection, and make decisions about future practice. Instead, robust workplace-based assessment requires the integration of different types of assessments involving multiple observations by multiple observers in varying contexts. Because learning is not linear, these multiple assessments may cause confusion when a trainee with generally positive assessments in one context performs poorly in another context. CCCs must determine how to make summative decisions with variation in workplace-based

[a] Personal communication Stephen Gauthier and David Taylor.

assessment, considering the upcoming tasks the trainee will face, their agility to work in various contexts of practice, with associated risks, and the support available for development (for more details see Chapter 21).

Although programmatic assessment emphasizes collecting many observations, the quality of assessment is not necessarily driven by the quantity of assessments. One observation by an experienced clinician who is trained in assessment and knows the trainee well can be more trustworthy than several observations by junior faculty who are not acquainted with the trainee and have little time or motivation for trainee assessment.[24] In competency-based education, success is measured by demonstrating performance and ability, not just the number of performances nor amount of time in training. Programs should evaluate what types, frequency and modes of assessment will best support decision-making in summative evaluations for their profession, practice, and context, and find a balance between quantity and quality.

Subjectivity and bias in observational judgment

Workplace-based assessment focuses on the contextual competence of trainees. Unlike much of the assessment of canonical competence, determining the contextual competence of trainees requires expert judgment—the opinion of experienced professionals who can appreciate the importance of their judgments, evaluate performance in context, and facilitate reflection and discussion with the trainee for growth (see Chapter 2 for a discussion of this multilayered competence model). One expert's judgment, based on their personal clinical and supervisory experiences, will show similarities but also differences with other experts' judgments. In other words, experts develop opinions that are both meaningfully 'subjective' and highly relevant.[25] This subjectivity is characterized by differences with other experts, which in the past has been considered 'error variance' or 'bias.' Valuing subjectivity also means acknowledging that some judgments cannot be fully expressed in numerical scales.[26,27] CCCs should, therefore, take into account both rating of readiness for autonomy and supportive narrative information, and at the same time acknowledge that contextual competence implies the ability to work in particular contexts, which may require different knowledge and skills that cannot always be characterized as generally 'right' or 'wrong.'

On the other hand, unwanted bias, or subjectivity that stems from prejudice that is unrelated to the proficiency of the trainee or readiness for a decrease in supervision, must be avoided. Psychometrically this is regarded as 'construct-irrelevant variance.'[28] The remaining legitimate subjective judgment must be retained. A recent AI analysis of narrative feedback highlighted the presence of unintended bias,[29] underscoring the need for observer vigilance and the importance of specifically addressing unconscious bias when training observers to give feedback. Although individual supervisors might find it hard to recognize their own bias,[30] the exchange of subjective judgments in a team, such as a CCC, may help to keep unwanted bias off the table.

Holistic evaluation of trainees

Most ES rating forms contain both numbers and words because numbers alone lack contextual detail. Narrative information can be distinguished in brief comments generated by direct observation, and more elaborate narratives, such as those generated by multisource feedback procedures (see Chapter 17). Together, integrated and synthesized with ratings, they provide the necessary story-type information needed to inform decisions made by CCCs. These committees need to take various professional attributes into account, besides clinical and technical proficiency, to allow for entrustment decisions. The A RICH framework provides an overview of these attributes in five categories: agency, reliability, integrity, capability, and humility.[31] The recommendation is not to translate the A RICH framework into a rating scale but to consider these attributes when writing narrative comments.

Words captured on entrustment rating forms serve two distinct purposes: (a) summatively, they contribute toward promotion decisions for trainees, and/or (b) formatively, they provide developmental feedback to trainees.[32] Word choice in narrative comments is important and should be aligned with the primary purpose of the assessment event, which should be clarified with the trainee beforehand.

A challenge of combining entrustment ratings and narrative text within a program of assessment is the accumulation of an overwhelming volume of data. This is where technology, with e-portfolios and mobile tools, may be of great help by assisting with data collection and aggregation to provide accessible overviews of trainee development. For more information see Chapter 20. And not everything needs to be documented. If supervisors concisely document narrative information, they also have time for undocumented, psychologically safe, oral communication with trainees.

Feedback

High-quality, meaningful feedback may be enhanced by a focus on EPAs and ES scales. However, trainee and supervisor perspectives may differ. The benefit of ES scales from a supervisor's perspective stems from the connection of direct observation in the workplace with a decision about readiness for autonomy. The trainee perspective may be complicated by blurring the value of feedback for further growth and development with judgment decisions about competence, the more traditional view of assessment.[33]

It is important to agree on the purpose of an observation followed by feedback. Since the latter should help a trainee improve, the search and focus on inadequacies, which does not directly feed intrinsic motivation[34] should be avoided. This can turn workplace-based assessment events into stressful and burdensome moments. Since giving and receiving feedback is a complex interpersonal process, supervisors and trainees need training (see Chapter 23).

A useful starting point is a definition of helpful feedback, which frames it as a 'supportive conversation that clarifies the trainee's awareness of their developing competencies, enhances their self-efficacy for making progress, challenges them to set objectives for improvement, and facilitates their development of strategies to enable that improvement to occur.'[35] Considering that entrustment decisions may also be informed by interprofessional feedback, guidelines for such feedback may be taken into account (Table 19.3).

Table 19.3: Guidelines for interprofessional feedback using the Westerfeld framework.[36]

Open, respectful	Participants are open to each other's input and communicate respectfully
Relevant	Agreed-upon goals for observed performance (e.g., EPAs)
Timely	Feedback is given in a phase of learning (hours or days, not months)
Dialogical	The conversation reflects a two-way communicative exchange
Responsive	The feedback is adapted to specific context at stake
Sense making	Feedback is explored and elaborated as needed to help trainees make sense of it
Actionable	Feedback contributes to its usability and leads to concrete action plans

Other useful feedback models are ask-and-tell approaches, self-assessment with encouragement and direction, or coaching (R2C2: relationship–reaction–content–coaching) frameworks.[37] While frameworks are useful to structure feedback conversations, there is no quick fix to generate helpful feedback that fulfills the promise of assessment for learning. A persistent complaint heard in clinical education is a lack of true constructive feedback, a complaint that should force supervisors to remain attentive toward a genuine interest in trainee development and progression toward entrustment. Supervisors need to consider the nature of effective communication with varying personalities and develop an understanding of how feedback is given and received.

Conclusion

Entrustment–supervision scales are useful for several reasons. They force observers to think about trainee readiness for patient care activities, support CCCs in making decisions about trainees' progress and summative entrustment, and serve as a focus for feedback to trainees. They also inform trainees about what is expected of them to achieve more autonomy and less supervision. Trainees have the responsibility to work on their progress in autonomy and reflect on it. Self-reflection by trainees helps supervisors understand what major gaps or problems are limiting trainees from achieving greater autonomy. ES scales are needed for making decisions about trainees' progress but scales alone are not enough. Narrative information gives much-needed depth and rich information to support such decisions. Finally, in the everyday workplace environment it is also critical to cherish the regular occurrence of undocumented, psychologically safe, oral communication in daily activities between supervisors and trainees.

Competing interests

The authors declare that they have no competing interests.

References

1. Norcini J, Burch V. Workplace-based assessment as an educational tool: AMEE guide no. 31. *Med Teach.* 2007;29(9):855–871. DOI: https://doi.org/10.1080/01421590701775453
2. Crossley J. Validity and truth in assessment. *Med Educ.* 2013;47(12):1152–1154. DOI: https://doi.org/10.1111/medu.12317
3. Crossley J, Johnson G, Booth J, Wade W. Good questions, good answers: construct alignment improves the performance of workplace-based assessment scales. *Med Educ.* 2011;45(6): 560–569. DOI: https://doi.org/10.1111/j.1365-2923.2010.03913.x
4. Weller JM, Misur M, Nicolson S, et al. Can I leave the theatre? A key to more reliable workplace-based assessment. *Br J Anaesth.* 2014;112(6):1083–1091. DOI: https://doi.org/10.1093/bja/aeu052
5. ten Cate O, Schwartz A, Chen HC. Assessing trainees and making entrustment decisions: on the nature and use of entrustment–supervision scales. *Acad Med.* 2020;95(11):1662–1669. DOI: https://doi.org/10.1097/ACM.0000000000003427
6. Rekman J, Gofton W, Dudek N, Gofton T, Hamstra SJ. Entrustability scales: outlining their usefulness for competency-based clinical assessment. *Acad Med.* 2016;91(2):186–190. DOI: https://doi.org/10.1097/ACM.0000000000001045
7. Gofton WT, Dudek NL, Wood TJ, Balaa F, Hamstra SJ. The Ottawa Surgical Competency Operating Room Evaluation (O-SCORE): a tool to assess surgical competence. *Acad Med.* 2012;87(10):1401–1407. DOI: https://doi.org/10.1097/ACM.0b013e3182677805

8. Rekman J, Hamstra SJ, Dudek N, Wood T, Seabrook C, Gofton W. A new instrument for assessing resident competence in surgical clinic: the Ottawa Clinic Assessment Tool. *J Surg Educ*. 2016;73(4):575–582. DOI: https://doi.org/10.1016/j.jsurg.2016.02.003
9. ten Cate O, Chen HC, Hoff RG, Peters H, Bok H, van der Schaaf M. Curriculum development for the workplace using entrustable professional activities (EPAs): AMEE guide no. 99. *Med Teach*. 2015;37(11):983–1002. DOI: https://doi.org/10.3109/0142159X.2015.1060308
10. ten Cate O, Schumacher DJ. Entrustable professional activities versus competencies and skills: exploring why different concepts are often conflated. *Adv Health Sci Educ Theory Pract*. 2022;27(2):491–499. DOI: https://doi.org/10.1007/s10459-022-10098-7
11. ten Cate O, Jarrett JB. *Would* I trust or *will* I trust? The gap between entrustment determinations and entrustment decisions for trainees in pharmacy and other health professions. *Pharmacy (Basel)*. 2023;11(3). DOI: https://doi.org/10.3390/pharmacy11030107
12. Postmes L, Tammer F, Posthumus I, Wijnen-Meijer M, van der Schaaf M, ten Cate O. EPA-based assessment: clinical teachers' challenges when transitioning to a prospective entrustment–supervision scale. *Med Teach*. 2021;43(4):404–410. DOI: https://doi.org/10.1080/0142159X.2020.1853688
13. Schumacher DJ, Michelson C, Winn AS, Turner DA, Martini A, Kinnear B. A realist synthesis of prospective entrustment decision-making by entrustment or clinical competency committees. *Med Educ*. December 13, 2023. DOI: https://doi.org/10.1111/medu.15296
14. Jonker G, Ochtman A, Marty AP, Kalkman CJ, ten Cate O, Hoff RG. Would you trust your loved ones to this trainee? Certification decisions in postgraduate anaesthesia training. *Br J Anaesth*. 2020;125(5):e408-e410. DOI: https://doi.org/10.1016/j.bja.2020.07.009
15. ten Cate O. Managing risks and benefits: key issues in entrustment decisions. *Med Educ*. 2017;51(9):879–881. DOI: https://doi.org/10.1111/medu.13362
16. Chen HC, van den Broek WES, ten Cate O. The case for use of entrustable professional activities in undergraduate medical education. *Acad Med*. 2015;90(4):431–436. DOI: https://doi.org/10.1097/ACM.0000000000000586
17. Jarrett JB, Goliak KL, Haines ST, Trolli E, Schwartz A. Development of an entrustment-supervision assessment tool for pharmacy experiential education using stakeholder focus groups. *Am J Pharm Educ*. 2022;86(1):8523. DOI: https://doi.org/10.5688/ajpe8523
18. Zwischenberger JB, Hatchett SP, Rahman NA, Chadha P, Sebok-Syer SS, George BC. Implementing workplace-based assessments at scale: The SIMPL approach. *Ann Surg Open*. 2023;4(4):e353. DOI: https://doi.org/10.1097/AS9.0000000000000353
19. Weller JM, Castanelli DJ, Chen Y, Jolly B. Making robust assessments of specialist trainees' workplace performance. *Br J Anaesth*. 2017;118(2):207–214. DOI: https://doi.org/10.1093/bja/aew412
20. Bryant BH, Anderson SR, Brissette M, et al. Leveraging faculty development to support validation of entrustable professional activities assessment tools in anatomic and clinical pathology training. *Acad Path*. 2024;11(2):100111. DOI: https://doi.org/10.1016/j.acpath.2024.100111
21. Hatala R, Ginsburg S, Gauthier S, Melvin L, Taylor D, Gingerich A. Supervising the senior medical resident: entrusting the role, supporting the tasks. *Med Educ*. 2022;56(12):1194–1202. DOI: https://doi.org/10.1111/medu.14883
22. Sandhu G, Thompson-Burdine J, Nikolian VC, et al. Association of faculty entrustment with resident autonomy in the operating room. *JAMA Surg*. 2018;153(6):518–524. DOI: https://doi.org/10.1001/jamasurg.2017.6117
23. van der Vleuten CPM, Norman GR, De Graaff E. Pitfalls in the pursuit of objectivity: issues of reliability. *Med Educ*. 1991;25:110–118.
24. Kulasegaram K, Paradis E. Better data ≫ Bigger data. *Med Teach*. 2014;36(11):1008–1009. DOI: https://doi.org/10.3109/0142159X.2014.917761

25. ten Cate O, Regehr G. The power of subjectivity in the assessment of medical trainees. *Acad Med.* 2019;94(3):333–337. DOI: https://doi.org/10.1097/ACM.0000000000002495
26. van Enk A, ten Cate O. 'Languaging' tacit judgment in formal postgraduate assessment: the documentation of ad hoc and summative entrustment decisions. *Perspect Med Educ.* 2020;9(6):373–378. DOI: https://doi.org/10.1007/s40037-020-00616-x
27. Cook DA, Kuper A, Hatala R, Ginsburg S. When assessment data are words: validity evidence for qualitative educational assessments. *Acad Med.* 2016;91(10):1359–1369. DOI: https://doi.org/10.1097/ACM.0000000000001175
28. Thomas MH, Steven MD. Construct-irrelevant variance in high-stakes testing. *Educ Meas Issues Pract.* 2004:17–27.
29. Gin BC, ten Cate O, O'Sullivan PS, Boscardin C. Assessing supervisor versus trainee viewpoints of entrustment through cognitive and affective lenses: an artificial intelligence investigation of bias in feedback. *Adv Health Sci Educ Theory Pract.* February 23, 2024. DOI: https://doi.org/10.1007/s10459-024-10311-9
30. Holmboe ES, Osman NY, Murphy CM, Kogan JR. The urgency of now: rethinking and improving assessment practices in medical education programs. *Acad Med.* 2023;98(8S): S37–S49. DOI: https://doi.org/10.1097/ACM.0000000000005251
31. ten Cate O, Chen HC. The ingredients of a rich entrustment decision. *Med Teach.* 2020;42(12):1413–1420. DOI: https://doi.org/10.1080/0142159X.2020.1817348
32. Ginsburg S, Watling CJ, Schumacher DJ, Gingerich A, Hatala R. Numbers encapsulate, words elaborate: toward the best use of comments for assessment and feedback on entrustment ratings. *Acad Med.* 2021;96(7S):S81-S86. DOI: https://doi.org/10.1097/ACM.0000000000004089
33. Schut S, Maggio LA, Heeneman S, van Tartwijk J, van der Vleuten C, Driessen E. Where the rubber meets the road - an integrative review of programmatic assessment in health care professions education. *Perspect Med Educ.* 2021;10(1):6–13. DOI: https://doi.org/10.1007/s40037-020-00625-w
34. ten Cate OTJ. Why receiving feedback collides with self determination. *Adv Health Sci Educ Theory Pract.* 2013;18(4):845–849. DOI: https://doi.org/10.1007/s10459-012-9401-0
35. Lefroy J, Watling C, Teunissen PW, Brand P. Guidelines: the do's, don'ts and don't knows of feedback for clinical education. *Perspect Med Educ.* 2015;4(6):284–299. DOI: https://doi.org/10.1007/s40037-015-0231-7
36. Tielemans C, de Kleijn R, van der Schaaf M, van den Broek S, Westerveld T. The Westerveld framework for interprofessional feedback dialogues in health professions education. *Assess & Eval in Higher Educ.* 2023;48(2):241–257. DOI: https://doi.org/10.1080/02602938.2021.1967285
37. Liakos W, Keel T, Ellen Pearlman R, Fornari A. Frameworks for effective feedback in health professions education. *Acad Med.* 2023;98(5):648. DOI: https://doi.org/10.1097/ACM.0000000000004884

CHAPTER 20

Addressing practical and conceptual challenges in workplace-based assessment

Daniel Nel, Adrian P. Marty, Sonia Frick, Marije P. Hennus, Machelle Linsenmeyer

Abstract

Despite its recognized importance in ensuring clinical competence, implementing and sustaining workplace-based assessment (WBA) in EPA-based programs faces various obstacles, including validity concerns, time constraints, administrative burdens, and a perceived lack of formative value. To overcome these challenges, the chapter proposes several strategies. First, it emphasizes the role of EPAs and entrustment in streamlining the WBA process, making it more time-efficient and relevant to real-world clinical practice. Second, the chapter advocates for interprofessional collaboration in WBA, highlighting the importance of incorporating input from diverse health care professionals who regularly interact with trainees. Additionally, the chapter explores the tension between formative and summative assessment in WBA, emphasizing the importance of creating a safe environment for both trainees and supervisors. By shifting the focus from high-stakes assessments to continuous learning conversations, stakeholders can optimize each assessment situation for learning while supporting trainee autonomy. Furthermore, the chapter discusses the role of technology in addressing the perceived assessment burden associated with WBA. By leveraging mobile applications, e-portfolios, and data analytics, technology can provide efficient means for data collection, storage, analysis, and visualization, ultimately enhancing the effectiveness of WBA in health care education. Lastly, the chapter considers strategies for implementing WBA in low-resource settings, highlighting the importance of local feasibility and resource adaptation. By simplifying assessment tools, leveraging low-cost tech platforms, and col-

How to cite this book chapter:
Nel D, Marty AP, Frick S, Hennus MP, Linsenmeyer M. Addressing practical and conceptual challenges in the implementation of workplace-based assessment. In: ten Cate O, Burch VC, Chen HC, Chou FC, Hennus MP. (Eds). *Entrustable Professional Activities and Entrustment Decision-Making in Health Professions Education*, Chapter 20, pp. 237–247. [2024] London: Ubiquity Press. DOI: https://doi.org/10.5334/bdc.t

This chapter uses cross-references to other chapters of the same book. For those who read this chapter as a standalone publication: all cross-references can be found at: https://doi.org/10.5334/bdc

laborating with colleagues from varying resource levels as well as different low-resource areas, low-resource settings can overcome barriers to WBA implementation and ensure the development of competent health care professionals tailored to their specific contexts.

Authors

- Daniel Nel, MD, MMEd. Groote Schuur Hospital and University of Cape Town, South Africa. Correspondence: danielnel87@gmail.com
- Adrian P. Marty, MD, MME. University Hospital Balgrist, Zurich, Switzerland.
- Sonia Frick, MD. Limmattal Hospital, Schlieren, Zurich, Switzerland.
- Marije P. Hennus, MD, PhD, MSc Clin Ed. University Medical Center Utrecht, Utrecht, the Netherlands.
- Machelle Linsenmeyer, EdD. West Virginia School of Osteopathic Medicine, Lewisburg, West Virginia, USA.

Introduction

Workplace-based assessment (WBA) is becoming increasingly crucial for ensuring and confirming clinical competence in trainees. However, a seemingly sound educational initiative does not always translate into something that is feasible in real-life practice. Perceptions of trainees and supervisors toward WBA have been mixed, with multiple conceptual and practical challenges identified that hinder its optimal implementation. The primary objective of this chapter is to offer a clearer perspective on overcoming these challenges and facilitating the realization of WBA. Special emphasis will be placed on how this process can be facilitated by entrustable professional activities (EPAs) and entrustment.

Limitations in the validity argument

A number of issues with the implementation of WBA are related to limitations in the validity argument. Although the validity argument for *entrustment decision-making* based on EPAs is discussed in more detail in Chapter 5, this chapter would be incomplete without mentioning some of the practical challenges and how they influence the validity argument of WBA. Table 20.1 summarizes some of the challenges that need to be addressed in WBA, in the context of Kane's validity model (for a deeper discussion, see Chapter 5).[1]

In terms of scoring, supervisors are frequently confused about the high stakes/low stakes conundrum related to the dual-purpose use of WBA. In addition, many do not understand how to judge a trainee's performance using WBA tools or how to provide high-quality feedback, and often lack the time or the interest to be adequately trained (such as frame of reference and performance dimension training). In terms of generalization, although multiple EPA ratings should give a clearer picture of a trainee's competence, this may result in a high assessment quota that is required per trainee. With service pressures and the busyness of a clinical workspace, EPAs may not be observed frequently enough to enable trustworthy high-stakes decision-making. In terms of extrapolation, although workplace-based assessments are grounded in authentic clinical

Table 20.1: How the validity argument in WBA can be undermined by practical challenges: some examples.

Inferences in Kane's validity model[1,2]	Purpose of the inference	Examples of practical challenges to be solved
Scoring	Judgment and scoring of observed performance should reflect the quality of this performance	Observers (often clinicians as raters) who do not understand well how to judge and report trainee performance and have little time or interest to be trained; tools used are not construct-aligned to a discipline
Generalization	Multiple scores of similar EPAs should provide a fair picture of EPA required competence	High assessment quota required; however, EPAs are infrequently observed
Extrapolation	EPA required competence should hold across all possible or relevant contexts	EPAs are observed in one context or by one observer only
Implications (consequences)	The summative decision of entrustment is warranted, as associated risks are acceptable	Summative decisions are made in a too simplified manner, leading to substandard performance with little supervision; assessment burden on students, supervisors, and educational system

situations, if this occurs in one training or clinical context only, it may not necessarily translate to the practice situation or a different context a trainee may find themselves in. Finally, in terms of implications or consequences, summative decisions may be made in too simplified a manner under duress from service delivery pressures or due to inadequate or low-quality assessment data for proper high-stakes decision-making. In addition, there are also unintended consequences on the trainees, the faculty, and the educational system from an assessment that requires significant input and may add to the administrative burden for all concerned.

These unintended consequences can be considered more broadly in light of the consensus framework for good assessment, which include the following criteria: validity or coherence, reproducibility or consistency, equivalence, feasibility, educational effect, catalytic effect, and acceptability.[3] The assessment burden introduced may limit the feasibility and acceptability of WBA. In addition, faculty and trainees often do not find that the perceived value of the assessment outweighs this burden, as the learning conversation or feedback may not be of sufficient value to overcome the requirements for completion. Potential solutions to address these and other practical concerns are discussed in the following sections.

Human resources in the clinical teaching environment

Critics of WBA often highlight its time-consuming nature, which translates into increased costs and adds to the administrative burden within an already-demanding work environment. Additionally, skeptics question the value of WBAs, citing a lack of demonstrated improvement in patient outcomes. This prompts the fundamental question: why invest time and resources into WBA? A succinct response to such skepticism echoes a quote often attributed to Abraham Lincoln: 'If you think education is expensive, try ignorance.' While this might seem clichéd, the underlying objective should be to cultivate competency efficiently, addressing the obstacles—money, time, administration—that hinder this process.

Despite the academic roots of medical professions, their real-world application unfolds in practical workplace settings. The pivotal task is to transfer theory into practice, emphasizing the importance of supervision and feedback in the workplace. Regularly employing WBAs within the structured framework of EPAs has proven to be remarkably time-efficient, averaging just three minutes per instance.[4] This diminishes the argument of time constraints. Furthermore, the assessment workload can be distributed among various stakeholders, including patients, nurses, and student peers, provided they grasp their own role, that of the trainee, and the WBA concept. To facilitate this process, EPA-related entrustment–supervision scales for WBA articulate a concept familiar to all teachers, one they have implicitly used throughout their careers—entrustment, assigning the responsibility for doing something to someone.[5] Emphasizing this point helps alleviate the common fear of something new and challenging. However, it is not necessarily straightforward for supervisors to explicitly elaborate an entrustment decision, and faculty development focusing on this process is important.[6]

In addition to assessor training, the increased emphasis on WBAs demands ongoing education for all involved parties to prevent assessment overload and subsequent stress. If trainees and supervisors do not perceive the benefits of WBA to outweigh the effort required, they may lose the motivation to participate. Establishing a cadre of 'champions' with dedicated time for introducing, teaching, and supervising the WBA process within an institution is crucial. These individuals must be well versed in the challenges of a feedback and assessment culture, addressing issues such as peer comparison, time pressures, overcontrol, and unrealistic expectations.[7] In addition to developing a core team or champions, specific WBA meetings for all supervisors and trainees explicitly showing the benefits within an institution, especially the educational value, can facilitate the positive impact of WBAs and serve to increase buy-in.

Gathering interprofessional input

Working, learning, and collaborating in an interprofessional team are indispensable for achieving safe, effective, and sustainable health care.[8] While multisource feedback (see Chapter 17 for more details) has demonstrated high reliability, validity, and feasibility in evaluating trainees,[9] the incorporation of interprofessional direct observation for WBA remains uncommon.[10] This discrepancy is particularly notable in postgraduate medical education, where trainees may have more frequent and intense interactions with nonphysician team members than with senior physician supervisors.[11] The reliance on a single assessor, typically a supervisor, may not be as defensible as incorporating input from diverse professional perspectives.[12]

Overcoming the scarcity of interprofessional WBA involves addressing practical and conceptual challenges. First, recognizing and highlighting the benefits and value of interprofessional input is crucial. This is especially pertinent when identifying and engaging a diverse range of assessors, including supervisors, nurses, physician assistants, dietitians, and other health care professionals that collaborate with the trainee on a regular basis. Furthermore, attending to the challenges associated with disparate professional perspectives, potential reluctance, and divergent opinions on competency is imperative.

To help establish a robust interprofessional assessment process, faculty development initiatives should extend beyond mono-professional supervisors to deliberately include all interprofessional stakeholders. Creating a standardized and seamless assessment process is pivotal, as is overcoming logistical hurdles such as ensuring access to digital platforms and addressing limited participant experience. In addition, legal considerations necessitate clear delineation of accountability and responsibility among the interprofessional team. For instance, how should the clinical competency committee (CCC), as the decision-making group responsible for evaluating trainees' progress in their specialty, value and utilize entrustment decisions made by interprofessional colleagues regarding their own trainees? Building trust and aligning expectations are essential in this context, requiring careful consideration to ensure a cohesive and effective decision-making process within the CCC. Finally, financial implications, particularly in regions linking remuneration to assessment outcomes, demand a balanced approach that ensures accuracy without compromising the assessment process's integrity.

By centering on interprofessional collaboration, WBA has the potential to become a more inclusive and effective tool in health professions education. This approach promotes a comprehensive and contextually relevant evaluation of trainee performance, contributing to the evolution of a more robust and holistic health care workforce.

The formative–summative tension

'Assessment drives learning'—well, not necessarily. When it comes to WBA there are some challenges to be aware of in order to optimize every assessment situation for learning. Collectively, a portfolio of WBAs can be used to make summative decisions regarding progress or promotion. However, on a spectrum from formative to summative, individual WBAs should be located in the formative corner. But, even if it is called 'formative,' from the trainee's perspective just using the term 'assessment' might create anxiety.[13] In addition, if done infrequently, the assessment situation might feel like a summative test. As a result, trainees might only ask for a WBA if they are already proficient in a specific task (EPA); they fear getting a 'bad mark.' In a culture where each assessment is perceived as a high-stakes event, much of the trainee's energy goes into impression management instead of actual learning.[14] On the supervisors' side, similar challenges exist as they might feel hesitant to use the lower spectrum of a performance scale because it might negatively impact a trainee's career or their relationship.[15]

In order to address these challenges in implementing WBA, the focus should shift to reducing stress and anxiety, and decreasing the perceived stakes as much as possible (for both trainees and supervisors). Every system of assessment needs to be absolutely transparent about the purpose of WBAs and how the data points are used to inform entrustment decisions of trainees. There is always some stake, even in formative assessment situations and especially if aggregated in an e-portfolio.[16] Instead of using the terms 'formative' and 'summative,' terms such as 'low-stakes' and 'high-stakes' or a 'continuum of stakes' may be used, as is described in programmatic assessment.[17] In addition, it may be recommended to avoid the term 'assessment' altogether, and instead call them 'observations' of performance in the workplace. Thus, rather than seeing it as an assessment, a workplace observation can be considered a perfect starting point for a 'learning conversation.' Trainees and supervisors should initiate frequent WBAs or 'observations' for facilitating learning from the first day of training until certification (and not just at the end). Using only the narrative descriptions of the entrustment–supervision scale in assessment tools (like 'direct supervision') emphasizes the clinical relevance of the rating, while using quantitative scales or levels at any point may still feel to the trainee like they are getting marked and that this should be avoided. In addition, no pass/fail decision or high-stakes decision should be made based on one single WBA.

If we succeed in our quest of decreasing trainee anxiety by carefully designing and communicating a system of assessment that is building on a growth mindset,[18] we can, for trainees, truly optimize each assessment situation for learning. In addition, for supervisors, we can make our way toward autonomy-supportive teaching styles that fosters students' intrinsic motivation to learn.[19]

Ideal vs reality

Although multiple observations are required to provide a fair picture of a trainee's competence, there needs to be a practical sampling approach that provides sufficient evidence of progress and feedback opportunities, without becoming burdensome for both the trainee and the supervisor. Overambitious assessment requirements may lead to trainee and supervisor dissatisfaction and a 'tick-box' mentality, with WBA losing its formative and summative potential.[20] Insufficient opportunities for granting autonomy in training may also arise due to legal and regulatory constraints, coupled with concerns about patient safety.[21] In particular, supervisors may not always trust the assessments of their colleagues, especially for higher-risk tasks like procedures.

Addressing these challenges may occur either in the context of establishing a new WBA strategy or refining an existing one. An essential starting point is gathering input from both supervisors and trainees to determine feasibility, including the number of required observations in a given time period and the selection of tasks or EPAs for assessment. Forming a stakeholder team, with or without surveys of the rest of the trainee and supervisor body, may facilitate this process, with feedback collection occurring iteratively during implementation. It is also valuable to examine what others have done and what principles they used to design their strategies, including barriers and facilitators identified to implementation and integration. However, it is essential to consider these insights in the light of the local context and adjust them based on local experience. In addition, the activities for assessment in the workplace (i.e., EPAs) should be mapped to curricular outcomes and the attributes of a successful graduate, as required by the relevant institution or regulatory body. Commencing with simplicity and gradual progression cannot be overemphasized. Starting with a few EPAs or a very low number of initial observations or both is advisable, and these can be progressively increased as feasibility is demonstrated and greater buy-in is achieved.

Multiple studies have defined minimum observation quotas for accurate assessments, but reliance on psychometrics should be balanced with subjective decision-making by a competence committee, emphasizing trust in trainees, supervisors, and in their high-stakes decision-making.[22] In terms of autonomy, the use of prospective entrustment decisions are advised. Whereas retrospective scales report the actual supervision provided during an activity, prospective entrustment decisions require an estimation of the student's readiness for a specific level of supervision, focusing on future performance.[23] This means that they carry more weight and may have a greater influence on decisions regarding autonomy provision.[23] While entrustment decisions may not directly impact supervision levels in all contexts, they can lead to advancement within training, with senior roles carrying increased responsibility and autonomy. Though changing regulatory and legal frameworks is challenging, in some settings the trustworthiness of a competence committee's prospective entrustment decisions, based on multiple EPA observations from multiple supervisors, may enable trainees to legally assume more senior roles and thus experience greater autonomy in training.

Technology solutions to address practical challenges

WBA has challenges and limitations for which technological solutions could serve as a resource to overcome. Examples of challenges are: (a) competing clinical demands that interfere with the time available for faculty to complete assessments; (b) the need for the collection of multiple data points to support a decision regarding readiness; (c) the analysis and visualization of data points to support both self-reflection, progression decisions, and program evaluation; and (d) the security and confidentiality of data. In the past, assessment data has been collected in paper form. While the paper-based method of data collection has benefits (e.g., more comprehensive feedback), it makes the collection, storage, analysis, presentation, and security of a large number of data points cumulatively and across time less effective.[24]

In looking to the future, it has been noted that technology such as mobile applications and dashboards or e-portfolios (if designed correctly) can provide efficient means to collect data immediately following a clinical interaction and allow instantaneous storage of data for analysis and further review in aggregate and across time. In addition to the efficiency in the collection, storage, and cumulation of data, technology also offers further ways for trainees and institutional entities (e.g., programs, directors, clinical competency committees, or institution administrators) to use the data. Trainees can benefit from seeing their progress across time and against other trainees, and from reviewing the feedback from each assessment as they consider their accomplishments and gaps toward unsupervised practice. Institutions can use the data more effectively for overall and longitudinal analysis. For example, CCCs, which are limited in their time to review trainee progress, can quickly see data displayed in multiple ways (e.g., individual data points, longitudinal progression, individual against aggregated group data) as they consider the next steps for a trainee. Regarding program evaluation, technology allows expansion from analysis of a trainee to broader perspectives of curriculum and the program (e.g., review of data by level of supervision for each EPA, looking at EPAs by program or specialty). Finally, it can provide a mechanism for digital 'badging' (electronically showing the qualifications for scope of practice of a trainee).[25]

While technology certainly has benefits, it also has important considerations such as cost, design, security and data safety, Wi-Fi coverage and networks, legal and ethical issues, reporting, standardization, disinfecting or sanitizing devices, and training and support. These issues and considerations are extensively discussed in the literature by experts who have implemented technologies to support WBA.[24,26,27]

Strategies in low-resource countries or areas

Although low-resource countries or regions encounter similar but often intensified challenges as those experienced in high-resource areas, some challenges are unique to resource-limited settings. In many low-resource environments, limited human resources and a high disease burden create service delivery pressure for clinicians, translating into less time for educational activities and fewer available human resources for initiatives like WBA.[28] Cultural dynamics as well as underdeveloped assessment systems and medical education departments may provide additional difficulties.[29] Further limiting factors include the cost of information technology platforms to make WBA user-friendly in the workplace, as well as the limited availability of Wi-Fi or cell phone data coverage. Low-resource settings may struggle to implement WBA strategies designed for high-income settings, with some concluding they lack the resources for WBA implementation altogether.[30]

Addressing these challenges in low-resource settings requires a focus on feasibility within that specific context. This involves the lowest possible assessment burden for busy clinicians and the use of extremely simple tools, ensuring quick observation capture and minimal disruption to the clinical workflow. Local design of low-cost tech platforms for WBA, such as using Google packages, RedCap, or commercially available survey software, is possible. Paper-based systems, even in low-resource settings, are discouraged owing to their multiple limitations.[26] Implemented tech platforms should ideally have low data requirements or cache features for data syncing when data coverage is available. While guidance on EPA selection and description for WBA from other contexts is helpful, it is crucial for low-resource settings to ensure that EPA selection is appropriate and that the resultant assessment requirements are feasible to implement locally. Examples of strategies to improve feasibility include selecting a limited core group of EPAs (with or without 'elective' EPAs that are optional to be assessed) or opting for fewer, broader EPAs; both resulting in a lower assessment burden (see Chapter 9 for more details). In addition, the definition of EPAs by experts in a particular setting allows curricula to be aligned to train graduates who are fit for purpose in that specific context. For some countries, particularly from the Global South, this presents an opportunity to transform and decolonize their curricula through the process of EPA selection and implementation. To ensure greatest feasibility, including the perspective of the lowest-resourced area in a particular context is needed when selecting national EPAs. Low-resource settings can also seek assistance from colleagues in well-resourced environments with experience in WBA implementation, but must take care to ensure the advice is feasible. As local expertise grows, a community of practice within a low-resource setting may facilitate the exchange of ideas and strategies for overcoming resource restrictions. Finally, although collaboration between areas with varying resource levels holds significant value, collaboration among different low-resource areas is important, which may facilitate the sharing of potential solutions or even collectively addressing development costs.

Conclusion

Whether it is a new WBA strategy being implemented or an existing one being refined, challenges are inevitable. It is imperative for drivers of educational change to understand what they can do to limit the magnitude and shorten the duration of the initial period of disarray that inevitably follows the introduction of change. This chapter highlights many such strategies that can be used to create a more supportive external environment, as well as to address some of the cognitive and other internal barriers to WBA implementation (summarized in Table 20.2 below). In addition, we have discussed how EPAs and the concept of entrustment may assist in achieving this goal. We hope that this information empowers those who are embarking on an implementation journey or encourages those who feel that the challenges are too great to overcome.

Table 20.2: Practical and conceptual challenges to WBA and strategies to overcome them.

Challenge	Strategies
Assessment burden for busy clinicians	• Use EPA-based assessments with simple tools that include entrustment–supervision scales • Distribute the load through interprofessional involvement • Ensure continuous education of all involved parties • Establish 'champions' with dedicated time for introducing and supervising WBA process • Arrange WBA meetings for all supervisors and trainees showing local progress and stressing benefits to individuals and the team
Scarcity of interprofessional WBA	• Ensure faculty development initiatives include all interprofessional stakeholders • Create a standardized and seamless assessment process, including digital platform • Ensure clear delineation of accountability, legal responsibility, and remuneration
Tension between formative and summative purposes in WBA	• Avoid term 'assessment'—instead use 'observations' of performance in the workplace/'WBO' • Use only narrative descriptions of the entrustment–supervision scale in assessment tools • Completely avoid numbers or 'levels' in rating scales • Ensure transparency about purpose of WBAs and how data points are used for high-stakes decision-making
Tension between educational ideals and reality of work-place environment	• Get local input from both supervisors and trainees to determine feasibility, especially regarding assessment quotas • Start with a few EPAs and/or a very low number of initial observations, then build up • Examine the literature to learn from the mistakes and successes of others • Continuously seek feedback from all participants during implementation and adjust as necessary
Logistics of continuous data collection in the workplace, and need to aggregate for later use	• Avoid paper-based system • Use mobile/smartphone-based applications to capture individual observations • Use e-portfolios for trainees to review own progress • Develop digital dashboards to aid competence committee view and analyze aggregated data points
Resource restrictions in lower-income countries/contexts	• Ensure lowest possible assessment burden • Use of extremely simple tools • Local design of low-cost tech platforms • Incorporate low data requirements or cache features for data syncing when data coverage is available • Ensure EPA selection is appropriate and feasible locally

Competing interests

The authors declare that they have no competing interests.

References

1. Kane MT. An argument-based approach to validity. *Psychol Bull.* 1992; *112*(3), 527–535. DOI: https://doi.org/10.1037/0033-2909.112.3.527
2. Cook DA, Brydges R, Ginsburg S, Hatala R. A contemporary approach to validity arguments: a practical guide to Kane's framework. *Med Educ.* 2015;49(6):560–575. DOI: https://doi.org/10.1111/medu.12678

3. Norcini J, Anderson MB, Bollela V, et al. 2018 consensus framework for good assessment. *Med Teach.* 2018;40:1102–1109. DOI: https://doi.org/10.1080/0142159X.2018.1500016
4. Cheung K, Rogoza C, Chung AD, Kwan BYM. Analyzing the Administrative Burden of Competency Based Medical Education. *Can Assoc Radiol J.* 2022;73(2):299–304. DOI: https://doi.org/10.1177/08465371211038963
5. ten Cate O. When I say … entrustability. *Med Educ.* 2020;54(2):103–104. DOI: https://doi.org/10.1111/medu.14005
6. Gingerich A. What if the 'trust' in entrustable were a social judgement? *Med Educ.* 2015;49(8):750–752. DOI: https://doi.org/10.1111/medu.12772
7. Ott MC, Pack R, Cristancho S, Chin M, Van Koughnett JA, Ott M. "The Most Crushing Thing": Understanding Resident Assessment Burden in a Competency-Based Curriculum. *J Grad Med Educ.* 2022;14(5):583–592. DOI: https://doi.org/10.4300/JGME-D-22-00050.1
8. Stalmeijer RE, Varpio L. The wolf you feed: challenging intraprofessional workplace-based education norms. *Med Educ.* 2021;55(8):894–902. DOI: https://doi.org/10.1111/medu.14520
9. Donnon T, Al Ansari A, Al Alawi S, Violato C. The reliability, validity, and feasibility of multisource feedback physician assessment: a systematic review. *Acad Med.* 2014;89(3):511–516. DOI: https://doi.org/10.1097/ACM.0000000000000147
10. van Keulen SG, de Raad T, Raymakers-Janssen P, Ten Cate O, Hennus MP. Exploring Interprofessional Development of Entrustable Professional Activities For Pediatric Intensive Care Fellows: A Proof-of-Concept Study. *Teach Learn Med.* 2024;36(2):154–162. DOI: https://doi.org/10.1080/10401334.2023.2200760
11. Sonnenberg LK, Pritchard-Wiart L, Hodgson CS, Yu Y, King S. Assessment of Resident Physicians' Communicator and Collaborator Competencies by Interprofessional Clinicians: A Mixed-Methods Study. *Teach Learn Med.* 2017;29(4):392–401. DOI: https://doi.org/10.1080/10401334.2017.1301817
12. van der Vleuten CP, Schuwirth LW, Scheele F, Driessen EW, Hodges B. The assessment of professional competence: building blocks for theory development. *Best Pract Res Clin Obstet Gynaecol.* 2010;24(6):703–719. DOI: https://doi.org/10.1016/j.bpobgyn.2010.04.001
13. Schut S, Driessen E, van Tartwijk J, van der Vleuten C, Heeneman S. Stakes in the eye of the beholder: an international study of learners' perceptions within programmatic assessment. *Med Educ.* 2018;52(6):654–663. DOI: https://doi.org/10.1111/medu.13532
14. Huffman BM, Hafferty FW, Bhagra A, Leasure EL, Santivasi WL, Sawatsky AP. Resident impression management within feedback conversations: A qualitative study. *Med Educ.* 2021;55(2):266–274. DOI: https://doi.org/10.1111/medu.14360
15. McQueen SA, Petrisor B, Bhandari M, Fahim C, McKinnon V, Sonnadara RR. Examining the barriers to meaningful assessment and feedback in medical training. *Am J Surg.* 2016;211(2):464–475. DOI: https://doi.org/10.1016/j.amjsurg.2015.10.002
16. Watling CJ, Ginsburg S. Assessment, feedback and the alchemy of learning. Med Educ. 2019;53(1):76–85. DOI: https://doi.org/10.1111/medu.13645
17. Schuwirth LW, Van der Vleuten CP. Programmatic assessment: From assessment of learning to assessment for learning. *Med Teach.* 2011;33(6):478–485. DOI: https://doi.org/10.3109/0142159X.2011.565828
18. Richardson D, Kinnear B, Hauer KE, et al. Growth mindset in competency-based medical education. *Med Teach.* 2021;43(7):751–757. DOI: https://doi.org/10.1080/0142159X.2021.1928036
19. Reeve J, Cheon SH. Autonomy-supportive teaching: its malleability, benefits, and potential to improve educational practice. *Educ Psychol.* 2021;56(1):54–77. DOI: https://doi.org/10.1080/00461520.2020.1862657
20. Massie J, Ali JM. Workplace-based assessment: a review of user perceptions and strategies to address the identified shortcomings. *Adv Health Sci Educ Theory Pract.* 2016;21(2):455–473. DOI: https://doi.org/10.1007/s10459-015-9614-0

21. ten Cate O, Jarrett JB. Would I Trust or Will I Trust? The Gap between Entrustment Determinations and Entrustment Decisions for Trainees in Pharmacy and Other Health Professions. *Pharmacy (Basel)*. 2023;11(3):107. Published 2023 Jun 18. DOI: https://doi.org/10.3390/pharmacy11030107
22. Hodges B. Assessment in the post-psychometric era: learning to love the subjective and collective. *Med Teach*. 2013;35(7):564–568. DOI: https://doi.org/10.3109/0142159X.2013.789134
23. Postmes L, Tammer F, Posthumus I, Wijnen-Meijer M, van der Schaaf M, ten Cate O. EPA-based assessment: Clinical teachers' challenges when transitioning to a prospective entrustment-supervision scale. *Med Teach*. 2021;43(4):404–410. DOI: https://doi.org/10.1080/0142159X.2020.1853688
24. Young JQ, Sugarman R, Schwartz J, McClure M, O'Sullivan PS. A mobile app to capture EPA assessment data: Utilizing the consolidated framework for implementation research to identify enablers and barriers to engagement. *Perspect Med Educ*. 2020;9(4):210–219. DOI: https://doi.org/10.1007/s40037-020-00587-z
25. ten Cate O. How can entrustable professional activities serve the quality of health care provision through licensing and certification? *Can Med Educ J*. 2022;13(4):8–14. DOI: https://doi.org/10.36834/cmej.73974
26. Marty AP, Linsenmeyer M, George B, Young JQ, Breckwoldt J, Ten Cate O. Mobile technologies to support workplace-based assessment for entrustment decisions: Guidelines for programs and educators: AMEE Guide No. 154. *Med Teach*. 2023;45(11):1203–1213. DOI: https://doi.org/10.1080/0142159X.2023.2168527
27. George BC, Bohnen JD, Schuller MC, Fryer JP. Using smartphones for trainee performance assessment: A SIMPL case study. *Surgery*. 2020;167(6):903–906. DOI: https://doi.org/10.1016/j.surg.2019.09.011
28. Frenk J, Chen L, Bhutta ZA, et al. Health professionals for a new century: transforming education to strengthen health systems in an interdependent world. *Lancet*. 2010;376(9756):1923–1958. DOI: https://doi.org/10.1016/S0140-6736(10)61854-5
29. Atta K. Bridge to trust: EPAs and the cultural odyssey in Pakistan's medical training. *Journal of University Medical & Dental College*. Epub ahead of print November 27, 2023. DOI: https://doi.org/10.37723/jumdc.v14i4.973
30. Ras T, Stander Jenkins L, Lazarus C, et al. 'We just don't have the resources': supervisor perspectives on introducing workplace-based assessments into medical specialist training in South Africa. *BMC Med Educ*. 2023;23(1):832. DOI: https://doi.org/10.1186/s12909-023-04840-x

CHAPTER 21

Clinical competency committees in an entrustable professional activity-based curriculum and assessment system

Robert Englander, Jacqueline de Graaf, Karen E. Hauer, Gersten Jonker, Daniel J. Schumacher

Abstract

Competency-based education (CBE) in the health professions is grounded in teaching and assessing the requisite competencies to develop professionals prepared to meet the health care needs of the public and provide high-quality and safe patient care. As such, the outcome of education is the demonstrable competence of graduates in patient care. A curriculum and assessment framework based on entrustable professional activities (EPAs) provides excellent scaffolding for ensuring this outcome. The system is dependent, however, on its ability to support grounded, credible, and summative decisions regarding granting or withholding trainee progression through a program and awarding of increased autonomy (i.e., less supervision) in patient care.

In this chapter, we begin by defining a clinical competency committee (CCC) and establishing its roles. We then provide a rationale for the group structure of a CCC as best suited to make the grounded, credible, and summative decisions required in an EPA-based curriculum and assessment system. Next, we explore more deeply the central role of a CCC—'what' it does. Then we address the 'how' of running a CCC, that is, the strategies to help CCCs function optimally, including issues of CCC structure and process. Finally, we explore some of the common pitfalls, misconceptions, and limitations regarding CCCs and suggest some mitigating strategies to overcome them.

How to cite this book chapter:

Englander R, de Graaf J, Hauer KE, Jonker G, Schumacher DJ. Clinical competency committees in an entrustable professional activity framework for curriculum and assessment. In: ten Cate O, Burch VC, Chen HC, Chou FC, Hennus MP. (Eds). *Entrustable Professional Activities and Entrustment Decision-Making in Health Professions Education*, Chapter 21, pp. 249–258. [2024] London: Ubiquity Press. DOI: https://doi.org/10.5334/bdc.u

Authors

- Robert Englander, MD, MPH. University of Illinois College of Medicine; Chicago, Illinois, USA. Correspondence: rengland@uic.edu
- Jacqueline de Graaf, MD, PhD. Radboud University Medical Center, Nijmegen, the Netherlands.
- Karen E. Hauer, MD, PhD. University of California San Francisco, San Francisco, California, USA.
- Gersten Jonker, MD, PhD. University Medical Center Utrecht, Utrecht University, Utrecht, the Netherlands.
- Daniel J. Schumacher, MD, PhD. Cincinnati Children's Hospital Medical Center/University of Cincinnati College of Medicine, Cincinnati, Ohio, USA.

Introduction

Competency-based education (CBE) in the health professions is grounded in teaching and assessing the requisite competencies to develop professionals who are prepared to meet the health care needs of the public and provide high-quality and safe patient care.[1] As such, the outcome of education is the demonstrable competence of graduates in patient care.

Clinical faculty make judgments on trainees' development, progress, and readiness to perform essential tasks of the profession. Decisions to delegate tasks, called summative entrustment decisions, should be based on grounded trust, that is, trust based on essential and longitudinal experience with the trainee and preceded by sufficient observation and pertinent data to qualify the trainee to act with a decreased level of supervision.[2] While in some programs those decisions are made by individual supervising faculty, in most programs summative decisions are made by a collective of supervising faculty and, in some committees, staff engaged in assessment as well. There are several names given to these committees. In some jurisdictions, the term clinical competency committee (CCC) is used. In programs using entrustable professional activities (EPAs) as the framework for their curriculum and assessment, these committees are often called entrustment committees. For the purposes of this chapter, we will collectively refer to these committees as CCCs.

A CCC can be defined as a group of individuals involved in trainee education and assessment responsible for making effective and credible judgments of trainee performance based on the review and interpretation of multiple aggregated assessments and then deliberately deciding on progression and entrustment of patient care tasks.[3–6] The primary tasks of the CCC are thus to make grounded, credible, and summative decisions on granting or withholding trainee progression through the program and on awarding increased autonomy (i.e., less supervision) in patient care. Summative decisions can therefore: (a) recognize attainment of a milestone within a phase of education or training; (b) provide permission to proceed to the next phase of training; or (c) provide entrustment decisions regarding EPAs, potentially allowing the learner to perform the EPA with decreased supervision. The entrustment decisions may also be accompanied by a statement of awarded responsibility (STAR).[7] A STAR provides formal documentation that a trainee has met the threshold for a given EPA to carry that EPA out unsupervised (in the case of a resident or fellow trainee) or with indirect supervision (in the case of an undergraduate trainee). Through these decisions, a CCC ultimately contributes to the primary purposes of competency-based education—educational accountability to the public and the learner.

Many programs use EPA assessments for formative feedback as well, and may engage a CCC in that formative feedback, reviewing trainee performance on EPAs and providing feedback to the trainee without rendering high-stakes decisions.[8] As an example, a CCC may use EPA assessment data formatively in an early meeting where trainee data is insufficient to make a summative entrustment decision but can be fed back to the trainee to provide guidance on opportunities to advance in the performance of the EPA toward entrustment. CCCs can also provide formative feedback through curricular suggestions to trainees, such as a rotation that might be advantageous, based on gaps the CCC identifies through the aggregate assessment data.

A summary of potential tasks, that have been ascribed to CCCs, besides making summative decisions about entrustment and trainee progress and associated feedback, include[3–6,9]:

1. identifying both suboptimal performance or dyscompetence (i.e., less than expected ability in one or more domains of competence in a certain context and at a defined stage of education or practice[10]) and performance exceeding expectations in trainees;
2. providing program directors with a transparent, rich, holistic group perspective on trainee performance;

3. providing trainees with credible and actionable feedback;
4. formulating remediation interventions and tailored training opportunities for learners who require them, or referring the learners to another entity such as a remediation or clinical coach;
5. evaluating program effectiveness and identifying weaknesses in curriculum or program of assessment;
6. providing feedback to those overseeing the program of assessment on the focus and quality of workplace-based assessments.

This chapter focuses on the role of CCCs in EPA assessment and entrustment decisions. Specifically, we explore the 'why' behind the critical nature of CCCs in implementing a curriculum and assessment system with EPAs, what evidence is used by CCCs to inform group decisions, and how a CCC operates. Finally, we explore some of the pitfalls, limitations, and misconceptions surrounding CCCs and offer some mitigating strategies.

Why do we need clinical competency committees in an EPA-based curriculum and assessment system?

An EPA-based curriculum and assessment system requires summative decisions about: (a) learners' ability to perform the EPAs with decreased levels of supervision; (b) learners' overall progress in the program; and (c) learners' overall trustworthiness. Programs that use EPAs as curricular building blocks and for learner assessment generate large amounts and varied types of data on learner performance. Making the high-stakes decisions, therefore, requires a process to synthesize and interpret these data. Synthesis involves more than just averaging entrustment scores or compiling all narrative comments. In fact, because the attainment of competence is a nonlinear developmental process, the learner's trajectory over time is considerably more important than any average rating, and longitudinal review of performance is essential. This process also involves human judgment to interpret and synthesize data and is vulnerable to bias. We submit that high-stakes decision-making in health professions education and training is thus optimally done by a group such as a CCC, the members of which can provide varying perspectives on the longitudinal view of the learner's trajectory, ensure defensible decisions, and mitigate bias.

Group decision-making within a CCC is important because, in general, groups make better decisions than individuals acting alone.[5] A group process that is well designed and implemented using recommendations for effective group procedures can generate greater buy-in to decisions among members, learners, the program, and the public. Group decision-making done well affords multiple benefits compared to decision-making by a single individual. The interactions among group members during meetings serve as real-time faculty development to build a shared mental model of expected trainee performance. Discussing what evidence pertains to the EPAs and what evidence demonstrates a trainee's achievement at a given level of entrustment promotes a shared understanding and interpretation of the data among members.[11] This shared understanding of expected development of trainees allows for earlier recognition by the CCC of trainees who are missing learning experiences or not progressing as expected. Early identification creates opportunities for intervention, such as adjusting learning experiences or strengthening feedback on certain skills or competencies. Group decision-making is thus a critical core component of programmatic assessment in CBE.[12]

One additional benefit to the group process designed to make determinations of individual trainee's progress is that it also generates insights about the program as a whole. A high-functioning CCC contributes to the overall quality of assessment and education by affording regular review of trainee outcomes both between and within phases of education and training.[13] Committee members can identify strengths or gaps of the curriculum and learning experiences and recommend adjustments to improve the content or quality of training.

With this understanding of the 'why' behind the use of CCCs in CBE in general and specifically in a CBE program that utilizes EPAs as the framework for curriculum and assessment, we turn to the 'nuts and bolts' of what a CCC does and how it best functions.

What does a CCC do?

The central role of all CCCs is to review aggregate evidence over time regarding trainees' performance in executing the EPAs, and to decide when a trainee has reached a predetermined level of entrustment to allow increased autonomy and advancement within or beyond an educational or training program. In general, that level of entrustment is at the indirect supervision level for undergraduate medical students advancing to residency, and unsupervised practice for residents moving to practice or fellowship.[14] In some countries, however, trainees move directly from undergraduate medical education to practice. Similarly, in many health professions, trainees move from a prelicensure undergraduate program directly to unsupervised practice. In these cases, trainees need to be entrusted at the level of unsupervised practice prior to graduation for those EPAs that they will be performing in practice.

In addition to reviewing data regarding trainee performance of EPAs, data that speak to the trainee's trustworthiness, in particular the ability to know one's limits and seek help, are central to a CCC's making sound entrustment decisions.[15,16] One published review of the literature suggests that there are five components of trustworthiness: Agency (proactive toward work, team, safety, personal development); Reliability (conscientious, predictable, accountable, responsible); Integrity (truthful, benevolent, patient-centered); Capability (specific knowledge, skills, experience, situational awareness), and Humility (recognizes limits, asks for help, receptive to feedback). Together, these factors allow for 'A RICH' entrustment decision.[17] For these reasons, CCCs making entrustment decisions perform best when they collect and use information about these factors in their deliberations.

In addition to these central roles, as noted above, some CCCs may also engage in: identifying trainees with both suboptimal performance and performance exceeding expectations; providing program evaluation based on aggregate data; providing trainees with formative, actionable feedback; formulating remediation interventions and tailored training opportunities for learners who require them; referring the learners to a remediation or clinical coach; and providing feedback to those overseeing the program of assessment on the focus and quality of workplace-based assessments.

How do CCCs function best?

An important first consideration in the optimal function of a CCC starts with the formation of the group. The CCC should have a chair with excellent knowledge of the education or training program and the assessment system. This individual is often a program or assessment leader. The membership of CCCs is also a critical factor in the group's function. Diversity of the membership in personal identities, specialty affiliation within a health profession, other health professionals, nonclinical members (e.g., PhDs), patients, trainees, and representatives of other training programs can enhance the CCC functioning, leading to better-informed or more defensible decisions than individuals acting alone or in a homogeneous group.[5,18,19] Diversity of the membership is also one of the primary strategies for mitigation of bias in assessment. CCCs should also include direct supervisors of trainees.[20]

Consistent membership, the ability to remove members, having a clear leader, and having administrative support are also important components for optimal CCC function.[19]

The literature also offers several structure and process considerations for the work of CCCs to optimize entrustment decisions in an EPA-based curriculum. First, they should follow evidence-based group decision-making practices.[21,22] CCCs need structured procedures for reviewing and interpreting learner performance information and generating decisions.[23] This approach should include processes for how consensus is reached, including means for conflict resolution either between committee members or between conflicting data points.[18,20,21,24–26] CCCs also need the time, energy, space, and engagement to complete their work with an eye toward maintaining a reasonable workload.[13,18,19,21] Achieving these goals may require completing prereviews of trainees before CCC meetings.[13,18,27]

Strategies to engage all group members in discussion and encourage information sharing maximize the wisdom of the group and can mitigate bias.[5] For example, the chair should use intentional meeting facilitation strategies such as encouraging junior members to speak first and inviting disparate opinions.[28] Appointing someone to serve in a role to monitor for bias or offer counter-arguments and varied interpretations is another strategy for optimizing engagement, leveraging diverse opinions, and minimizing bias.[20] CCCs must similarly mitigate against groupthink, in which the desire to maintain harmony within the group overrides members' willingness or ability to speak up when a decision may be erroneous, harmful, or incomplete.[29] Social loafing arises when group members over-rely on others in the group and contribute less effort than if they were working alone.[30]

The optimal CCC meeting frequency is unclear. It will often depend on the volume of learners and the number of committee members. Higher volumes of learners will require more frequent meetings, often reviewing a subset of those learners at each meeting.[15] Higher volumes of committee members may make logistics more difficult but may also allow for a subset of committee members to form a quorum for any given meeting. The literature suggests a minimum of at least two meetings per year,[18] but quarterly[27,31,32] or even monthly[19] meetings have also been suggested. Not surprisingly, small programs have reported that the work of the CCC is easier, with more time to devote to reviewing each trainee.[18]

Faculty development for CCC members is also important.[18,26,33] Important aspects of faculty development include the development of common mental models for key functions of EPAs,[26,33] for what development looks like for individual EPAs,[19] and for what entrustment should and does mean.[34] Furthermore, if the CCC is making decisions at transition points, such as between medical school and residency, a common mental model for the entrustment–supervision level needed for transition is important.[27]

Finally, the way data are presented to CCC members is critical. Data visualization can be used to offset CCC members' cognitive load and help enable entrustment decision-making.[13,17,18,25–27,31,32,35,36] Dashboards that enable data visualization should be intuitive, contextualized, fast, and accessible.[35] Well-organized learner EPA performance data strengthen members' access to learner information and ability to interpret the data, optimizing their high-stakes decision-making.

Pitfalls, limitations, and misconceptions of CCCs

A full discussion of CCCs in an EPA-based curriculum and assessment system would not be complete without laying out and understanding the key pitfalls, limitations, and misconceptions. These are presented in Table 21.1 with some potential mitigating strategies.

Table 21.1: Pitfalls, misconceptions, and limitations regarding CCCs.

Potential pitfall, misconception, or limitation	Potential mitigating strategies
Pitfall: ignoring potential sources of bias in the CCC process	1. Ensure diversity of the CCC members (e.g., on issues of identity, specialty, phase of education/training, nonphysician members) 2. Faculty and trainee development on the evidence that suggests a trainee merits entrustment/advancement 3. Structured procedures for reviewing and interpreting learner performance information and generating decisions 4. Avoid having each member prepare for one trainee, precluding group deliberations. 5. Standard approach to data presentation
Pitfall: inadequate engagement of trainee in the process[37]	1. Standardized process for engaging trainees, transparent to both CCC members and trainees 2. A priori clarity around what trainee data is to be used by the CCC in decision-making, including data on trustworthiness 3. Standard process for trainee self-assessments on the EPAs that requires them to attest to their self-perceived readiness for entrustment 4. Involvement of trainees in a portion of the CCC meeting to present their self-assessment 5. Standard process for post-CCC meeting feedback (written and oral) to the trainee, including CCC findings and decisions and any plans for follow-up
Misconception: 'one size fits all.' CCCs will need to vary depending on the type of trainees they are assessing (e.g., where on the education–training–practice continuum the trainee is), the volume of trainees, and the volume of EPAs	1. Adjust meeting frequency to ensure ability to discuss each trainee's progress on the EPAs (i.e., ensure time allotted matches the workload) 2. Adjust size of CCCs to ensure engagement of all members 3. Adjust number of CCCs to accommodate increased trainee volume (for example, a program with four trainees per year might have a single CCC, while an undergraduate student body of 250 students/year might require several CCCs)
Misconception: the CCC is only for struggling trainees	1. Ensure discussion of all trainees at the same intervals and allow sufficient time to provide feedback on EPA-based decisions and progress to each trainee. (Note: This does not mean that a CCC must review every trainee at every meeting!)
Limitation: CCCs are time-consuming	1. Optimize administrative support, such as premeeting aggregation of data, intra-meeting notetaking, and post-meeting provision of written feedback 2. Develop a reward system for participation (such as counting toward promotion and tenure) 3. Create term limits for committee membership, when possible, to share the time commitment across faculty
Limitation: CCCs may be both an entrustment body and a promotion body simultaneously	1. Ensure roles are clear a priori regarding the decision-making expectations for entrustment on EPAs and for advancement across phases of training 2. Identify potential conflicts of interest a priori and determine standard processes for conflict resolution

Conclusion

The goal of CBE in the health professions is to produce trainees competent to meet the needs of the public. Ensuring competence requires decisions regarding trainees' capacity to perform in the clinical environment, and EPAs create an entrustment framework for the decision-making process. Such decisions are best served through the group process of clinical competency committees to ensure the fidelity of the process to all the stakeholders, including faculty, staff, trainees, and patients.

Competing interests

The authors declare that they have no competing interests.

References

1. Frenk J, Chen L, Bhutta ZA, et al. Health professionals for a new century: transforming education to strengthen health systems in an interdependent world. *Lancet.* 2010;376(9756):1923–1958. DOI: https://doi.org/10.1016/S0140-6736(10)61854-5
2. ten Cate O, Hart D, Ankel F, et al. Entrustment decision-making in clinical training. *Academic Medicine.* 2016;91(2):191–198, February 2016. DOI: https://doi.org/10.1097/ACM.0000000000001044
3. Andolsek K, Padmore J, Hauer KE, Ekpenyong A, Edgar L, Holmboe E. *(ACGME) Clinical Competency Committees. A Guidebook for Programs.* 3rd ed. Accreditation Council for Graduate Medical Education; 2020.
4. Ekpenyong A, Padmore JS, Hauer KE. The purpose, structure, and process of clinical competency committees: guidance for members and program directors. *J Grad Med Educ.* 2021;13(2S):45–50. DOI: https://doi.org/10.4300/JGME-D-20-00841.1
5. Hauer KE, Cate OT, Boscardin CK, et al. Ensuring resident competence: a narrative review of the literature on group decision-making to inform the work of clinical competency committees. *J Grad Med Educ.* 2016;8(2):156–164. DOI: https://doi.org/10.4300/JGME-D-15-00144.1
6. Pack R, Lingard L, Watling CJ, Chahine S, Cristancho SM. Some assembly required: tracing the interpretative work of clinical competency committees. *Med Educ.* 2019;53(7):723–734. DOI: https://doi.org/10.1111/medu.13884
7. ten Cate O. Nuts and bolts of entrustable professional activities. *J Grad Med Educ.* 2013;5(1):157–158. DOI: https://doi.org/10.4300/JGME-D-12-00380.1
8. Amiel J, Ryan MS, Andriole DA, Whelan AJ. *Core Entrustable Professional Activities for Entering Residency: Summary of the 10-School Pilot, 2014–2021.* AAMC; 2022.
9. Rowland K, Edberg D, Anderson L, Wright K. Features of effective clinical competency committees. *J Grad Med Educ.* 2023;15(4):463–468. DOI: https://doi.org/10.4300/JGME-D-22-00756.1
10. Frank JR, Snell LS, Cate OT, et al. Competency-based medical education: theory to practice. *Med Teach.* 2010;32(8):638–645. DOI: https://doi.org/10.3109/0142159X.2010.501190
11. Edgar L, Jones MD Jr, Harsy B, Passiment M, Hauer KE. Better decision-making: shared mental models and the clinical competency committee. *J Grad Med Educ.* 2021;13(2 Suppl):51–58. DOI: https://doi.org/10.4300/JGME-D-20-00850.1
12. Van Melle E, Frank JR, Holmboe ES, et al. A core components framework for evaluating implementation of competency-based medical education programs. *Acad Med.* 2019;94(7):1002–1009. DOI: https://doi.org/10.1097/ACM.0000000000002743

13. Pack R, Lingard L, Watling C, Cristancho S. Beyond summative decision-making: illuminating the broader roles of competence committees. *Med Educ.* 2020;54(6):517–527. DOI: https://doi.org/10.1111/medu.14072
14. Englander R, Flynn T, Call S, et al. Toward defining the foundation of the MD degree: core entrustable professional activities for entering residency. *Acad Med.* 2016;91(10):1352–1358. DOI: https://doi.org/10.1097/ACM.0000000000001204
15. Schumacher DJ, Michelson C, Winn AS, Turner DA, Elshoff E, Kinnear B. Making prospective entrustment decisions: knowing limits, seeking help and defaulting. *Med Educ.* 2022;56(9):892–900. DOI: https://doi.org/10.1111/medu.14797
16. Schumacher DJ, Michelson C, Winn AS, Turner DA, Martini A, Kinnear B. A realist synthesis of prospective entrustment decision-making by entrustment or clinical competency committees. *Med Educ.* Dec 13, 2023;doi:10.1111/medu.15296
17. ten Cate O, Chen HC. The ingredients of a rich entrustment decision. *Med Teach.* 2020;42(12):1413–1420. DOI: https://doi.org/10.1080/0142159X.2020.1817348
18. Acai A, Cupido N, Weavers A, et al. Competence committees: the steep climb from concept to implementation. *Med Educ.* 2021;55(9):1067–1077. DOI: https://doi.org/10.1111/medu.14585
19. Schumacher DJ, Schwartz A, Zenel JA Jr, et al. Narrative performance level assignments at initial entrustment and graduation: integrating EPAs and Milestones to improve learner assessment. *Acad Med.* 2020;95(11):1736–1744. DOI: https://doi.org/10.1097/ACM.0000000000003300
20. Chan T, Oswald A, Hauer KE, et al. Diagnosing conflict: conflicting data, interpersonal conflict, and conflicts of interest in clinical competency committees. *Med Teach.* 2021;43(7):765–773. DOI: https://doi.org/10.1080/0142159X.2021.1925101
21. Chahine S, Cristancho S, Padgett J, Lingard L. How do small groups make decisions? A theoretical framework to inform the implementation and study of clinical competency committees. *Perspect Med Educ.* 2017;6(3):192–198. DOI: https://doi.org/10.1007/s40037-017-0357-x
22. ten Cate O, Balmer DF, Caretta-Weyer H, Hatala R, Hennus MP, West DC. Entrustable professional activities and entrustment decision-making: a development and research agenda for the next decade. *Acad Med.* 2021;96(7S):S96-S104. DOI: https://doi.org/10.1097/ACM.0000000000004106
23. Duitsman ME, Slootweg IA, van der Marel IC, et al. Group assessment of resident performance: valuable for program director judgment? *J Grad Med Educ.* 2019;11(4 Suppl):118–124. DOI: https://doi.org/10.4300/JGME-D-18-01069
24. Brown DR, Moeller JJ, Grbic D, et al. Entrustment decision-making in the core entrustable professional activities: results of a multi-institutional study. *Acad Med.* 2022;97(4):536–543. DOI: https://doi.org/10.1097/ACM.0000000000004242
25. Brown DR, Warren JB, Hyderi A, et al. Finding a path to entrustment in undergraduate medical education: a progress report from the AAMC Core Entrustable Professional Activities for Entering Residency Entrustment Concept Group. *Acad Med.* 2017;92(6):774–779. DOI: https://doi.org/10.1097/ACM.0000000000001544
26. Brown DR, Moeller JJ, Grbic D, et al. Comparing entrustment decision-making outcomes of the core entrustable professional activities pilot, 2019–2020. *JAMA Netw Open.* 2022;5(9):e2233342. DOI: https://doi.org/10.1001/jamanetworkopen.2022.33342
27. Murray KE, Lane JL, Carraccio C, et al. Crossing the gap: using competency-based assessment to determine whether learners are ready for the undergraduate-to-graduate transition. *Acad Med.* 2019;94(3):338–345. DOI: https://doi.org/10.1097/ACM.0000000000002535
28. Kinnear B, Warm EJ, Hauer KE. Twelve tips to maximize the value of a clinical competency committee in postgraduate medical education. *Med Teach.* 2018;40(11):1110–1115. DOI: https://doi.org/10.1080/0142159X.2018.1474191

29. Janis L. Groupthink. *IEEE Engineering Management Review*. 2008;36(1): 36–36. DOI: https://doi.org/10.1109/EMR.2008.4490137
30. Simms A, Nichols T. Social loafing: a review of the literature. *Journal of Management Policy and Practice*. 2014;15(1):58.
31. de Graaf J, Bolk M, Dijkstra A, van der Horst M, Hoff RG, ten Cate O. The implementation of entrustable professional activities in postgraduate medical education in the Netherlands: rationale, process, and current status. *Acad Med*. 2021;96(7S):S29-S35. DOI: https://doi.org/10.1097/ACM.0000000000004110
32. Hobday PM, Borman-Shoap E, Cullen MJ, Englander R, Murray KE. The Minnesota method: a learner-driven, entrustable professional activity-based comprehensive program of assessment for medical students. *Acad Med*. 2021;96(7S):S50-S55. DOI: https://doi.org/10.1097/ACM.0000000000004101
33. Carraccio C, Martini A, Van Melle E, Schumacher DJ. Identifying core components of EPA implementation: a path to knowing if a complex intervention is being implemented as intended. *Acad Med*. 2021;96(9):1332–1336. DOI: https://doi.org/10.1097/ACM.0000000000004075
34. Favreau MA, Tewksbury L, Lupi C, et al. Constructing a shared mental model for faculty development for the core entrustable professional activities for entering residency. *Acad Med*. 2017;92(6):759–764. DOI: https://doi.org/10.1097/ACM.0000000000001511
35. Thoma B, Bandi V, Carey R, Mondal D, Woods R, Martin L, Chan T. Developing a dashboard to meet competence committee needs: a design-based research project. *Can Med Educ J*. 2020;11(1):e16-e34. DOI: https://doi.org/10.36834/cmej.68903
36. Warm EJ, Carraccio C, Kelleher M, Kinnear B, Schumacher DJ, Santen S. The education passport: connecting programmatic assessment across learning and practice. *Can Med Educ J*. 2022;13(4):82–91. DOI: https://doi.org/10.36834/cmej.73871
37. Hall J, Oswald A, Hauer KE, et al. Twelve tips for learners to succeed in a CBME program. *Med Teach*. 2021;43(7):745–750. DOI: https://doi.org/10.1080/0142159X.2021.1925233

SECTION E

Implementation

CHAPTER 22

Managing curriculum reform in the transition to competency-based education using entrustable professional activities

Fremen Chihchen Chou, Siobhan Fitzpatrick, David R. Taylor, Adrian P. Marty, Mabel Yap, Harm Peters

Abstract

Curriculum reform in health professions education is essential to address evolving societal expectations for healthcare. Competency-based education (CBE), advocated by leaders in healthcare such as the Lancet Commission and the World Health Organization, aims to bridge the gap between traditional training in the health professions and modern healthcare needs. This chapter outlines a comprehensive approach to curriculum reform, emphasizing the integration of change management for the human aspects and project management for the technical aspects, to ensure successful implementation. Drawing from different models, five essential themes to manage curriculum reform emerge: communication, iterative design, leadership, teamwork, evaluation and refinement.

The transition to a CBE program based on entrustable professional activities (EPAs) necessitates a major curriculum reform that can be considered a systemic overhaul. This process involves planning, implementing, and monitoring changes while preparing and supporting stakeholders to embrace and sustain these changes. This chapter utilizes Van Melle's core components framework of CBE to set the blueprint for an EPA-based curriculum, guiding the development of EPAs as training outcomes, creat-

How to cite this book chapter:

Chou FC, Fitzpatrick S, Taylor DR, Marty AP, Yap M, Peters H, Managing curriculum reform in the transition to CBE using EPAs. In: ten Cate O, Burch VC, Chen HC, Chou FC, Hennus MP. (Eds). *Entrustable Professional Activities and Entrustment Decision Making in Health Professions Education*, Chapter 22, pp. 261–274. [2024] London: Ubiquity Press. DOI: https://doi.org/10.5334/bdc.v

This chapter uses cross-references to other chapters of the same book. For those who read this chapter as a standalone publication: all cross-references can be found at: https://doi.org/10.5334/bdc

ing tailored instruction and learning experiences to foster competency acquisition, and establishing programmatic assessment to inform entrustment progression. By leveraging international experiences and ensuring contextualization and localization, this chapter provides a robust framework to navigate the complexities of transitioning to CBE. The chapter concludes by presenting a practical, step-by-step method for managing curriculum reform through the phases of initiation, implementation, and sustainability. The principles and strategies outlined offer valuable insights for educational leaders, program directors, and policymakers aiming to effectively align education with healthcare practice.

Authors

- Fremen Chihchen Chou, MD, PhD. School of Medicine, China Medical University and China Medical University Hospital, Taichung, Taiwan. Correspondence: fremen.chou@gmail.com
- Siobhan Fitzpatrick, BA, MA. World Health Organization, Geneva.
- David R. Taylor, MD, MHPE. Queen's University, Kingston, Ontario, Canada.
- Adrian P. Marty, MD, MME. University Hospital Balgrist, University of Zurich, Zurich, Switzerland.
- Mabel Yap, MBBS, MSc, PhD. Ministry of Health Singapore and National University Health System, Singapore.
- Harm Peters, MD, MHPE. Charité – Universitätsmedizin Berlin, Berlin, Germany.

Contextualizing curriculum reform in modern health professions education

Societal expectations of healthcare have expanded significantly over the past few decades, reflecting the increasingly complex and multifaceted health needs of populations.[1] Traditional curricular models in health professions education (HPE), characterized by rigid, analytical, and process-oriented designs, have not adequately adapted to these heightened expectations.[2,3] This not only leaves graduates unprepared for the complex realities of modern healthcare practice but also places patients at risk due to the misalignment between HPE and healthcare needs.[3–5] Consequently, leaders in healthcare globally, including the Lancet Commission and the World Health Organization, are advocating for a shift toward competency-based HPE to address these needs.[2,6,7]

Entrustable professional activities (EPAs) can bridge the current gap between CBE and healthcare delivery. EPAs, as units of professional practice, are conferred on learners upon demonstrating requisite competence, emphasizing the provision of professional work as the outcome of education. A curricular design incorporating EPAs provides a practice-oriented approach to operationalizing the premise of CBE. EPAs provide a framework for sequenced progression through training focused on practice-based outcomes. They can tailor teaching and learning activities to the development of competencies and assess competence through professional activities and entrustment decisions.[3,8,9] With EPAs, CBE more effectively integrates education and healthcare as an interdependent system by aligning and optimizing their delivery, thus better addressing existing gaps.[3,4] EPAs' strength in healthcare education is the translation of competencies into tangible, easy-to-communicate building blocks for curriculum transformation, fostering a gradual increase of professional autonomy, responsibility, and accountability.[9,10]

Frameworks for curriculum reform

The transition to or implementation of an EPA-based CBE program represents an educational paradigm shift and can be clearly characterized as major curriculum reform.[10] The changes required for curriculum reform of this scope extend beyond learning objectives, curricular content, teaching methods, assessment approaches, and learning resources. They also involve support areas such as governance structures, administration, facilities, teacher training, evaluation, quality assurance, and, importantly, the underpinning philosophy of learning, the curriculum's goals, and the culture of education.[11–13] The complexity of this type of change brings numerous potential pitfalls and requires that project leaders use a strategic approach.[14] While most of the principles discussed in the following sections apply to managing any major curriculum reform, this chapter contextualizes the reform in the transition to CBE and highlights the roles of using EPAs.

There is no single established approach or framework to manage major curriculum reform successfully.[10] In practice, it involves a blend of the two closely related concepts of project management and change management (Table 22.1). Project management refers to the more technical aspects of curriculum reform. It involves the planning, implementing, and monitoring of projects to achieve specific goals within a set timeframe.[15] Change management focuses on the human side of the reform. It involves communicating, preparing, supporting, and helping individuals, teams, and organizations to cocreate, embrace, and implement change at macro, meso, and micro levels.[15]

Drawing from the different models for project management and change management, five essential themes for managing curriculum reform become apparent[13,24]:

Communication: Build understanding, consensus, and ownership of the change among trainees, faculty, governance structures, administrators, communities, and other stakeholders.

Iterative design: Introduce change effectively through pilots with an iterative design process, based on continuous feedback, anticipating and addressing potential challenges.

Table 22.1: Key characteristics of project management and change management in curriculum reform.

Area	Project management	Change management
Models and frameworks	• PDSA (plan, do, study, act) cycle[16] • Strengths, weaknesses opportunities, threats (SWOT) analysis[17] • Agile management framework[18] • Design thinking (empathize, define, ideate, prototype, test)[19]	• Kotter's eight steps (see example in Table 22.2)[20] • Roger's diffusion of innovation theory[21] • Lewin's three-stage model of freeze–defreeze–freeze[22] • ADKAR (awareness, desire, knowledge, ability, reinforcement) model[23]
Strategies and tasks	• Define the scope and goals • Establish the governance structure • Analyze and allocate resources • Manage time and time as a resource[13] • Establish and manage communication channels • Pilot and sequence implementation • Monitor performance, including quality control • Identify and manage risks • Close the project	• Make the need for change tangible • Analyze readiness for change • Analyze and engage the stakeholders • Provide opportunities for cocreation, coproduction to support buy-in • Facilitate the local adaptation of the change (glocalization) • Communicate with all involved (upward and downward) • Deal with resistance and threats • Provide training and support (empower) • Evaluate for early and continuous refinement and quality improvement • Sustain the change

Leadership: Navigate the power dynamics and politics essential for change implementation and sustainability.

Teamwork: Leverage the often-limited available time and resources for maximum impact by engaging champions from various stakeholders and forming a functional project management team.

Evaluation and refinement: Continuously assess and adapt curricular elements to sustain change, ensuring constructive alignment both within the elements and with the underpinning philosophy.

It is important to note that these elements of the management of change in HPE, though introduced here in a linear fashion for ease of understanding, do not follow a strict sequence when practiced in the real world. They may unfold in parallel or iteratively following an order that suits the specific situation, illustrating the complexity and nature of change within HPE. Major curriculum reforms regard time as a resource rather than only a goal to be attained, and should be planned over years, not months.[13,24]

As we move from traditional models to CBE frameworks with EPAs, what begins with minor curriculum changes—such as introducing a new assessment method—reflects incremental steps toward major curriculum reform. These small steps contribute to a shift toward a fundamentally different educational paradigm. Thus, managing change in the transition toward CBE with EPAs requires a well-coordinated approach between incremental change and overarching reform. Each step or adjustment must be carefully orchestrated, understanding that it contributes to a larger transformation. This discussion offers a roadmap for navigating this complex process, ensuring that each change, no matter how small, aligns with the ultimate goal of a reformed, more effective HPE system.

Using the core components framework to set the blueprint for an EPA-based curriculum

To initiate EPA-based curriculum reform, it is crucial to see both 'the forest' and 'the trees.' A holistic vision is necessary to sustain the momentum of change, utilizing change management strategies that focus on *people* management. At the same time, detailed, actionable steps are necessary for implementation, requiring *project* management. The integration of project management and change management, with alignment of actions, is imperative to facilitate both organizational and cultural change.[2,11,13]

Visualizing the whole picture of the curricular blueprint for an EPA-based curriculum is crucial to the development of detailed project management plans. Van Melle's core components framework for the implementation and evaluation of CBE elaborates its operationalization and supporting philosophy.[8] In this model, the five components include 'outcome competencies' framing the designed 'sequenced progression' in a local program context, to guide the development of 'competency-focused instruction,' 'tailored learning experiences,' and 'programmatic assessment.'[8] This core components framework delineates the alignment of curricular elements in CBE and can serve as the blueprint when preparing for major curriculum reform.

First, a defined and elaborated set of EPAs as the outcome of training operationalizes the competencies required for practice and allows for backward curricular design (start with the end in mind). The sequence of learning in the curriculum could be established by setting the expected trajectory of supervision level and the application of nested EPAs (see Chapter 10).[9,25] Second, this work is followed by the development of teaching or instructional methods and designed learning experiences to facilitate the acquisition of competencies required to practice the EPAs. This includes the application and extension of canonical competence and the development of contextual competence, aiming to support increasing autonomy as trainee competence grows (see Chapter 2). Third, the curriculum needs to create a programmatic approach to assessment embedded within the instructional and learning activities. This assessment informs the progression of entrustment as trainees move through their trajectory of legitimate participation in the community of healthcare professionals. These dimensions of curricular design need to be considered and balanced in detailed project management plans. Hall et al. reported a case study in Canada where an imbalance occurred due to an overemphasis on programmatic assessment; the granularity of assessments undermined the curriculum reforms of competency-focused instruction and tailored learning experiences.[26]

A proven approach to curriculum reform is to strategically leverage international experiences and literature—standing on the shoulders of giants. Borrowing relevant EPA definitions or assessment tools can be beneficial, but this global wisdom *must* undergo a process of contextualization and localization, or 'glocalization,' to ensure cultural appropriateness and linguistic consensus, as suggested by Chou et al.[27] Comprehensive projects such as Ireland's internship EPA initiative, which underwent eight stages from establishing a local consensus on EPA templates to stakeholder development and international benchmarking, illustrate the process and value of 'glocalization.'[28] The significance of such an initiative lies not only in developing and implementing a comprehensive set of EPAs but also in its thorough process to foster buy-in, ownership of change, as well as faculty and key stakeholder development.

Managing curriculum reform in three phases

The curriculum reform involving the implementation of EPA-based CBE, like any other major curriculum reform, generally proceeds through three sequential and interrelated phases: initiation, implementation, and sustainability.[10] Maaz et al. provides an example how project and change management strategies were applied through these phases in a large European medical university transitioning its undergraduate education program to CBE using EPAs as the foundation.[10] Each phase has important goals, which should reflect a cohesive change management strategy. Table 22.2 illustrates the potential guiding questions of managing changes in EPA-based curriculum reform with Kotter's eight-step model,[20] mapped onto the three phases of curriculum reform, with key features of these three phases from a change management perspective.

Table 22.2: Phases and potential guiding questions of managing changes in EPA-based curriculum reform.

Phases and functions in change management	Kotter's eight steps for leading change as an exemplary model	Guiding questions
Initiation phase: Creating the climate for change	**1. Create a sense of urgency**	• What's the problem with current practice? • What is the burning platform? • Why EPAs and why now? • What are the opportunities? • Where can we reduce friction?
	2. Form a powerful coalition	• Who can contribute to the curriculum development process or effect change—faculty, academic leadership, patients, communities, and learners? • Will there be a working group? • Who can champion the agenda?
	3. Develop a strategic vision	• Where do we want to go from here? • How do we collaborate to draft what the EPAs might be? • What changes are needed—assessment, learning activities, or physical spaces? • Will this be a curriculum change or curriculum reform?
Implementation phase: Engaging and enabling the organization	**4. Communicate the vision**	• What are the processes or strategies to communicate with various stakeholders?
	5. Enable action	• What are the opportunities to get involved? • How can you or someone else lead the change? • To what extent do stakeholders involved have a say in action? • What resources are needed? • How can these resources be leveraged? • What faculty training is needed? • What time will it take to support and enable change?
	6. Produce short-term wins	• What will the short-term win look like? • What is its role in overall reform? • How and when should it be celebrated?
Sustainability phase: Refining and sustaining the change	**7. Build on the change**	• What has been achieved? • How can we continuously improve? • What is the next step?
	8. Create a new culture	• Are the changes fit for the purpose of the reform? • What are the differences (underpinning philosophy of learning and education outcome) between the reform and original curriculum?

Elaborating on the Kotter model, and based on the experiences of the authors and the literature, we suggest paying attention to 11 key components in these three phases of curricular change management (Table 22.3), elaborated below.

Initiation phase

Communicating the sense of urgency for curriculum reform. Essential preparation for curriculum reform must include actions that create readiness for change and inspire individuals and groups to engage in the transition toward an EPA-based curriculum.[12,20] This includes creating a sense of urgency, presenting an appealing vision of the future curriculum, and fostering confidence that these changes can be achieved.[21] Emphasizing ongoing challenges in patient safety and quality of care can highlight the need to better prepare graduates for a rapidly evolving healthcare landscape.[6] Additionally, there is a critical need for alignment and integration between healthcare and education systems.[3,5] EPAs' strengths in providing an outcome of education that is directly tied to the readiness of graduates to perform the work of the profession demonstrates how the proposed change can bring this alignment.

Building the project team and the vision. Two important goals in the initiation phase include reaching an agreement on the blueprint for the new EPA-based curriculum (the vision) and establishing a project management team.[10,29] The project management team should preferably be recruited from within the organization and include a mix of expertise in education (curriculum development, CBE, and EPAs), clinical practice, and project and change management. In addition, learners should also be included as full team members. This core team relieves the larger faculty from the substantial structural and content-related work that curriculum reform requires, minimizing the impact on patient care, research, and teaching responsibilities.[10,29] Framing and communicating the strategic vision to stakeholders become central responsibilities for this team. An important early task of the project team is to position the initiative visibly within the faculty, providing transparency around important aspects of the project including governance, decision-making processes and policies, curriculum planning, and planned implementation.

Success in curriculum reform requires open, transparent, and ongoing dialogue—aiming to demonstrate, not just assert, the need for change by 'showing the gaps' in current practices. This process should reveal and clarify curricular challenges, allowing a shared vision and main strategy to emerge through discussion. For instance, Jonker et al. opened a public dialogue on certification decisions in postgraduate training with the question 'Would you trust your loved ones to this

Table 22.3: Eleven components of curricular change management to pay attention to.

Initiation phase	• Communicating the sense of urgency for curriculum reform • Building the project team and the vision
Implementation phase	• Setting up a standardized planning process • Piloting and implementing sequentially • Communicating and listening • Providing space for discussion and engaging a large body of faculty • Involving trainees at many levels • Creating opportunities for codesign and for empowerment • Anticipating resistance to change • Celebrating successes
Sustainability phase	• Program evaluation and continuous quality improvement

trainee?'[30] Transparent discussion can facilitate the development of a shared vision for curricular changes by expanding ownership and building a shared mental model about the underlying principles of CBE, thereby reducing barriers and fostering longevity. Addressing the question 'What's in it for me with EPAs?' can create opportunities for engagement in codesign and cocreation with various stakeholders.[31]

Another key is the active and visible support of faculty leaders, either as change leaders[20] in managing and directing the change toward EPAs or as sponsors by providing support, resources, and advocacy. It also necessitates support and ownership across multiple levels of the institution, encompassing individuals in senior leadership positions, faculty, and those involved in curriculum delivery.[13] Crucially, the engagement of trainees and patients who are impacted by the curriculum reform fosters the effectiveness and acceptability of implementation. Ignoring them can lead to negative consequences for curriculum reform and adoption. Through engaging various stakeholders, building a shared mental model for change, and recognizing champions, a powerful coalition emerges.

Implementation phase

The most labor- and resource-intensive part of major curriculum reform is the implementation phase.[10] An estimation for the duration of this phase is to add at least one year to the duration of the curriculum (i.e., a minimum of six years for a five-year curriculum plan, even once the plan and the desired outcomes have been agreed upon). The greater the gap between the existing and the future program, the more resources will be needed. Successful implementation cannot be taken for granted and includes the possibility of failure and reverting to the previous situation.[12] Below are key activities and strategies to manage implementation.

Setting up a standardized planning process. This helps to work out the details of the curriculum blueprint for each part of the new curriculum.[10] This process should outline who participates in the planning process, their roles, and who chairs the planning group, including the procedure for their election. Policies around decision making and conflicts of interest are important to prevent problems that can easily emerge in these groups. Simplicity helps. For example, holding meetings on the same day, time, and location can enable better attendance. Start with a bottom-up perspective (what do people in the planning group want to contribute?), match this with the curriculum blueprint for the respective time block, and finalize the process using a discursive top-down process. Achieving consensus should be the main decision-making principle. Formal, written procedures should be put in place in advance to manage conflicts and define what constitutes consensus (majority, absence of 'no' votes, quorum, etc.). In addition to addressing the 'who' and the 'how,' it is crucial to consider 'what' needs to be done at different stages ('when') of developing and implementing an EPA-based curriculum. The literature provides numerous examples detailing the tasks required at various stages.[10,28] For instance, Chapter 9 offers comprehensive approaches to identifying and elaborating EPAs in the early stages to prepare for curriculum reform. As previously mentioned, time should be regarded as a resource rather than merely a goal to be attained in major curriculum reforms.[13] Planning should span years, not months.[13] Figure 22.1 illustrates an example of a planning scheme across multiple years, created early in the process and used to monitor the project's progress and ensure it remains on track.

Piloting and implementing sequentially. Both approaches allow the identification of potential problems or challenges on a smaller scale before reforms are rolled out across the entire curriculum, enabling iterative adjustments based on feedback from the real-world context.[10] It can also build confidence in the organization that the intended changes can be managed. Piloting with a smaller group of trainees, with a single module, and/or implementing sequentially will make it more likely that the reforms will be successful in the long term through the accumulation of granular short-term wins that make the intended goals seem achievable.

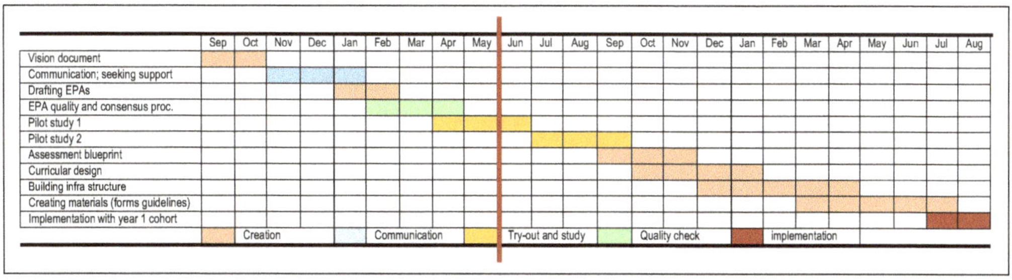

Figure 22.1: Example of a project planning scheme for curriculum development.

Supporting information technology is considered a key factor for the success of CBE.[13] Continuous piloting is necessary for the alignment of information systems and adjustments during the practical implementation of CBE. Through iterative improvements, these efforts can eventually lead to a seamless experience in the workplace learning environment. For example, conducting assessments, providing feedback, and generating learning records should not overly disrupt the workflow or create excessive additional burdens.[32] Only through such repeated refinements can the reform become integrated into daily practice.

Communicating and listening. A key task of the project team is to communicate actively and effectively about the progress of the change process through multiple channels, ensuring listening, reflection, and adaptation to insights gained.[10,24] Establishing communication channels for dialogue, listening, and information dissemination is essential to ensure stakeholder buy-in, support, and engagement. In addition to these project-specific communication initiatives, conventional communication channels such as email, blogs, and faculty or departmental announcements should also be leveraged.

Providing space for discussion and engaging a large body of faculty. Open planning sessions (or 'townhall' sessions) increase transparency in the organization and provide space for discussion.[10,12] This facilitates the development of shared views about the reform process, the diffusion of the curriculum reform concept within the host organization, and the future expectations of faculty members involved in delivering the program. In addition, all stakeholders should have the opportunity to weigh the need for reform against the effort required, considering the consequences both for patient care and for their own practice. The implementation of EPAs should translate educational reform directly into improved patient care. Developing this understanding, relaying expectations, and responding to concerns facilitate the ongoing implementation work. The participation of faculty members in these open planning sessions is an important, natural, and efficient faculty development process. Formal faculty development planning is also a key task in the implementation stage.[13] Faculty development should further expand to stakeholder development, encompassing leaders, trainees, and administrators. (For details on faculty and stakeholder development, see Chapter 23.)

Involving trainees at many levels. Trainees are experts in their own learning experience and how the current and new curricula are experienced in action.[10] Their insights can help identify gaps and redundancies. They often bring fresh ideas for tackling problems and improving the new curriculum, including alignment of intended, taught, learned, and assessed content. Involving trainees at multiple levels of curriculum reform, including in the development of the curriculum blueprint, in the project team, and in block planning groups, which, for example, organize the curriculum into thematic modules, promotes ownership of both their own learning and the new curriculum. By involving trainees, we ensure that their rights and responsibilities are appropriately balanced in the workplace.[13] This not only fosters trainee buy-in but also ensures the feasibility of the EPA-based curriculum. It prevents overly idealistic designs from leading to unexpected, nonideal strategies on the part of the trainees.[33]

Creating opportunities for codesign and for empowerment. Engaging teaching faculty and trainees in decision making about processes and outcomes should build on opportunities to codesign the change.[10] This allows insights from their experiences, which can actively shape the proposed change. It promotes their buy-in and helps to manage resistance. Coownership can be facilitated by giving many of them active roles and responsibilities as formal members or chairs of the block planning groups or for individual teaching courses.[10] Planning meetings should include regular faculty development activities related to the change process and the teaching of the new curriculum to empower those involved in this process.

Anticipating resistance to change. Resistance to change is normal and should be expected.[10,21] It need not be feared and must not be ignored. Many of the strategies mentioned above will help mitigate resistance from faculty members, especially when their concerns are heard and addressed in subsequent discussions and decisions. Identifying the source of resistance is crucial, as solutions for issues related to cost and effort differ from those stemming from a lack of ownership of the change.

One major resistance to CBE and EPA-based curricula is the challenge around assessments, observation, and feedback in the workplace, including competing clinical demands, workflow, supervisor-trainee interaction, and 'assessment burnout.'[32,33] Chapter 20 addresses practical and conceptual challenges in workplace-based assessment.

Celebrating successes. Major curriculum reform is a long-term endeavor with uncertain outcomes for many involved. Openly recognizing and celebrating early and ongoing achievements fosters confidence that change can be managed and maintains commitment and motivation throughout the process.[20] It will also maintain the commitment and motivation of those involved in the ongoing process of changing the entire curriculum.

Sustainability phase

Program evaluation and continuous quality improvement. Key factors contributing to the sustainability of the change process include: (a) departments maintaining their valued role in teaching and (b) demonstrating that the intended new outcomes are achieved by trainees and, where that is not evident, that programs are positioned to respond and adapt.[10] These factors facilitate the new curriculum structures, establishing themselves as the new standard operating procedures. This in turn allows for continuous adaptation and improvement through regular program evaluation and continuous quality improvement measures[5] (see Chapter 24 for details about program evaluation and continuous quality improvement). While the role of the project team gradually fades, they will have laid the foundation for this phase during the implementation phase, namely the tasks and strategies related to the buy-in, cocreation, and empowerment of the teaching faculty and learners involved in the EPA-based curriculum and its delivery.

It is important to view CBE as a dynamically evolving, iteratively improving concept.[3] Thus, the new curriculum will never be 'finished,' and curriculum change should be seen as a constant state, requiring a curriculum development group or department. The philosophies, concepts, and practices associated with the new curriculum will lead to a change in organizational culture.[34] This takes time as it involves collective learning and unlearning old habits and beliefs. The literature includes examples of curriculum reform for EPA-based programs.[10,35,36] Box 22.1 presents one example of curriculum reform in postgraduate education in Asia, demonstrating the application of change management and project management strategies and principles discussed in this chapter, and offering valuable reflections for future directions.

Box 22.1: Case study: 12-year journey of transitioning to competency-based emergency medicine residency training in Taiwan.

Overview

In 2011, a medical professor's newspaper editorial questioning the value of emergency medicine specialty training prompted action. Clinician educators in the Taiwan Society of Emergency Medicine (TSEM) formed a coalition to reform training with a CBE approach. In 2012, the TSEM Education Committee proposed a five-year curriculum reform plan, using milestones and EPAs to operationalize competence outcomes. Milestones guided canonical competencies and provided supervisor feedback, while end-of-training EPAs structured contextualized competencies.

By 2013, a CBE taskforce, including leaders from 80% of Taiwan's emergency medicine training programs, was established. Bimonthly meetings using consensus methods resulted in shared mental models and iteratively developed EPAs and milestones. The principle of 'glocalization' increased clinical teacher involvement and fostered local ownership,[27] with national surveys generating candidate professional activities for EPAs. This led to seven EPAs as a framework, and the development of curricula and assessment tools for underdeveloped competencies, such as delivering bad news.

The initial five-year plan was extended to eight years for preliminary completion. The TSEM continued to evaluate and plan for subsequent phases, including an attempt to link specialty licensure with competency-based training, implementing national mid-term residency assessments, developing a national competency-based assessment and learning system, and promoting clinical competency committees. Periodic consensus forums led by international scholars fostered sustainable reform and cultural change.

Analysis

This 12-year journey encompassed strategies from the initiation, implementation, and sustainability phases discussed in this chapter, achieving initial success and positioning TSEM as a leader in the CBE transition in Taiwan. However, challenges remain, such as insufficient trainee and patient involvement and maintaining momentum after the initial success. Assessment has often overshadowed the development of tailored curricula and learning experiences. Robust information systems are crucial for effective CBE implementation, yet national systems have faced limitations in meeting local training program needs. The initial success of this journey demonstrates effective change management strategies, but ongoing challenges must be addressed to ensure sustained progress with continuous quality improvement.

Acknowledgments

This chapter draws substantially from a paper published in *Medical Teacher*.[10] ChatGPT 4o aided in sentence editing.

Competing interests

The authors declare that they have no competing interests.

References

1. Farrell TW, Greer AG, Bennie S, Hageman H, Pfeifle A. Academic health centers and the quintuple aim of health care. *Acad Med.* 2023;98(5):563–568. DOI: https://doi.org/10.1097/ACM.0000000000005031
2. Frenk J, Chen L, Bhutta ZA, et al. Health professionals for a new century: transforming education to strengthen health systems in an interdependent world. *Lancet.* 2010;376(9756):1923–1958. DOI: https://doi.org/10.1016/S0140-6736(10)61854-5
3. Holmboe ES. Competency-based medical education and the ghost of Kuhn: reflections on the messy and meaningful work of transformation. *Acad Med.* 2018;93(3):350–353. DOI: https://doi.org/10.1097/ACM.0000000000001866
4. O'Brien BC, Reed DA. Exploring the intersections of education and healthcare delivery using a clinical learning environment framework. *J Gen Intern Med.* 2019;34(5):654–656. DOI: https://doi.org/10.1007/s11606-019-04929-4
5. Holmboe ES, Kogan JR. Will any road get you there? Examining warranted and unwarranted variation in medical education. *Acad Med.* 2022;97(8):1128–1136. DOI: https://doi.org/10.1097/ACM.0000000000004667
6. Irby D. Educating physicians for the future: Carnegie's calls for reform. *Med Teach.* 2011;33(7):547–550. DOI: https://doi.org/10.3109/0142159X.2011.578173
7. World Health Organization. *Global Competency and Outcomes Framework for Universal Health Coverage.* World Health Organization; 2022. Accessed March 4, 2024. https://www.who.int/publications/i/item/9789240034662
8. Van Melle E, Frank JR, Holmboe ES, et al. A core components framework for evaluating implementation of competency-based medical education programs. *Acad Med.* 2019;94(7):1002–1009. DOI: https://doi.org/10.1097/ACM.0000000000002743
9. ten Cate O, Chen HC, Hoff RG, Peters H, Bok H, van der Schaaf M. Curriculum development for the workplace using entrustable professional activities (EPAs): AMEE guide no. 99. *Med Teach.* 2015;37(11):983–1002. DOI: https://doi.org/10.3109/0142159X.2015.1060308
10. Maaz A, Hitzblech T, Arends P, et al. Moving a mountain: practical insights into mastering a major curriculum reform at a large European medical university. *Med Teach.* 2018;40(5):453–460. DOI: https://doi.org/10.1080/0142159X.2018.1440077
11. Reis S. Curriculum reform: Why? What? How? And how will we know it works? *Isr J Health Policy Res.* 2018;7(1):30. DOI: https://doi.org/10.1186/s13584-018-0221-4
12. Bank L, Jippes M, Scherpbier AJJA, FeddeScheele. Change management support in postgraduate medical education: a change for the better. In: Tsoulfas G, ed. *Medical and Surgical Education—Past, Present and Future.* InTech eBooks; 2018. DOI: https://doi.org/10.5772/intechopen.72113
13. Nousiainen MT, Caverzagie KJ, Ferguson PC, Frank JR, ICBME Collaborators. Implementing competency-based medical education: what changes in curricular structure and processes are needed? *Med Teach.* 2017;39(6):594–598. DOI: https://doi.org/10.1080/0142159X.2017.1315077
14. Dagnone JD, Taylor D, Acker A, et al. Seven ways to get a grip on implementing competency-based medical education at the program level. *Can Med Educ J.* 2020;11(5):e92-e96. DOI: https://doi.org/10.36834/cmej.68221
15. Creasey T. Change management and project management: a side by side comparison. Prosci, Inc. 2021. Accessed February 28, 2024. https://www.prosci.com/blog/change-management-and-project-management-comparison
16. Christoff P. Running PDSA cycles. *Curr Probl Pediatr Adolesc Health Care.* 2018;48(8):198–201. DOI: https://doi.org/10.1016/j.cppeds.2018.08.006

17. Teoli D, Sanvictores T, An J. SWOT analysis. In: *StatPearls*. StatPearls Publishing; 2023.
18. Desai M, Tardif-Douglin M, Miller I, et al. Implementation of agile in healthcare: methodology for a multisite home hospital accelerator. *BMJ Open Qual.* 2024;13(2):e002764. Published 2024 May 27. DOI: https://doi.org/10.1136/bmjoq-2024-002764
19. Deitte LA, Omary RA. The power of design thinking in medical education. *Acad Radiol.* 2019;26(10):1417–1420. DOI: https://doi.org/10.1016/j.acra.2019.02.012
20. Kotter J, Rathgeber H. Our iceberg is melting: changing and succeeding under any conditions. Penguin Random House LLC; 2005.
21. Sanson-Fisher RW. Diffusion of innovation theory for clinical change. *Med J Aust.* 2004;180(S6):S55–S56. DOI: https://doi.org/10.5694/j.1326-5377.2004.tb05947.x
22. Burnes B. Kurt Lewin and the planned approach to change: a re-appraisal. *J. Manag. Stud.* 2004;41(6):977–1002.
23. Shepherd ML, Harris ML, Chung H, Himes EM. Using the awareness, desire, knowledge, ability, reinforcement model to build a shared governance culture. *JNEP.* 2014;4(6):90.
24. Gale R, Grant J. AMEE medical education guide no. 10: managing change in a medical context: guidelines for action. *Med Teach.* 1997;19(4):239–249. DOI: https://doi.org/10.3109/01421599709034200
25. ten Cate O, Taylor DR. The recommended description of an entrustable professional activity: AMEE guide no. 140. *Med Teach.* 2021;43(10):1106–1114. DOI: https://doi.org/10.1080/0142159X.2020.1838465
26. Hall AK, Rich J, Dagnone JD, et al. It's a marathon, not a sprint: rapid evaluation of competency-based medical education program implementation. *Acad Med.* 2020;95(5):786–793. DOI: https://doi.org/10.1097/ACM.0000000000003040
27. Chou FC, Hsiao CT, Yang CW, Frank JR. 'Glocalization' in medical education: a framework underlying implementing CBME in a local context. *J Formos Med Assoc.* 2022;121(8):1523–1531. DOI: https://doi.org/10.1016/j.jfma.2021.10.024
28. O'Dowd E, Lydon S, O'Connor P, Boland J, Offiah G, Byrne D. The development of a framework of entrustable professional activities for the intern year in Ireland. *BMC Med Educ.* 2020;20(1):273. DOI: https://doi.org/10.1186/s12909-020-02156-8
29. de Graaf J, Bolk M, Dijkstra A, van der Horst M, Hoff RG, ten Cate O. The implementation of entrustable professional activities in postgraduate medical education in the Netherlands: rationale, process, and current status. *Acad Med.* 2021;96(7S):S29-S35. DOI: https://doi.org/10.1097/ACM.0000000000004110
30. Jonker G, Ochtman A, Marty AP, Kalkman CJ, ten Cate O, Hoff RG. Would you trust your loved ones to this trainee? Certification decisions in postgraduate anaesthesia training. *Br J Anaesth.* 2020;125(5):e408-e410. DOI: https://doi.org/10.1016/j.bja.2020.07.009
31. Luke K. Twelve tips for managing change in medical education. *MedEdPublish.* 2021;10(1). DOI: https://doi.org/10.15694/mep.2021.000053.1
32. Bentley H, Darras KE, Forster BB, Sedlic A, Hague CJ. Review of challenges to the implementation of competence by design in post-graduate medical education: what can diagnostic radiology learn from the experience of other specialty disciplines? *Acad Radiol.* 2022;29(12):1887–1896. DOI: https://doi.org/10.1016/j.acra.2021.11.025
33. Gauthier S, Braund H, Dalgarno N, Taylor D. Assessment-seeking strategies: navigating the decision to initiate workplace-based assessment. *Teach Learn Med.* Published online June 29, 2023. DOI: https://doi.org/10.1080/10401334.2023.2229803
34. Franz A, Peters H. Diving beneath the surface of major curriculum reform using Bourdieu's field theory. *Med Educ.* Published online December 4, 2023. DOI: https://doi.org/10.1111/medu.15288

35. Mejicano GC, Bumsted TN. Describing the journey and lessons learned implementing a competency-based, time-variable undergraduate medical education curriculum. *Acad Med.* 2018;93(3S):S42-S48. DOI: https://doi.org/10.1097/ACM.0000000000002068
36. ten Cate O, Graafmans L, Posthumus I, Welink L, van Dijk M. The EPA-based Utrecht undergraduate clinical curriculum: development and implementation. *Med Teach.* 2018;40(5):506–513. DOI: https://doi.org/10.1080/0142159X.2018.1435856

CHAPTER 23

Faculty development for implementation of an EPA-based program

Josephine Boland, H. Carrie Chen, Fremen Chihchen Chou, Jean A. Fitzpatrick, Sonia Frick

Abstract

Faculty development, trainee orientation and stakeholder engagement are essential elements of change management in the implementation of EPAs. An effective strategy addresses stakeholder needs over the various stages of planning, piloting, and implementation of EPAs. It encompasses faculty and all other stakeholders, i.e., clinical supervisors and assessors, non-workplace-based teaching faculty, coaches or advisers for trainees' portfolios, members of clinical competence committees, administrators, program directors and other leaders. Best practices involve engaging with stakeholders as essential partners working toward a shared vision, building a sense of a community of practice, planning a range of activities in a continuous, dynamic, and enabling process, and including trainee development alongside faculty development.

This chapter introduces evolving conceptions of faculty development and identifies key principles and strategies to guide the design of an effective plan. A range of approaches is outlined from passive to active, with various modes of delivery including face-to-face and hybrid and self-directed learning. Factors to consider are discussed and the significance of context is acknowledged. The importance of resourcing faculty and other stakeholders and the need to make a business case supported by ongoing evaluation are highlighted. Three examples of strategies in practice illustrate some key ideas. An analysis of the specific needs of different stakeholder groups, with potential approaches and a directory of accessible digital resources to support faculty development, trainee orientation, and engagement with other stakeholders, is also provided.

How to cite this book chapter:
Boland J, Chen HC, Chou FC, Fitzpatrick J, Frick S. Faculty development for implementation of an EPA-based program. In: ten Cate O, Burch VC, Chen HC, Chou FC, Hennus MP. (Eds). *Entrustable Professional Activities and Entrustment Decision-Making in Health Professions Education*, Chapter 23, pp. 275–291. [2024] London: Ubiquity Press. DOI: https://doi.org/10.5334/bdc.w

This chapter uses cross-references to other chapters of the same book. For those who read this chapter as a standalone publication: all cross-references can be found at: https://doi.org/10.5334/bdc

Authors

- Josephine Boland, MSc, EdD. Medical education consultant, Galway, Ireland. Correspondence: josephinea.boland@gmail.com
- H. Carrie Chen, MD, PhD. Kaiser Permanente Bernard J. Tyson School of Medicine, Pasadena, California, USA.
- Fremen Chihchen Chou, MD, PhD, School of Medicine, China Medical University and China Medical University Hospital, Taichung, Taiwan.
- Jean A. Fitzpatrick, PT, PhD, MHS. Vagelos College of Physicians & Surgeons, Columbia University, New York, USA.
- Sonia Frick, MD, MME. Spital Limmattal, Switzerland. University of Zurich, Zurich, Switzerland.

Introduction

The implementation of an EPA-based framework for health professions education requires a change in educational practices and culture that is beyond that often needed with typical curricular innovations. An EPA-based curriculum involves an interactive, intensive teaching, learning, and assessment culture that may be new to many of the members of the institution. A key element of change management is faculty development and the orientation of any other stakeholder groups, including trainees, managers, and administrative personnel. The vital importance of engagement and consultation with the wider stakeholder community is addressed in Chapter 22. Faculty development is described as all activities that health professionals pursue to improve their knowledge, skills, and behaviors as teachers and educators, as leaders and managers, and as researchers and scholars in both individual and group settings.[1] For the purpose of this chapter, other key stakeholders (such as trainees and administrators) are included in the discussion. Faculty development, while essential, is an often-underappreciated aspect of curricular reform.[2] Most challenging, arguably, is the cultural change required for the adoption of new practices including the impetus for change and the value of the proposed innovation. Many stakeholders may need to shift from the educational paradigm in which they were trained (for example, the shift from using proficiency scales and scoring rubrics to entrustment–supervision scales) and adapt their practices to support a curriculum that provides learning activities allowing assessment of the EPAs, with a focus on entrustment. Educational programs must allocate resources toward the faculty development that will support implementation of change not just in the curriculum but in stakeholder practices.

Moving to EPA-based training will involve changes in both curricular and assessment structures. First, outcome expectations are defined by a focus on units of work that may be entrusted to a competent trainee rather than on the competencies of a trainee. It relies heavily on the concept of entrustment and links decisions around the entrustment and supervision of trainees to assessment, longitudinal progression, and achievement of outcomes. This has consequences for how clinical supervisors and clinical sites engage with trainees. First, supervising clinicians need to be able to talk to trainees about trust and entrustment and use EPA descriptions to guide learning and teaching. Second, trainees need be proactive about identifying their EPA-specific learning needs, negotiating experiences, seeking feedback, gathering evidence of attainment of EPAs, and accepting greater responsibility when ready.[3] Stakeholders must understand data from assessments and believe that they are credible, meaningful, and useful, and that the processes used are acceptable.[4] Curricular alignment of the EPAs with the training program must be visible and understandable to faculty and trainees alike. Faculty development must be defined for, and promoted to, an institution's members in a manner that clearly connects with its capacity to contribute to organizational change.[5] Moreover, they must have confidence in the process used to support EPA-based training and assessment, including summative entrustment decision-making. Table 23.1 shows, as an example, changes to be anticipated in culture and prac-

Table 23.1: Changes in culture and practice required.

Common changes in culture and practice when implementing EPAs and WBA	
For supervisors	**For trainees**
• Adopt a shared understanding of standards depicted in EPAS descriptions • Increase direct observations of trainee in the performance of EPAs • Apply the concept of entrustment decisions to assessment and feedback • Promote a trainee growth mindset through awarding of increased responsibility • Make time for teaching and assessment in the clinical day • Use new technologies to support the EPA-based curriculum	• Adopt a growth mindset to achieve entrustment for a greater responsibility • Be proactive in seeking and responding to feedback • Collaborate actively with supervisors • Share responsibility for collecting evidence of competence • Use new technologies to support the EPA-based curriculum

tice for supervisors and trainees. While many of these conditions may be in place in contexts where workplace-based assessment is already embedded, an EPA framework can bring additional challenges and responsibilities for supervising faculty and trainees. This chapter provides a general overview of key principles in faculty development, important for successful implementation of curricular interventions with examples specific to changes needed for an EPA-based curriculum.

Faculty development: for whom?

Fundamentally, development of faculty and other stakeholders is about supporting the implementation and management of change.[5] Implementation science provides a valuable framework to apply evidence-based faculty development approaches while also ensuring attention to drivers that promote and reinforce change.[6] Implementation science focuses on the uptake and incorporation of change into regular practice and outlines the importance of considering key drivers that support and sustain transformative change within an educational program. It also highlights the importance of gaining consensus on the need for change, which in turn requires a clear articulation of the rationale on the part of those leading it. Another valuable aspect of implementation science is the attention to context and how initiatives need to be adjusted to local contexts to be successful. An effective program of faculty development in a particular context aims for a shared vision for change, an understanding of the concept and language of EPAs, and a sense of responsibility to achieve that change.[7] A shared understanding of an EPA-based curricular system is critical, and includes trainees as a key stakeholder for change; hence, we include considerations for trainee development.[8] While the terminology used for stakeholder groups and roles may vary with context, we include eight groups: (a) clinical supervisors, (b) non-workplace-based teaching faculty, (c) trainees, (d) portfolio advisers and coaches, (e) clinical competency committee members, (f) program directors and other educational leaders, and (g) administrative personnel. Champions are an important category and can be recruited from within several of these groups (e.g., supervisors, trainees, administrators). The prior educational experience and their expectations are unlikely to be homogenous for each stakeholder group. Nonetheless, the needs of each group are generally described below and further addressed later in this chapter.

Faculty development: conceptions, principles, and strategies

Conceptions

There have been many conceptions of faculty development in recent decades. One is a deficit model suggesting they need to be 'developed' with new knowledge or skills. In recent decades, however, there has been increasing attention to faculty development as the building of an empowered 'community of practice.'[9] A community of practice has been defined by Lave and Wenger as a group of people who share a common concern or a passion for something they do, or learn how to do as they interact regularly.[10,11] This latter conception of faculty development highlights the need for a continuous and dynamic process where faculty enable each other's development. Faculty development should therefore aim to empower all stakeholders as members of the same community of practice, raise awareness of the value each stakeholder plays, and actively involve them as essential partners from the earliest stages of the change process including discussions on development and implementation.

Guiding principles for the development of a faculty development strategy

The establishment of a strategy for faculty development is highly context-specific. Those responsible for designing and implementing it need to respond to local conditions, opportunities,

Table 23.2: Stakeholder groups defined.

(a) Clinical supervisors
These include all frontline clinical supervisors (e.g., faculty, senior trainees) who are responsible for teaching, conducting workplace-based assessments, and making ad hoc entrustment decisions. They do not need to know how to write an EPA but they need to appreciate how they were derived. They need to be able to observe effectively, give feedback, use the entrustment–supervision scale and understand what the levels mean. They need to appreciate the concept of trust and be aware of the factors that may influence entrustment decisions. See Chapters 17–19 for an elaboration of workplace-based assessment to support entrustment decision-making.
(b) Non-workplace-based teaching faculty
These are faculty who have the important role of teaching classroom courses, developing intentional learning activities including simulation exercises to prepare for patient care, and instructing trainees in nonclinical settings. They need to know the content of the EPAs. While they do not have responsibility for conducting workplace-based assessment, they need to be aware of how their trainees will be assessed in the workplace. They can help introduce the concept of trust and hold trainees accountable for the factors that enable entrustment (e.g., agency, reliability, integrity, capability, humility).
(c) Trainees
Trainees need to be properly oriented to their role in an EPA-based system. They need to have s ufficient understanding of EPAs to be agents in their own learning and help support the behavioral change required of both clinical supervisors and themselves. They need to know what factors enable and impact entrustment and what they will be assessed on.
(d) Portfolio advisers and coaches
Advisers and coaches provide guidance to trainees to promote their professional growth, which requires establishing trusting and supportive relationships with trainees. They need to know how to interpret data within a portfolio, monitor progress, advise on progress toward achievement of EPAs, and mediate the outcomes of multisource feedback. They may be required to provide a report to a clinical competence committee.
(e) Clinical competency committee (CCC) members
These individuals need to understand and synthesize information from multiple sources, identify patterns of performance to determine a broad picture of a trainee's progression, and make summative entrustment decisions. The chair of a CCC has a particularly important role in ensuring equitable and consistent procedures. See Chapter 21 for the role and functions of a CCC.
(f) Program directors and other educational leaders
This group needs to be able to provide a sound and compelling vision and rationale for change when leading that change. They need to be able to facilitate the acquisition of new skills and inspire changes in behavior for others. They are centrally involved in planning the faculty development strategies and may be helpful in identifying and procuring needed resources.
(g) Administrative personnel
These individuals play an important role in providing logistical support to program directors and trainees. They have a key role in the management of the IT infrastructure to support workplace-based assessment and are responsible for pulling together all the assessment data that is collected for clinical competency committees.

and constraints. The work by Van Schaik et al. can provide useful guidance for the development of an accessible and adaptable strategy to support implementation of EPAs.[2] While Van Schaik's paper is concerned with 'faculty' in the conventional sense, the points are equally valid for other stakeholders and for the effective orientation of trainees, which is optimally done as a paired activity with members of faculty.

- *Create a blueprint* to inform the design and implementation of faculty development activities. This involves identifying the target group or groups with a plan that covers the various stages involved from piloting to implementation and consolidation.
- *Build on existing resources*, networks, and communities. Some faculty development activities can tap into training activities and resources already available internally or externally (e.g., training on how to give effective feedback).
- *Target different needs* and competence levels for different stakeholders utilizing a repertoire of activities, with flexible and adaptable opportunities, which optimize relevance for individual faculty members.
- *Encourage co-creation* in the workplace to involve all stakeholders in the development and continuous improvement of new strategy, workflows, and processes.
- *Promote collaboration* between practicing clinical supervisors and health profession educators to significantly enhance the design and delivery of faculty development. The involvement of credible peers has a powerful impact, when combined with external expertise.
- *Tap into faculty's intrinsic motivation* for professional development, following the principles of self-determination theory, supporting autonomy, competence and relatedness. Intrinsic motivation is augmented if there is a sense of interconnectedness and engagement. This approach may be complemented with some strategies that tap into extrinsic motivation, such as recognition and rewards.
- *Develop curriculum leaders, champions and faculty developers.* Faculty development to support curricular reform needs to be sustained, to ensure maintenance of skills and practices, and to accommodate new faculty. Champions can also be recruited from among the trainees, and recent graduates of the program.
- *Evaluate for continuous improvement.* This is essential and should encompass the impact on both the faculty and the trainees they teach and the quality of the training program. Evidence from evaluation can justify the continued investment in faculty development.

Instituting a faculty development program that extends over time is of particular relevance for EPAs, where implementation may be phased over a period of time. Changes in practice need to be reinforced and sustained, especially where new roles are concerned in an EPA-based system, such as portfolio advisers, champions, and CCC members. Steinert et al.[12] caution against an overreliance on formal structured approaches such as workshops and short courses and advocate a move to methods that involve experiential learning in the workplace that include guided reflection, peer coaching, and mentoring – a function that champions could help serve. Recommendations from the Core AAMC EPAs pilot in the US provide an example of using more experiential faculty development strategies and of creating a community of practice of all who teach and assess the EPAs.[7] These include pairing faculty development and trainee orientation to better inculcate a culture of shared entrustment, reciprocal feedback-seeking behaviors, and meaningful trainee–educator partnerships. They also recommend aligning assessment skill development with initiatives to enhance clinical skills and creating multiple opportunities for deliberate practice after self-assessment training, which resulted in reduced variability in faculty assessments of trainees. Box 23.1 shows an example derived from another pilot using the AAMC Core EPAs.[13]

Modes of delivery

A blueprint for faculty development will need a range of strategies and activities. It is possible to identify a range of modes of delivery from the relatively passive, such as written material to more active approaches requiring deeper engagement as seen in Figure 23.1,[14] which is not an exhaustive list.

Box 23.1: Strategies in practice – Example A: Faculty development for the Educating Pediatricians Across the Continuum project in the USA.

Background

The Association of American Medical Colleges (AAMC) in the Unites States ran a competency-based education pilot called EPAC (for Education in Pediatrics across the Continuum) at four different institutions including the University of California San Francisco (UCSF). The pilot program used an EPA framework for student assessment and advanced students from medical school to postgraduate training based on achievement of a specified level of entrustment on the AAMC 13 core EPAs. What is unique about this program from a faculty development perspective is that it only involved a small subset of students (approximately four annually) and the faculty who worked with or supervised those students. These faculty, along with the rest of the students and faculty, were still part of the regular curriculum using traditional assessments. Even though the program primarily impacted faculty in the pediatrics department, the EPAC students also worked with faculty in other departments.

Elements of the faculty development strategy at UCSF

Because the EPAC students would be rotating through multiple departments, UCSF ensured that all stakeholders were aware of the program and bought into the rationale for a competency-based education pilot. These stakeholders understood that the students would be assessed using a different (i.e., EPA) framework, but they were not expected to have literacy around EPAs. Because of the relatively few supervising clinicians involved in the pilot, a strategy was employed using students as the drivers of change. Faculty development efforts focused on two groups: the local leaders of and students in the EPAC program.

The local EPAC program leaders received intensive faculty development to ensure that they understood EPA principles and how these principles applied to the curriculum and assessment at the institution. They functioned as EPA champions among institutional leaders and other faculty, and could be engaged in the competency committees that made summative advancement decisions. The local leaders also provided ongoing development of the EPAC students.

Primary efforts went into the development and engagement of the EPAC students. By ensuring that the EPAC students fully understood the 13 core EPAs, how to use the entrustment–supervision scale, and the program's expectations of them, the students became partners in faculty development and drivers of curricular change. They were able to faculty-develop the small group of supervising clinicians working with and assessing them. The students made sure their supervising clinicians understood the core EPAs and how to use the scale, and pointed out opportunities for observation and assessment related to each of the EPAs. Additional questions or concerns that the students did not feel equipped to address were referred to the local leaders. Students pushed the faculty for actionable feedback that would allow them to gain further autonomy. They corrected the faculty when faculty were tempted to grade-inflate by reminding the faculty that the entrustment–supervision scale was not a proficiency rating scale but a supervision scale and that they should not be provided with less supervision before they are ready. This strategy not only empowered the students; it also allowed for a very targeted and experiential approach to the faculty development of supervising clinicians with few additional resources.

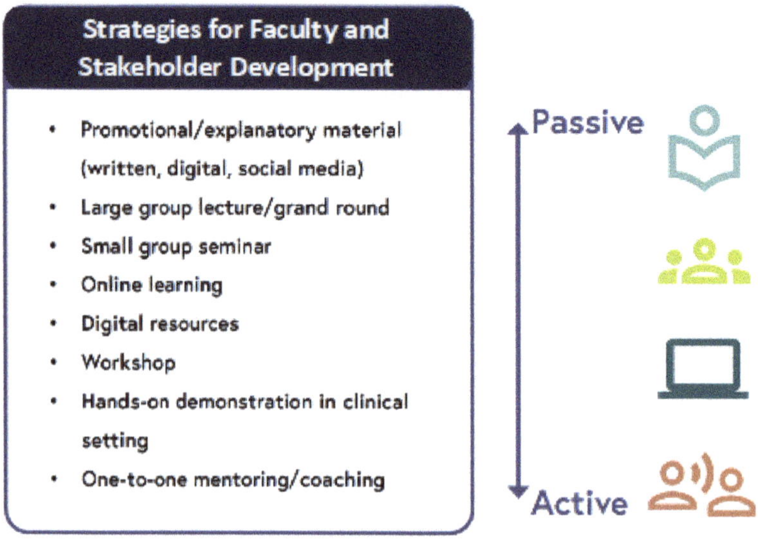

Figure 23.1: Strategies for faculty development.[14]

Materials that explain the innovation have a place and can reach a large audience, especially with the advent of social media. Traditionally, faculty development has been commonly envisioned as *events* that bring people together in a room, for face-to-face engagement.[1] As noted above, faculty should have opportunities to learn through facilitated skills practice and collegial approaches are important in setting standards and developing a shared mental model of expectations in trainees' performance of EPAs. While these face-to-face activities are extremely valuable, alternative approaches that harness other methodologies should be considered. Use of remote synchronous or asynchronous learning, independent learning, new communication technologies, and digital resources allow increased logistical flexibility and support different learning preferences.[15] New communication technologies can replicate many of the active learning features of the face-to-face workshop. Digital resources, such as explanatory animations and demonstrations of good practice in the workplace, can be incorporated into workshops and made available for just-in-time self-directed learning.

Factors to consider in designing a faculty development strategy

A range of factors need to be considered when devising an overall strategy for faculty development.[16] The list of factors in Table 23.3 has been compiled on the strength of the insights and experience of those engaged in EPA implementation. What is needed will vary significantly depending on the scale of faculty development, the stage of rollout of EPAs, and the level of familiarization and experience with CBE and WBA. A strategic choice to be made is whether faculty development is mandatory or optional. Is it aimed only at faculty who are willing to undertake WBA, or are all faculty expected to do it? Are only those who are trained regarded as legitimate or qualified assessors? While compulsory faculty development or the requirement of teaching qualifications for specific roles can help ensure key stakeholders are trained, one caution is that they may be difficult to enforce and unlikely to meet development goals if implemented without attention to resources and the environment.[17] Challenges experienced by faculty for participating in optional faculty development (e.g., lack of time) also exist for compulsory faculty development.[18] Implementation decisions related to all of the factors above will inform the approach.

Table 23.3: Factors to consider when planning faculty development.

Factors to consider	Think of
1. Scale	Program, regional, national
2. Stage of roll out the process	Preparation, piloting, implementation
3. Familiarization with CBE/WBA	Nature and scale of change involved
4. Whom to target	All or self-selected, mandatory or optional
5. Target group	Their particular needs
6. Aims and objectives	Expected effectiveness
7. Content and topics to be included	What is most useful for the target group
8. Activities	What will participants do; active learning
9. Format and group size	Large/small; online/face-to-face/hybrid
10. Venue	Where is most accessible for participants
11. Materials and space	Room, handouts, technology
12. Preparation by participants	Flipping the classroom; readings, questions
13. Evaluation of effectiveness	Reaction, learning, behavior, result
14. Follow up activities	Addition activities, support groups
15. Promoting engagement	Communication, rewards and recognition
16. Timing	Planning a series of opportunities scheduled over time
17. Delivered by	Insiders, outside expertise, peers
18. Resources	Making a business case
19. Expertise	A balance of internal and external expertise

Needs assessment and potential approaches

The design of faculty development requires clarity about each group's training needs (new knowledge, skills, practices), specific aims and objectives for training, and strategies to sustain the changes after initial development.[16] Based on this needs analysis, the next step is to select appropriate methodologies for each target group. Table 23.4 summarizes new knowledge, skills, and attitudes needed by each target group and potential approaches.[a] The degree of overlap in the needs of different groups is significant, as indicated in the first row in Table 23.3: knowledge, skills, attitudes, and potential approaches common for all groups.

In addition to conducting needs analyses for various stakeholders, one must consider that enabling and constraining factors, and challenges and opportunities are very context-specific.[16] Particular cultural traits of the profession or the institution (e.g., a reputation for innovation, commitment to education, or desire to lead curriculum reform) may prove pertinent as something that can be used for leverage. Similarly, it is important to anticipate common issues that may arise in one's specific context for each stakeholder group.

[a] This table was inspired by the yield of a break-out group exercise in the International Online Ins and Outs of EPAs course (www.epa-courses.nl) across 10 deliveries of the course. This is not intended as an exhaustive list.

Table 23.4: Suggested needs and approaches for various stakeholder groups.

	Knowledge, skills, and attitudes needed	Potential approaches
Common for all groups	• the rationale for change to CBE • concept of EPAs and entrustment • entrustment–supervision levels and scales • learner factors enabling entrustment (e.g., the A RICH framework) • operationalizing the EPA program in one's context • how to use the technology for the system • a growth mindset • engaging in team work	• common presentations • blended/hybrid learning • a way to respond to issues e.g., hotline, champions • FAQ section on the program website • continued attention and reinforcement • interdisciplinary and interprofessional approaches
Clinical supervi-sors/asses-sors	• providing effective feedback • documenting workplace-based assessments • making time in the clinical day • coaching in the moment (e.g., SMART, RC2C techniques) • identifying opportunities for entrustment decisions • the 'big picture,' i.e., curriculum overview • what progression of trainee should look like • applying the A RICH criteria for trainee trustworthiness when carrying out assessments (i.e., agency, reliability, integrity, capability, and humility)[19] • address deficits/gaps for achieving the next level of entrustment	• workshops (roleplay, scenario discussion) • online learning (instructional, video demonstration) • role modeling • demonstrations • peer observation and feedback • mentoring • toolkits and guidelines (paper-based or online)
Non-work-place-based Teaching faculty	• know the EPA curriculum • aligning their teaching to the EPAs • rethinking professionalism in terms of the A RICH criteria • applying the A RICH criteria for trainee trustworthiness to nonclinical learning environments	• curriculum review meetings • workshops (e.g., on mapping learning activities to EPAs) • other methods, as for supervisors/assessors but with different focus
Trainees	• taking responsibility for their own learning • seeking feedback proactively • responding to feedback • identifying opportunities for entrustment decisions • negotiating entrustment decisions with supervisors • collecting and reviewing evidence of own progress in portfolio	• orientation process • workshops (roleplay/simulation, scenario discussions) • near peer teaching of new trainees by senior trainees
Portfolio advisers	• providing feedback to support ongoing trainee devel-opment • mentoring as an effective longitudinal coach • analyzing and synthesizing data points • recognizing when trainees are on track (or not) • identifying when support or remediation is necessary • reporting to CCC and program director	• regular meetings as a community of advisers • workshops (roleplay, scenario discussion) • online learning resources • role modeling by more experienced portfolio advisers • guidelines (paper-based or online)
CCC members	• understanding program outcome expectations and developmental trajectories • appreciating the importance of their role • understanding the entire assessment system including psychometrics, context, and validity of available data • analyzing and synthesizing assessment data • engaging effectively in meetings • group facilitation skills for sound decision-making (chair)	• workshops with mock CCC for practice of consensus decision-making • case studies • guidelines on procedures for CCCs (paper-based or online) • special training for the CCC chair

(Continued)

Table 23.4: Continued.

	Knowledge, skills, and attitudes needed	Potential approaches
Program directors/ leaders	• leading change management • undertaking curriculum development in health professions education • planning entire assessment system including understanding of psychometrics, context, and validity of data • planning delivery of the EPA-based curriculum • designing and planning remediation for underperforming students • developing approaches for accelerated students • demonstrating alignment of the EPA curriculum with accreditation requirements • planning and delivering faculty development • providing training in effective group facilitation for sound decision-making • tapping into internal and external resources • planning piloting and implementation	• access existing training programs o leadership training courses o EPA development and implementation courses (e.g., Ins and Outs course) • linking into relevant institutional, national and international networks • (Inter)national teamwork for creating the curriculum • peer consulting from existing and functional programs • develop supportive teams
Admin. personnel	• understanding the entire EPA program and assessment processes • supporting program director • organizational skills • directing all stakeholders to resources • preparing reports for CCCs • supporting users in use of technology • preparing accreditation reports	• briefing meetings • training in data management system

Resourcing faculty development

Faculty development is a significant investment and requires resources, as evident from each of the strategies in practice featured in this chapter. Faculty development programs are not just an investment in individuals; they are an investment in the health of the institution, especially so in the case of longitudinal programs.[20] Programs must promote engagement, utilize appropriate recognition and rewards where feasible, and include an evaluation process for effectiveness. Strategies for finding and engaging people who will buy into and commit to the new curriculum and faculty development efforts include identifying and rewarding early champions, harnessing the goodwill of early adopters and those with an interest in education, and involving outside expertise. Those planning faculty development need to be able to identify and tap into available resources inside and outside the institution and make a business case for additional resources to budget-holders. A sound business case involves identifying the problem, as well as alternatives and the ideal solution. It offers an executive summary for the project and outlines the resources needed with the project scope, risks, and a timeline. This can include resources for materials, activities, outside expertise, and protected time for stakeholder development. It is necessary to identify resources and facilities required and make a sound business case to those in control of funding for the faculty development strategy. Another effective strategy for resourcing faculty development is to partner internationally in the planning and resourcing of faculty development.[21] Whatever the source of the funding, however, there is a need for constant attention to the business model – sustainability being heavily influenced by costs of delivery and number of participants.

A significant ongoing resource need is protected time for supervisors and assessors to implement and sustain change. While this is a matter for contractual arrangements by the institution, the availability of protected time may impact on engagement with faculty development and successful change in practice. A strategy that was employed by Singapore's Ministry of Health is explained in Box 23.2.

Box 23.2: Strategies in practice – Example B: Singapore's cascade model of training with a multidisciplinary approach.

Background

EPAs were first introduced into the postgraduate year 1 medical training in Singapore in 2014. Following a pilot study for selected health care professions, EPAs were made mandatory for all residency programs by the Ministry of Health (MOH) in 2022. The implementation aimed to involve 50 medical disciplines across four years, undergraduate and advanced nurse training, and other undergraduate health care professional training (speech therapy, dietetics, physiotherapy, occupational therapy, diagnostic radiography, radiation therapy).

Elements of the faculty development strategy

Due to the large effort across multiple professionals, the Singapore MOH decided to use a cascade model of training the trainers. After sending a MOH team to the 'Ins and Outs of Entrustable Professional Activities' international course, their next step was to raise awareness for the need to change among faculty members and trainees through multiple communication channels, including town halls and education conferences at health care institutions. They identified stakeholders who were likely to be early adopters for the initial wave of training and invited external experts to lead workshops and help train MOH facilitators and early adopters. These MOH facilitators then provided supplemental in-house EPA workshops to additional stakeholders.

The MOH then conducted a series of in-depth specialty and institution-based training sessions using trained MOH and local facilitators from the targeted institution. Structured workshops on EPA development and EPA implementation were customized to each specialty based on their progress and with support from the local facilitators. Consultation sessions were embedded within the workshops to allow facilitators to exercise flexibility in the learning outcomes for respective specialties. The facilitators supported these specialties through their EPA development and implementation, gradually reducing their assistance as specialties became more independent.

The MOH also appointed and trained faculty members from each program to serve as EPA champions and change leaders. Embedded within the program and specialty, they could coordinate change efforts and were best equipped to assess risks, anticipate resistance, and remove obstacles unique to each specialties' context. This cascade approach of ongoing efforts to train new trainers as subject matter experts to roll out national-level faculty development initiatives will help to further reinforce the adoption and implementation of EPAs.

The MOH provided several resources using a faculty development framework. They provided funding for those attending the international course and for the engagement of external experts. They also resourced institutions to provide the trained MOH and local facilitators with protected time away from their clinical commitments to conduct workshops and guide programs. Certain individuals with a keen interest in faculty development were further supported to conduct nation-wide faculty development initiatives. The MOH also produced a comprehensive online faculty development package with resources to help the faculties in their implementation of EPAs. It includes a wide array of content ranging from EPA literature to case scenario videos and to practical tips when implementing EPAs on the ground, with links to digital resources (accessible at https://go.gov.sg/eparesourcepackage).

The value of digital resources

Many of the faculty development strategies outlined above can be effectively supported with the judicious use of appropriate digital resources such as narrated PowerPoint presentations, multimedia presentations, instructional videos, whiteboard animations, and demonstration videos of workplace-based assessment in practice.[22] They can be used effectively to reach large audiences and are important in providing a convincing rationale for the changes that will be required. Easily accessible whiteboard animations or video demonstrations can provide just-in-time learning opportunities for busy clinicians e.g., to view in advance of completing a WBA. Demonstration of how to provide effective feedback when conducting WBAs, in various clinical scenarios for different EPAs, can prove powerful tools in faculty development workshops. They can assist in the process of developing a shared mental model by prompting discussion of standards of performance expected at different levels of supervision for EPAs.

When utilizing digital resources, one of the choices to be made is whether to use those developed by others or to develop one's own, set in one's cultural and organizational context and clinical settings. There are several free-to-use online resources on how to give effective feedback which provide general guidance. More recently, specific resources have been created, and shared, to support the introduction of EPAs in specific contexts. They are included as separate resources in Chapter 25. Bespoke resources, developed specifically to explain the rationale in *one's own* context and demonstrate supervisors', assessors', and trainees' functioning in one's clinical environment, have the obvious advantage of being authentic, relatable, and credible for one's stakeholders. Box 23.3 provides an account of the process used to develop bespoke digital resources to support the introduction of EPAs and workplace-based assessment within the Internship in Ireland. Collaboration between institutions offers valuable opportunities to share the cost of developing digital resources that can be adapted for use in different professional contexts.

Box 23.3: Strategies in practice – Example C: Creating resources to support rollout of a national program: Internship in Ireland.

Background

A new national curriculum framework was developed in Ireland for the internship program – the first year of postgraduate medical training. The framework comprises three elements: (a) *knowing* (knowledge guides), (b) *doing* (seven EPAs), and (c) *being* (professional behaviors, values, and practices), and a system of programmatic assessment using new workplace-based assessment tools. In 2003, the Medical Council approved the EPA-based framework for implementation by intern training networks across the country (https://www.lenus.ie/handle/10147/638294).

Elements of a faculty development strategy

The Medical Intern Unit devised a strategy to support implementation nationally, including meetings with stakeholders to raise awareness using town hall meetings on zoom and in-person in hospital sites face-to-face workshops in hospital sites and creation of digital resources.

(*Continued*)

Creation of digital resources to support faculty development

The Medical Intern Unit created a set of digital resources for its use and for the use of intern training networks in a cascade model of training. These focused on the EPAs and the workplace-based assessment tools and were explicitly set in the context of intern training, carefully scripted, and professionally produced. They included multimedia presentations to explain the rationale for EPAs and describe the seven EPAs, instructional animations to explain how to conduct workplace-based assessments, and authentic videos to demonstrate WBA in practice.

Features of authentic video demonstrations

The videos were set in clinical settings with credible scenarios for internship training and were relatable for supervisors and trainees in that context. Learning goals were clearly established for each one and scenarios were developed by clinicians through a facilitated process. Scripts were written and peer-reviewed by clinicians and the demonstrations were acted by clinicians, trainees, and professional actors.

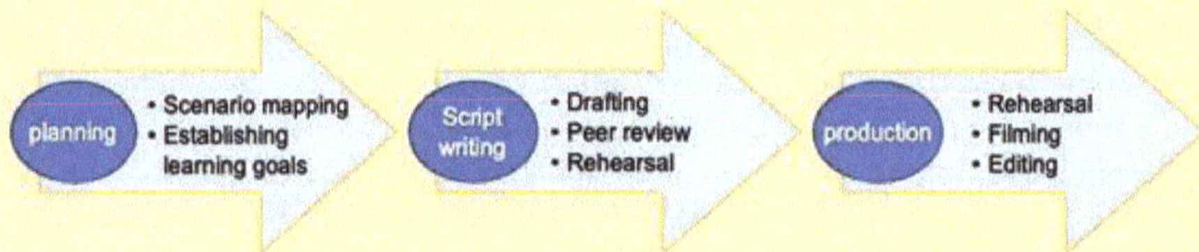

Tips for scripting authentic video demonstrations

(a) Think of three/four key messages for each one, (b) identify staging and props needed, (c) demonstrate best practice in the feedback conversation, (d) describe what the characters are feeling and how this might be expressed, and (e) make the script feel authentic for the audience.

The planning process

Given a defined budget for production of a digital resources, the steps taken were to:

1. create a matrix (of EPAs and WBA tools)
2. prioritize which EPAs to demonstrate
3. select which WBA tool to demonstrate for each EPA
4. select the supervision level for trainee performance in each video
5. recruit a team of practicing clinicians to draft scenarios, write scripts, and act in the videos
6. ensure diversity in the selection of clinicians/trainees/actors across the range of videos

Links to digital resources for presentations and animations: Introduction to EPAs, The 7 EPAs for the internship; How to do a case based discussion; How to do a case presentation; How to do a direct observation

Links to video demonstrations: Demo of a direct observation; Demo of direct observation of a clinical task; Demo of a case based discussion; Demo of a case presentation

The importance of evaluation

Appropriate and timely evaluation of faculty development is vital to inform future strategies and to demonstrate the value of faculty development in times of limited resources.[16] A range of evaluation methods will be required, from surveys to more longitudinal research, and a number of evaluation models exist. While not without its limitations, the Kirkpatrick model of training evaluation provides one potentially valuable framework for the design of evaluation with successive levels of evidence sought, from reaction, learning, and behavior to results.[23] Other approaches to evaluation include the CIPP framework, which provides an analytic basis for decision-making, focusing on context, input, process and product evaluation. While offering comprehensive insights, the CIPP model can be resource-intensive, demanding considerable time, personnel, and financial resources to conduct an extensive evaluation.[24] Moreover, it is claimed that evaluators may not deal with issues that go against the concerns of the decision maker. The logic model involves visual representation of the relationship between program inputs, activities, outputs and outcomes. One of the limitations of the logic model, however, is that programs (such as implementation of an EPA framework) are not necessarily linear and sequential. Each approach to evaluation has its strengths and limitations but they can usefully inform program design, implementation, and evaluation. More details about the various models for evaluation to achieve continuous quality improvement can be found in Chapter 24.

Conclusions

Implementing EPAs as a framework for competency-based education is a major change management process requiring ongoing faculty development. Effective needs assessment as an important first step involves determining what type of faculty development each stakeholder group needs in one's specific context. A successful faculty development strategy involves mapping out engaging activities over time for successive phases of piloting and implementation. An effective strategy also utilizes a range of approaches including face-to-face, blended/hybrid approaches, and self-directed learning. Clinical leadership and institutional commitment are key to effecting change and should be clearly visible to those engaging in faculty development. Faculty development needs to combine support from credible peers, external expertise, accessible resources, and flexible learning opportunities. It needs to be appropriately resourced, by making a sound business case for it to fund-holders. The development of bespoke digital learning resources can effectively support faculty development in workshop situations and for self-directed, just-in-time learning by supervisors and trainees. Opportunities exist, within and outside the institution, to collaborate with other bodies or international partners to share the cost of faculty development. Evaluation and review of the faculty development strategy is key to future planning and justifying the necessary investment of resources.

Competing interests

The authors declare that they have no competing interests.

Acknowledgments

Box 23.1: H. Carrie Chen (former site co-director of EPAC at UCSF). Box 23.2: M. Yap (Director, Professional Training and Assessment Standards Division, Ministry of Health, Singapore),

Box 23.3: Boland, J Geoghegan, R Jenkins, J Offiah, G: The power of authentic demonstrations when training health professionals in the conduct of workplace based assessment. 2023 AMEE Conference Workshop, Glasgow

References

1. Steinert Y, Mann K, Anderson B, et al. A systematic review of faculty development initiatives designed to enhance teaching effectiveness: a 10-year update: BEME guide no. 40. *Med Teach.* 2016;38(8):769–786. DOI: https://doi.org/10.1080/0142159X.2016.1181851
2. van Schaik SM. Accessible and adaptable faculty development to support curriculum reform in medical education. *Acad Med.* 2021;96(4):495–500. DOI: https://doi.org/10.1097/ACM.0000000000003804
3. Peters H, Holzhausen Y, Boscardin C, ten Cate O, Chen HC. Twelve tips for the implementation of EPAs for assessment and entrustment decisions. *Med Teach.* 2017;39(8):802–807. DOI: https://doi.org/10.1080/0142159X.2017.1331031
4. Norcini J, Anderson MB, Bollela V, et al. 2018 Consensus framework for good assessment. *Med Teach.* 2018;40(11):1102–1109. DOI: https://doi.org/10.1080/0142159X.2018.1500016
5. Jolly B. Faculty development for organizational change. In: Steinert Y, ed. *Faculty Development in the Health Professions: A Focus on Research and Practice.* Springer Netherlands; 2014: 119–137. DOI: https://doi.org/10.1007/978-94-007-7612-8_6
6. Bray MJ, Bradley EB, Martindale JR, Gusic ME. Implementing systematic faculty development to support an EPA-based program of assessment: strategies, outcomes, and lessons learned. *Teach Learn Med.* 2021;33(4):434–444. DOI: https://doi.org/10.1080/10401334.2020.1857256
7. Favreau MA, Tewksbury L, Lupi C, et al. Constructing a shared mental model for faculty development for the core entrustable professional activities for entering residency. *Acad Med.* 2017;92(6):759–764. DOI: https://doi.org/10.1097/ACM.0000000000001511
8. Lupi CS, Ownby AR, Jokela JA, et al. Faculty development revisited: a systems-based view of stakeholder development to meet the demands of entrustable professional activity implementation. *Acad Med.* 2018;93(10):1472–1479. DOI: https://doi.org/10.1097/ACM.0000000000002297
9. Steinert Y. Faculty development: from workshops to communities of practice. *Med Teach.* 2010;32(5):425–428. DOI: https://doi.org/10.3109/01421591003677897
10. Wenger E. *Communities of Practice: Learning, Meaning, and Identity.* Cambridge University Press; 1998.
11. Lave J, Wenger E. *Situated Learning: Legitimate Peripheral Participation (Learning in Doing: Social, Cognitive and Computational Perspectives).* 1st ed. Cambridge University Press; 1991:138.
12. Steinert Y, Mann K, Centeno A, et al. A systematic review of faculty development initiatives designed to improve teaching effectiveness in medical education: BEME guide no. 8. *Med Teach.* 2006;28(6):497–526. DOI: https://doi.org/10.1080/01421590600902976
13. Andrews JS, Bale JF, Soep JB, et al. Education in Pediatrics Across the Continuum (EPAC): first steps toward realizing the dream of competency-based education. *Acad Med.* 2018;93(3): 414–420. DOI: https://doi.org/10.1097/ACM.0000000000002020
14. Boland J, Offiah G. *Curriculum Framework for the Internship Programme in Ireland.* Health Service Executive; 2023.
15. Cook DA, Steinert Y. Online learning for faculty development: a review of the literature. *Med Teach.* 2013;35(11):930–937. DOI: https://doi.org/10.3109/0142159X.2013.827328
16. Silver I. Starting a faculty development program. In: Steinert Y, ed. *Faculty Development in the Health Professions: A Focus on Research and Practice.* Springer Netherlands; 2014:331–349. DOI: https://doi.org/10.1007/978-94-007-7612-8_16

17. Trowler P, Bamber R. Compulsory higher education teacher training: joined-up policies, institutional architectures and enhancement cultures. *International Journal for Academic Development*. 2005;10(2):79–93. DOI: https://doi.org/10.1080/13601440500281708
18. van Bruggen L, ten Cate O, Chen HC. Developing a novel 4-C framework to enhance participation in faculty development. *Teach Learn Med*. 2020;32(4):371–379. DOI: https://doi.org/10.1080/10401334.2020.1742124
19. ten Cate O, Chen HC. The ingredients of a rich entrustment decision. *Med Teach*. 2020;42(12):1413–1420. DOI: https://doi.org/10.1080/0142159X.2020.1817348
20. Gruppen LD. Intensive longitudinal faculty development programs. In: Steinert Y, ed. *Faculty Development in the Health Professions: A Focus on Research and Practice*. Springer Netherlands; 2014:197–216. DOI: https://doi.org/10.1007/978-94-007-7612-8_10
21. Friedman S, Cilliers F, Tekian A, Norcini J. International faculty development partnerships. In: Steinert Y, ed. *Faculty Development in the Health Professions: A Focus on Research and Practice*. Springer Netherlands; 2014:311–329. DOI: https://doi.org/10.1007/978-94-007-7612-8_15
22. Dyrbye LN, Bergene AL, Leep Hunderfund AN, Billings HA. Reimagining faculty development deployment: a multipronged, pragmatic approach to improve engagement. *Acad Med*. 2022;97(9):1322–1330. DOI: https://doi.org/10.1097/ACM.0000000000004688
23. Cahapay M. Kirkpatrick model: its limitations as used in higher education evaluation. *Int J Assess Tools Educ*. 2021;8(1):135–144. DOI: https://doi.org/10.21449/ijate.856143
24. Alkin MC. Evaluation roots. In: *Evaluation Roots*. SAGE Publications, Inc.; 2004:374–380. DOI: https://doi.org/10.4135/9781412984157.n25

CHAPTER 24

Advancing and sustaining excellence in EPA-based curricula

Machelle Linsenmeyer, Andrew K. Hall, Chien-Yu Jonathan Chen, María José López, Fremen Chihchen Chou

Abstract

The quality of health professions education is socially determined and closely linked to the quality of health care. Entrustable professional activities (EPAs) add strength to and operationalize curricula for competency-based education for health professions by focusing on both the patient and trainee, bringing health professions education together with patient care. This social accountability within an EPA-based curriculum emphasizes measurable enhancements to local health services through EPAs. As such, both external quality assurance (QA) and internal QA are crucial for implementing and improving an EPA-based program. External QA involves guidance from the regulating body regarding training policies, procedures, and practices. Internal QA entails self-auditing, utilizing mechanisms like program evaluation (PE) to monitor, evaluate, and improve the assessment and attainment of EPAs. Continuous quality improvement (CQI) can be used to augment PE by serving as a system for accountability and transparency. This section introduces the concepts of PE and CQI to be used within an EPA-based curriculum, models to support PE and CQI processes, examples of actual cases where PE and CQI were beneficial, and solutions to address challenges specific to EPA-based curricula.

Authors

- Machelle Linsenmeyer, EdD, FNAOME. West Virginia School of Osteopathic Medicine, Lewisburg, West Virginia, USA. Correspondence: alinsenmeyer@osteo.wvsom.edu

How to cite this book chapter:

Linsenmeyer M, Hall AK, Chen CY, López, M, Chou FC. Advancing and sustaining excellence in EPA-based curricula. In: ten Cate O, Burch VC, Chen HC, Chou FC, Hennus MP. (Eds). *Entrustable Professional Activities and Entrustment Decision-Making in Health Professions Education*, Chapter 24, pp. 293–301. [2024] London: Ubiquity Press. DOI: https://doi.org/10.5334/bdc.x

- Andrew K. Hall, MD, FRCPC, MMEd, DRCPSC. University of Ottawa, Ottawa, Ontario, Canada and Royal College of Physicians and Surgeons of Canada.
- C-Y Jonathan Chen, MD, PhD. School of Medicine, College of Medicine, Taipei Medical University, Taipei, Taiwan.
- María José López, MPsy, Ed. Esp. Medical Sciences Faculty, Cuyo National University, Mendoza, Argentina.
- Fremen C. Chou, MD, PhD. School of Medicine, China Medical University and China Medical University Hospital, Taichung, Taiwan.

Introduction

In the development of initiatives around entrustable professional activities (EPAs), one must consider strategies for program evaluation (PE) and continuous quality improvement (CQI). These concepts are slightly different but related. PE is defined as the systematic investigation of the quality of programs,[1] with multiple potential decision-making purposes, including accountability, knowledge generation, and program development.[2] PE involves collecting data (both quantitative and qualitative) and providing evidence to support results to answer specific questions, such as 'how do or will we know the "program" is working?' and 'is there credible evidence that the program contributed to achieving the desired results?' PE can be narrow in scope or examine larger questions of program direction, efficiency, feasibility, and viability, and it can seek to evaluate an entire training program or focus on specific elements of the program that may be new or need revision. In CQI, the focus is on looking beyond *what* is happening to *why* it is happening and how that fits into the greater scheme of successes and failures within the initiative. It asks questions like 'how are we doing?' and 'can we do better?'[3] CQI should be an ongoing, constant, and sustained approach used to achieve improved standards that will lead to better outcomes, efficiency, communication, reducing errors, and improving safety.[3,4] A CQI system adds several unique and important processes including acting upon data (from PE) to implement or improve processes, testing of program penetration/precision/consistency, testing of impact, and cost analysis or considerations. CQI provides a system of accountability and transparency to both internal and external stakeholders (e.g., consumers, partners, and regulating bodies). PE is fundamental to CQI, serving as part of the planning, feedback, and evidence used for decision-making. The capacity to do PE is a characteristic of a high-functioning CQI program. Therefore, developing CQI processes that incorporate solid strategies for PE will help ensure a continued driver for analysis and improvement of initiatives around EPAs.

Building on this foundation, the literature underscores the significance of establishing PE and CQI processes at the outset of initiatives to enhance educational outcomes.[5–8] These processes are crucial for effectively addressing challenges, such as the risk of implementing improvements only after problems have occurred, which can miss opportunities for immediate enhancement. They help maintain momentum and trust by clearly defining roles, setting up efficient data collection systems for quick problem identification and resolution, and reducing duplication of efforts by integrating these processes into existing assessment frameworks. Furthermore, it is important to establish mechanisms to keep all stakeholders well-informed about progress and procedures, ensuring ongoing community engagement and support for the initiatives.

By being very intentional about setting up PE and CQI processes at the beginning, an institution can engage in PE and CQI in a meaningful way that will ensure the desired impact and avoid unintended negative consequences. It is rare that initial implementations of educational innovations and programs 'get it right' from the start. Making conscientious efforts to set up mechanisms to identify potential issues as they occur leads to better outcomes. In fact, in the implementation of Competence-By-Design in Canada, introduced in 2017, the Royal College of Physicians and Surgeons of Canada's PE strategy was able to detect and respond to a host of unintended consequences of initial implementation, including negative impacts on resident wellness.[9] Other examples include the identification of curricular deficiencies that need to be addressed to ensure success in EPA assessments, such as the experience of the West Virginia School of Osteopathic Medicine, where a lack of opportunities for learners to perform oral presentations during clinical training—despite the requirement to be assessed on this essential EPA—led to curricular revisions to better ensure opportunities for direct assessment in clinical training.

Models of program evaluation and continuous quality improvement

Evidence-based CQI should be an ongoing cycle of collecting data and then testing, implementing, learning from, and revising solutions. Several models can be used for both CQI and PE. The PDSA cycle, devised by Deming, is a methodical four-step approach (plan–do–study–act) for continuous improvement by systematically integrating learning and knowledge acquisition through innovation or implementation.[10] The cycle starts with planning a goal and strategy, followed by implementing the plan, studying the outcomes to evaluate success or identify improvements, and finally acting on these insights to refine or expand the approach, thus initiating a new cycle of improvement. Most CQI models have roots in Deming's PDSA model.[10] For example, the CAPA-CAR model[11] (context–aim–plan–approval—collect–analyze–report) builds on Deming's PDSA model by expanding phases for considerations unique to curriculum and faculty, such as the context and approval phases. Other popular models place PDSA within a specific context to provide direction to the process. These include Lean,[12,13] which focuses on organizational improvement in the context of the patient and identifying poor quality and waste, and Six Sigma,[14] which emphasizes DMAIC (define–measure–analyze–improve–control), with a focus on reducing variations and defects. Depending on an institution's goals and findings from PE, one or more of these models may be useful in outlining an institution's CQI initiatives. Within CQI initiatives, specific steps can be supplemented by the logic models, PE models, and other evaluation methods noted in Table 24.1.

These models or frameworks can be explored to supplement phases of an institution's CQI initiative depending on the questions outlined for focus and review. The frameworks can support multiple types of evaluation and feed into an institution's CQI process. Types of PE include formative, developmental, process, outcome, economic, and impact evaluation.

Table 24.1: Example models or frameworks to support program evaluation and continuous quality improvement.

Frameworks or models	Explanation
Logic model[21,22]	A logic model is a tool commonly used in PE to build an understanding of how a program is supposed to work, that is, the relationship between the program components or process and the program outcomes. It links results and changes with inputs, activities, outputs, and outcomes.
Kirkpatrick framework[23]	It is used to evaluate the results of training and learning programs through four criteria: reaction, learning, behavior, and results. Recent discussions have proposed new thoughts on this framework related to EPA assessments in relation to patient outcomes.[24]
Rapid evaluation[25,26]	PE focused on capturing and providing timely evidence to engage in a process of evolutionary adaptation. Key steps: (a) description of the ideal implementation, or implementation as intended (b) measurement of stakeholder experiences, or implementation as enacted (c) proposed program adaptations based on an analysis of the ideal vs enacted implementation.
Realist evaluation[27,28]	Realist evaluation asks the questions: what works, for whom, in what circumstances, in what respects, to what extent, and why? It employs multiple methods of data collection and analysis, seeking to ensure an in-depth understanding of both the context of implementation and subsequent outcomes, considering the mechanisms by which the desired outcomes of an educational intervention are or are not experienced.
Experimental or quasi-experimental models[29]	These are used to determine cause and effect and support multiple designs such as intact-group design, time-series experimental design, and ex post facto experiment design.[2]
CIPP-I model[30]	This model expands the CIPP model[31] to include analysis of context, input, process, product, and impact.

Formative evaluation involves gathering evidence during implementation to understand strengths and weaknesses for improvement purposes, to ensure that a program or program activity is feasible, appropriate, and acceptable before it is fully implemented. It is a feasibility study that is usually conducted when a new program or activity is being developed or when an existing one is being adapted or modified.[15]

Developmental evaluation supports innovation development to guide adaptation to emergent and dynamic realities in complex environments. It is particularly suited for innovation, radical program redesign, replication, complex issues, and crises.[16]

Process evaluation determines whether an educational intervention or program has been implemented as intended, also known as the fidelity of implementations.[17]

Outcome evaluation measures program or intervention effects in the target population by assessing the progress in the outcomes or outcome objectives that the program is to achieve.[18]

Economic evaluation looks at the cost–benefit of the program, which could include cost analysis, cost-effectiveness evaluation, cost–benefit analysis, cost–utility analysis, value-based analysis, etc.[19]

Impact evaluation assesses program effectiveness in achieving its ultimate goals.[20]

How does this apply to EPAs initiatives? First, these models can be used to develop processes for continuous improvement in EPAs-based curriculum. One example is for the clinical competency committees (or equivalent body performing summative assessments) to support quality improvement efforts by recording comments in quality, scope, and practice that may need to be adjusted or changed in the curriculum, in the professional development of evaluators, in opportunities for assessments, in the expansion of views or evaluators with multiple views to broaden perspectives, etc. By presenting findings to end users (i.e., clinical competency committees, assessors, and learners/trainees), institutions can better understand variances, uncover possible factors causing issues, and discover viable solutions for improvement. Boxes 24.1, 24.2, and 24.3 provide example cases of CQI in EPA implementation initiatives in different countries.

Box 24.1: Rapid evaluation cycle at Queens University, Kingston, Ontario.

With the staged implementation of CBME and EPAs in the specialist Canadian Postgraduate Medical Education system by the Royal College of Physicians and Surgeons of Canada (starting in 2017),[32] it was imperative to understand the experience of early implementers and those who piloted EPAs prior to formal implementation. One such program was the emergency medicine training program at Queen's University in Kingston, Canada. Recognizing the need to engage in evaluation and for prompt broad sharing of lessons learned, program leadership coordinated with national education leaders to engage in a systematic rapid evaluation of program-level implementation post-implementation with a focus on both fidelity of implementation and the measurement of early outcomes.[26] After an explicit description of the ideal implementation, stakeholder focus groups and interviews were performed at three and nine months after implementation. Organized using the core components framework,[33] thematic analysis was conducted to understand stakeholder experiences, and the actual, or enacted, implementation was compared with ideal implementation to plan rapid adaptations. An example of an early lesson learned was clear concerns about the granularity of assessment with EPAs and a loss of the 'forest for the trees,' prompting the return of global feedback to supplement EPA-focused feedback. Additionally, there was detection of a lack of a shared mental model in the use of assessment tools and scales, resulting in significant variability and difficulty among frontline faculty assessors. The findings of this PE were shared broadly with the Canadian medical education community to help revise subsequent CBME/EPAs implementations. Further, this method of rapid evaluation has been further employed to evaluate the implementation of CBME by the Royal College of Physicians and Surgeons of Canada across multiple disciplines and institutions.[6]

Box 24.2: Implementing the continuous quality improvement cycle in CBME: the Taiwan experience.

To advance health care training programs toward EPA- and competency-based approaches, leaders from various institutions and specialties in Taiwan adopted the logic model. Since 2016, they have collaboratively investigated problems, created consensus, and designed tools and strategies for implementing a CQI cycle.

World Café workshops emerged as an appropriate tool to address initial challenges, which revealed the failure of the 'top-down' model in previous educational reforms. This innovative strategy facilitated connections among diverse perspectives, promoted the development of shared mental models, and served as a valuable platform for faculty development. As a result of this collaborative effort, Taiwan now boasts nationwide versions of EPAs for various postgraduate programs, including anesthesiology (2017), postgraduate general physicians (2018), emergency medicine (2019), otolaryngology–head and neck surgery (2021), and also undergraduate medical education (2024).

Furthermore, specialized evaluation toolkits were devised to address a second issue concerning the quality of implementation. A Competence Committee Checklist (2019), a Program Evaluation Committee Checklist (2021), and a Program Evaluation Checklist (2023) were introduced to bolster the effectiveness and integrity of the program's design and execution.

To alleviate the administrative load associated with organizing the competence committee and program evaluation committee, and to effectively implement the CQI cycle, some institutions have adopted Microsoft Power BI, using the vast educational data available from the clinical training e-portfolio platform as indicators for program quality. Data analysis with Power BI enabled a comprehensive and continuous review of various aspects such as the quantity and quality of courses delivered, faculty development, trainee performance, and feedback on areas like workplace-based assessments with EPAs.

Box 24.3: Continuous quality improvement under low resourced conditions: an Argentina experience.

CQI requires resources that are not always available. The undergraduate medical program of the Universidad Nacional de Cuyo, in Mendoza, Argentina, applies a quality assurance process with limited resources. The program has been externally evaluated four times in the last 20 years and was accredited every time. However, institutional concerns arose regarding the assessment system and the expected learning outcomes in the final mandatory practice (FMP) year of the program. Limited resources precluded them from having a dedicated team or person for CQI, and no technology was available for automated data collection and processing. Any annual CQI thus belongs to the work of already-busy teaching coordinators.

Within these limitations, the defined CQI goals remained to improve the specification of competencies and to develop an assessment system that is accepted by teachers and students, to warrant sustainability across time. Coordinators of the four main clerkships

(*Continued*)

played a key role in this CQI implementation under the decisive leadership of the director of FMP, and supported by education specialists and faculty development. Since 2017, five internal annual cycles of quality assessment (with a two-year COVID-19 pause) have focused on purpose definition, planning, change implementation, data collection, analysis, and purpose reformulation for the next academic year. Evaluation data included student assessment results, supervisor opinions through online surveys and face-to-face workshops, and student opinions collected by surveys.

In each cycle, steps toward the CQI goals were taken, based on the evaluation of the previous academic year. This model allowed those who provided evaluation input to witness change and feel ownership.

Informed by this formative evaluation and in the context of a new external evaluation, a new curriculum design was planned for 2025, with EPAs and assessment based on entrustment decision-making.

Table 24.2: Challenges of program evaluation and continuous quality improvement specific to EPA-based curricula.

Key factors	Challenges to be addressed
Money/resources	Establishing reasonable budgets (including all possible costs such as technology platforms, data analysts, funds to support focus groups, and so on) will ensure a projected amount of money to complete/support the initiative.
Dedicated person	A dedicated person or team (depending on size of programs) will help establish responsibility and ensure a point person with the skills and experiences necessary to carry out the initiatives.
Timeframe	A realistic timeline will help establish accountability for the PE and CQI initiatives.
Projects not sustainable	Consider breaking the initiative into smaller projects or phases, as needed. By breaking initiatives into smaller projects, an institution can build enthusiasm and energy from project to project while still pulling findings together from each project into an overall initiative.
Stakeholder buy-in	Buy-in is imperative. Ensure that stakeholders are included in the processes so that they are not resistant to the initiatives—providing professional development can help with buy-in.
PE and CQI alignment	Ensure that continuous quality improvement feeds into an institution's program planning so the institution can see and highlight the findings to action.
Leadership and culture	Institutions should ensure support and expertise in methods at the very top levels so that the culture is affected at all levels of the organization, not just the ground levels.
Data capture and visualization	Institutions can lessen the administrative load associated with organizing data for use by stakeholders (i.e., clinical competency committees), program evaluation committees, and for CQI processes by employing effective data capture and visualization systems.
Clear goals and objectives	Institutions should engage stakeholders to ensure cocreation of the programs(s) and processes related to EPAs for not only clarity of goals and objectives but also for buy-in.

Several challenges may come to light in thinking of PE and CQI specific to EPA-based curricula, especially in the area of time and resources to carry out initiatives. Table 24.2 introduces challenges that institutions should consider.

Conclusion

While defining quality can be subjective and ever-changing, as well as influenced by a multitude of factors both internally and externally, it is also imperative as a driver for improvement and mechanism to ensure success by identifying and overcoming challenges faced. Institutions must be thoughtful in creating the CQI (and PE) initiatives, remembering that a combination of tools, methods, and processes can be used and focusing on an organization's specific needs and goals. These CQI initiatives should be fully embraced as part of continued growth and development for both the curriculum or assessment program as well as faculty serving as teachers or evaluators in the system.

Competing interests

The authors declare that they have no competing interests.

References

1. Yarborough DB, Shulha LM, Hopson RK, Caruthurs FA. *The Program Evaluation Standards*. 3rd ed. Sage Publications; 2011.
2. Frye AW, Hemmer PA. Program evaluation models and related theories: AMEE Guide No. 67. *Med Teach*. 2012;34(5):e288-e299. DOI: https://doi.org/10.3109/01421 59X.2012.668637
3. Adams D. Quality improvement; part 1: instruction and overview. *BJA Education*. 2018;18(3):89–94.
4. Jamieson S. State of the science: Quality improvement of medical curricula—How should we approach it? *Med Educ*. 2023;57(1):49–56. DOI: https://doi.org/10.1111/medu.14912
5. Hedrick JS, Cottrell S, Stark D, et al. A review of continuous quality improvement processes at ten medical schools. *Med Sci Educator*. 2019;29(1):285–290. DOI: https://doi.org/10.1007/s40670-019-00694-5
6. Wong BM, Headrick LA. Application of continuous quality improvement to medical education. *Med Educ*. 2021;55(1):72–81. DOI: https://doi.org/10.1111/medu.14351
7. Bendermacher G, De Grave W, Wolfhagen I, et al. Shaping a culture for continuous quality improvement in undergraduate medical education. *Acad Med*. 2020;95(12):1913–1920. DOI: https://doi.org/10.1097/ACM.0000000000003406
8. Loper AC, Jensen TM, Farley AB, et al. A systematic review of approaches for continuous quality improvement capacity-building. *J Public Health Manag Pract*. 2022;28(2):E354-E361. DOI: https://doi.org/10.1097/PHH.0000000000001412
9. Hall AK, Oswald A, Frank JR, et al. Evaluating competence by design as a large system change initiative: readiness, fidelity, and outcomes. *Perspect Med Educ*. 2024;13(1):95–107. DOI: https://doi.org/10.5334/pme.962
10. Deming WE. *Out of the Crisis*. MIT Press; 2000. Also, see the Deming Institute website at: https://deming.org/explore/pdsa/. Accessed March 5, 2024.
11. Linsenmeyer, M. Curriculum and teacher evaluation. In: Dent J, Harden R, Hunt D, eds. *A Practical Guide for Medical Teachers*. 6th ed. Elsevier; 2021:419–427.
12. Womack JP, Jones DT. *Lean Thinking: Banish Waste and Create Wealth in Your Corporation*. 2nd ed. Free Press; 2003.
13. Smith I, Hicks C, McGovern T. Adapting lean methods to facilitate stakeholder engagement and co-design in healthcare. *BMJ*. 2020;368:m35.

14. Fereday S. *A Guide to Quality Improvement Methods.* Healthcare Quality Improvement Partnership; 2015.
15. Goldie J. AMEE education guide no. 29: evaluating educational programmes. *Med Teach.* 2006;28(3):210–224. DOI: https://doi.org/10.1080/01421590500271282
16. Patton M. *Developmental Evaluation Applying Complexity Concepts to Enhance Innovation and Use.* Guilford Press; 2010.
17. Century J, Rudnick M, Freeman C. A framework for measuring fidelity of implementation: a foundation for shared language and accumulation of knowledge. *Am J Eval.* 2010;31:199–218.
18. Van Melle E, Hall AK, Schumacher DJ, et al. Capturing outcomes of competency-based medical education: the call and the challenge. *Med Teach.* 2021;43(7):794–800. DOI: https://doi.org/10.1080/0142159X.2021.1925640
19. Rudmik L, Drummond M. Health economic evaluation: important principles and methodology. *The Laryngoscope.* 2013;123(6):1341–1347. DOI: https://doi.org/10.1002/lary.23943
20. Gertler PJ, Martinez S, Premand P, Rawlings LB, Vermeersch CM. *Impact Evaluation in Practice.* 2nd ed. World Bank Publications; 2016.
21. Frechtling J. *Logic Modeling Methods in Program Evaluation.* 1st ed. Jossey-Bass/Wiley; 2007.
22. Van Melle E. Using a logic model to assist in the planning, implementation and evaluation of educational programs. *Acad Med.* 2016;91:1464.
23. Kirkpatrick DI. Evaluation of training. In: Craig R, Mittel I, eds. *Training and Development Handbook.* McGraw Hill; 1967:87–112.
24. ten Cate O, Snell L, Carraccio C. Medical competence: The interplay between individual ability and the health care environment. *Med Teach.* 2010;32(3):669–675. DOI: https://doi.org/10.3109/0142159X.2010.500897
25. Gold M, Helms D, Guterman S. The Commonwealth Fund. Identifying, monitoring, and assessing promising innovations: Using evaluation to support rapid-cycle change. https://www.commonwealthfund.org/publications/issue-briefs/2011/jun/identifying-monitoring-and-assessing-promising-innovations-using. Published June 16, 2011. Accessed March 5, 2024.
26. Hall AK, Rich J, Dagnone JD, et al. It's a marathon, not a sprint: rapid evaluation of competency-based medical education program implementation. *Acad Med.* 2020;95(5):786–793.
27. Wong G, Greenhalgh T, Westhorp G, Pawson R. Realist methods in medical education research: what are they and what can they contribute? *Med Educ.* 2012;46:89–96. DOI: https://doi.org/10.1111/j.1365-2923.2011.04045.x
28. Graham AC, McAleer S. An overview of realist evaluation for simulation-based education. *Adv Simul.* 2018;3(13). DOI: https://doi.org/10.1186/s41077-018-0073-6
29. Stufflebeam DL, Shinkfield A. *Evaluation Theory, Models, & Applications.* Jossey Bass/John Wiley & Sons, Inc.; 2007.
30. Barber C, van der Vleuten C, Leppink J, Chahine S. Social accountability frameworks and their implications for medical education and program evaluation: a narrative review. *Acad Med.* 2020;95(12):1945–1954. DOI: https://doi.org/10.1097/ACM.0000000000003731
31. Stufflebeam DL. The CIPP model for evaluation. In: Kellghan T, Stufflebeam DL, eds. *International Handbook of Educational Evaluation.* Springer, Kluwer; 2003.
32. Frank JR, Karpinski J, Sherbino J, et al. Competence by design: a transformational national model of time-variable competency-based postgraduate medical education. *Perspect Med Educ.* 2024;13(1): in press.
33. Van Melle E, Frank JR, Holmboe ES, Dagnone D, Stockley D, Sherbino J; International competency-based medical education collaborators. A core components framework for evaluating implementation of competency-based medical education programs. *Acad Med.* 2019;94(7):1002–1009. DOI: https://doi.org/10.1097/ACM.0000000000002743

CHAPTER 25

Resources to support the development of EPA-based education

A major purpose of this book is to support educators with the development and implementation of EPA-based education. The idea arose from an international course that has been conducted several times per year since 2018. This course draws heavily on interactive workshops with exercises, using worksheets and other resource materials. This chapter provides specific resources from the course useful for educators, scholars, and faculty developers. Additional useful tools and references also have been included.

In this chapter we provide the following collection of resources and information:

- Glossary of EPA-related terminology
- Online resources to support faculty development on EPA frameworks and workplace-based assessment
- Bibliography of most of the literature published from 2005 to 2023 about EPAs and related concepts
- Tools and instructions for use in faculty development workshop exercises
- The EQual Rubric tool to evaluate the fit-for-purpose validity of entrustable professional activities

Glossary of EPA-related terminology

Throughout this book, many terms have been used that are either specific or directly linked to EPA-based education. We have included this glossary to support readers who may be new to these terms. Note, however, that terms are sometimes used in slightly different ways, even within this book by different author teams and across different chapters. In the overview below, we suggest a definition that can be used as a starting point to understand and describe EPAs, for curriculum

How to cite this book chapter:
ten Cate O, Burch VC, Chen HC, Chou FC, Hennus MP. (Eds). *Entrustable Professional Activities and Entrustment Decision-Making in Health Professions Education*, Chapter 25, pp. 303–314. [2024] London: Ubiquity Press. DOI: https://doi.org/10.5334/bdc.y

development and implementation, for assessment, for scholarship, etc. We do not claim that these are the only correct definitions, or even that all are the preferred ones. The book's index refers to chapters where these terms are used elsewhere, to provide further explanations and nuance, in addition to the references listed below the table.

Table 25.1: Glossary of terms related to entrustable professional activities and entrustment decision making.

Ad hoc entrustment decisions	Entrustment decisions situated in time and place, based on estimated trustworthiness of the trainee for a task, estimated risk of the situation, urgency of the job to be done, and suitability of this task at this moment for this trainee. They do not necessarily constitute a precedent for similar decisions in the future.
Core EPAs	All EPAs that every trainee in a program must master to successfully complete the program (term also used for AAMC-proposed EPAs for undergraduate medical education[1]).
CBE (competency-based education)	An outcomes-based approach to the design, implementation, assessment, and evaluation of medical education programs, using an organizing framework of competencies. CBE-HPE relates this to all health professions; CBME, CBVE are acronyms for medical and veterinary competency-based education, respectively, and other variants may be used for other professions.
Domains of competence	Broad areas of competence that constitute a general descriptive competency framework for a profession, such as described in the six-domain ACGME framework[2] or in the seven CanMEDS roles.[3]
Dreyfus stages	The five stages of learning for skill acquisition proposed by Dreyfus and Dreyfus: novice–advanced beginner–competent–proficient–expert,[4] sometimes extended with 'master'.
Elective EPAs	EPAs that, in addition to core EPAs that hold for all graduates, trainees may elect to supplement their personal EPA portfolio, and provide them with a specific profile at graduation.
Entrustment decisions	In an educational context, entrustment decisions are decisions to trust a trainee with an essential professional task or responsibility at a specified level of supervision.
Entrustment-based discussion (EBD)	The EBD is a 10- to 20-minute conversation between a supervisor and trainee, focused on risk assessment when anticipating an entrustment decision. It is completed either directly after an EPA has been performed or before an upcoming activity. The conversation checks the trainee's full understanding of the activity with its associated risks and assesses the trainee's readiness to act in unfamiliar situations with 'what would you do if...' questions.[5]
Entrustment determinations	When an actual entrustment *decision* with a clinical task cannot be made (e.g., for legal reasons), entrustment 'determination' is sometimes used as an alternate term. It is the difference between saying 'we *will* trust' and 'we *would* trust' ('...if we could').[6] Entrustment determinations instead of entrustment decisions render the use of EPAs less powerful.
EPA (entrustable professional activity)	A unit of professional practice or essential task of a discipline (profession, specialty, or subspecialty) that a trainee can be trusted to perform without direct supervision, once sufficient competence and readiness has been demonstrated. As EPAs reflect *professional* practice, EPAs are not created for education but education is created for EPAs.
Entrustable	The property of an activity that makes it suitable for entrustment to someone. Note that entrustable does not pertain to persons.[7]

(*Continued*)

Table 25.1: Continued.

Entrustment–supervision scale	Levels of supervision reflect increasing degrees of responsibility and entrustment and decreasing supervision. The original proposed levels range from 1 to 5, but several variations have been proposed, often with more granular levels in between. These levels constitute a scale that has been named an entrustment–supervision or ES scale.[8] See also: Supervision level.
Grounded trust	Grounded trust is trust based on essential and usually prolonged experience with the trainee and grounded in sufficient observations, leading to judgments that are shared among experts (the educational team or a clinical competency committee).[9]
Initial trust	Initial trust is trust based on first impressions, sometimes called swift trust or thin trust.[9]
Logic of EPAs	The categorization of EPAs used in a framework. Different logics have been used such as procedural EPAs, as well as those EPAs associated with disease entities, services, functions or a combination of these.[10]
Micro-assessment	Brief assessment of performance of an EPA, a nested EPA, or part of an EPA, proposed in surgery and happening in pre-, intra- or postoperative phases, lasting 45–90 seconds.[11]
Nested EPA	Small unit of professional practice meeting the EPA definition that is also part of a larger EPA to be entrusted later in training.[12]
Presumptive trust	Trust based solely on credentials, without prior interaction with the trainee. Prior credentials can be diplomas, the fame of the university where a degree was obtained, recommendations, etc.[9]
Prospective and retrospective assessment approaches	Most workplace-based assessments are retrospective: a report of what was observed ('the student did well'). A prospective approach to assessment looks toward the future ('this student is now [or not yet] ready for indirect supervision').[13]
Readiness for entrustment	Readiness is an alternative (and preferred) term for 'trustworthiness' to qualify a learner who passes the threshold of competence and suitability to execute an EPA.
A RICH ingredients for entrustment decisions	Agency, reliability, integrity, capability, and humility are five literature-based trainee features, or categories of features, that enable 'a rich' entrustment decision.[14]
Shaded independence	The status of a resident who is fully trusted with the core and breadth of the profession and allowed to act unsupervised while still in training.[15]
STAR	A STAR is a statement of awarded responsibility, resulting from a summative entrustment decision, usually to qualify for unsupervised practice of a specific EPA.[16]
Summative entrustment decision	Entrustment decision, grounded in sufficient observations and evaluations, and made by an educational program director or clinical competency committee, leading to certification (STAR) and privileging of the trainee to act with a specified level of supervision, for a specific EPA.
Supervision (in HPE)	The provision of guidance and support in learning and working effectively in health care by observing and directing the execution of tasks or activities to ensure that they are done correctly and safely, from a position of being in charge.[17]
Supervision level (1–5)	Amount of executive responsibility a clinical teacher has or assumes for a trainee's clinical activities, often expressed in levels of trainee responsibility. In the original five-level scale, the trainees may (1) observe only, (2) act under direct supervision, (3) act under indirect supervision, (4) act unsupervised, or (5) act as a supervisor for junior learners.[12]

(*Continued*)

Table 25.1: Continued.

	Note that, as long as the individual is still in training, level 4, the most critical level, still includes a formal 'distant supervision' (also called 'clinical oversight') until specialty certification has been granted. This also implies that a STAR for level 4 can, in rare cases, still be retracted.
Threshold of competence for an EPA	The stage in the development of a trainee that allows for the initial summative entrustment with the unsupervised practice of an EPA.
Transdisciplinary EPA	One EPA that would be applicable in different disciplines or specialties. The EPA may be elaborated, established, and identified for a specific professional domain, profession, or discipline that is being used in one or more other disciplines or professions. Alternatively, it may be a newly identified broad activity, applicable across several related specialties.[18]
Workplace-based assessment sources of information to support entrustment	
1. Direct observation	Focused observation of a trainee during a natural patient care activity in an authentic clinical setting, usually 10–20 minutes, followed by a few minutes of focused feedback.
2. Conversation	A 5- to 20-minute one-on-one discussion with a trainee to probe knowledge, understanding, reasoning, and/or decision making.
3. Longitudinal observation	The natural, unplanned observation of a trainee over time by collaborators and others (including patients) who have natural encounters with the trainee.
4. Product evaluation	Assessment of trainees through their output, that is artifacts resulting from patient care that does not require their direct presence during the assessment (for example, a discharge summary in the electronic health record, or a crown placed in dental training).

Online resources to support faculty development on EPA frameworks and workplace-based assessments

The internet hosts a wealth of video clips with explanations and instructions about EPAs and workplace-based assessment, from universities to conference reports and commercial sources. The overview below lists recommended resources that can be used for faculty development. They have been collected by the organizers of the international online course Ins and Outs of Entrustable Professional Activities in the period 2020–23 and supplement resources provided in Chapter 23.

Table 25.2: Online resources to support faculty development on EPA frameworks and WBA.

Source	EPAs explained	mins.	
Dutch Federation of Medical Specialists	EPA-based approach to individualizing the postgraduate training duration.	3'01	Link
Royal College of Physicians and Surgeons (Canada)	Explains the concept of entrustment and EPAs and how they are used in residency training.	5'11	Link
Internship program in Ireland	Provides an overview of the new framework, the rationale for change and what it means for interns and supervisors.	3'30	Link
CZO-Flex level for Postgraduate Nursing in the Netherlands	A Dutch national EPA project for workplace-based assessment, explaining supervision levels and flexible career opportunities for nurses and medical assistants.	2'09	Link

(*Continued*)

Table 25.2: Continued.

Source	EPAs explained	mins.	
Royal Australasian College of Physicians	Provides an overview of EPAs and how they are used in Australia.	7'35	Link
Association of Directors of Psychiatry Residency Training, USA	Five videos that explain the historical context for EPAs, rationale and process of change to CBME, defining EPAs, and connecting EPAs, competencies and milestones.	7'02	Link
Australian Pharmacy Council	Explains EPAs and how they support intern training in pharmacy.	8'47	Link
Medical Education Flamingo, Spain	Explains EPAs with examples and explains CanMEDS and ACGME competency frameworks.	5'24	Link
Queens University	Explains the EQual Rubric tool for evaluation of the quality of EPAs.	17'40	Link
Swiss hospitals	Three videos explaining EPAs and assessment (Chur, Laufenberg, Locarno).	8'24 8'48 7'57	Link
Source	**EPAs in specific contexts**	**mins.**	
Irish internship program	Describes each of the seven EPAs for the internship.	3'30	Link
HPC Pharmacy Group	Describes the concept of EPAs in hospital palliative care pharmacy education.	4'07	Link
University of Toronto PGME	EPAs in internal medicine.	3'28	Link
University of Toronto PGME	EPAs in anatomical pathology medicine.	4'09	Link
University of Toronto PGME	EPAs in general internal medicine.	4'07	Link
University of Toronto PGME	EPAs in psychiatry.	3'59	Link
University of Toronto PGME	EPAs in anaesthesia.	3'47	Link
University of Toronto PGME	EPAs in emergency medicine.	4'59	Link
Source	**Workplace-based assessment in an EPA framework**	**mins.**	
American Board of Pediatrics	Explains decision making in E/CCCs.	3'18	Link
Swiss Society of Nephrology	Explains EPA-based assessment with the prEPAred mobile app.	14'57	Link
Dutch PGME Federation	Explains entrustment decision making in teams.	3'35	Link
CZO Flex Level project in the Netherlands	Explains workplace-based assessment and entrustment decision-making using supervision levels for postgraduate nursing education.	3'03	Link
Dutch PGME training	Explains summative entrustment decisions from the trainee perspective.	2'54	Link
Dutch PGME training	Explains summative entrustment decision-making in pediatric training.	9'05	Link
Switzerland	Explains how to use the prepared mobile app.	4'14	Link
Irish internship program	Explains how to conduct a direct observation, have the feedback conversation and record the outcome.	2'40	Link
Irish internship program	Demonstrates how to conduct a direct observation of a procedure and give feedback using supervision levels.	6'12	Link
Irish internship program	Demonstrates how to conduct a direct observation of a clinical task and give feedback using supervision levels.	6'11	Link

(Continued)

Table 25.2: Continued.

Source	Workplace-based assessment in an EPA framework	mins.	
Irish internship program	Explains how to conduct a case-based discussion, have the feedback conversation, and record the outcome.	2'38	Link
Irish internship program	Demonstrates how to conduct a case-based discussion effectively, have feedback conversation, and record the outcome.	8'01	Link
Irish internship program	This animation explains how to conduct a case presentation, have the feedback conversation, and record the outcome.	2'40	Link
Irish internship program	This video demonstrates how to conduct a case presentation and give feedback using supervision levels.	6'02	Link
Radboud University Nijmegen	Example of EPAs in Dentistry in the Netherlands.	3'07	Link
American Association of Veterinary Medical Colleges	This website includes multiple CBVE Educational Videos and other resources (including about EPAs).	–	Link

Table 25.3: Links to 2024 clips used in the international online course In and Outs of EPAs.

YouTube Links	mins
1 Introduction to CBME and EPAs	15
2 Supervision and entrustment	14
3 Advanced topics in EPAs part I	16
4 Advanced topics in EPAs part II	15
5 Eight components of a full EPA description	19
6 Arriving at a defensible framework of EPAs for a program	15
7 UME curriculum development	11
8 PGME curriculum development	13
9 Factors affecting entrustment decisions	13
10 Workplace based assessment with EPAs	14
11 Entrustment based discussion	11
12 ePortfolios and mobile apps for EPAs	15
13 Summative entrustment decision making in teams	17
14 Faculty development for EPA-based education part I	15
15 Faculty development for EPA-based education part II	15
In addition: Instruction for use of the EQual tool	18

Bibliography of most of the literature about EPAs and related concepts

This overview aims to be comprehensive but does not imply recommendation of the articles or endorsement of their content. It is merely a categorization of publications, based on a PubMed search of articles including 'entrustable' or 'entrustment decision' in its title or abstract. There are limitations. A more elaborate systematic search may reveal more journal publications. The vast gray literature is not included. The publication titles may be copied and pasted into a search engine, such as Google Scholar, to find the abstracts or full texts. The bibliography can be downloaded here and has the current, following categories of literature. Note, the manual categorization of articles may have resulted in duplications across categories.

- General and introductory texts
- Literature reviews
- Identifying, defining, and validating EPAs
- EPAs for medical school and internship
- Assessment, entrustment decisions, and feedback
- Entrustment–supervision scales and their validity
- Clinical competency committees
- EPAs versus competencies and milestones
- EPAs, technology, portfolios, apps, and AI
- Supervision and autonomy
- General and theoretical aspects of entrustment
- Time variability
- Transitions to clerkship, residency, practice, continuous professional development
- Curriculum development; EPA implementation
- CBME and EPA language
- Learner perspectives
- Controversies and discussion
- Faculty development
- EPAs and interprofessional education
- EPAs for medical disciplines (categorized by specialty)
- EPAs for other health professions (categorized by profession)
- Specific EPAs elaborated
- EPAs for non-health care disciplines

Tools and instructions for faculty development workshop exercises

This section provides tools for faculty development activities to support the development and implementation of EPAs. While the activities resemble the types of activities conducted in the international online course Ins and Outs of Entrustable Professional Activities, their use requires experienced facilitation and dedicated participants groups. For those who have attended the course, these materials are now provided to allow attendees to conduct local faculty development efforts under the creative commons conditions of CC BY-NC-SA (used with credit to creator, used for noncommercial purposes only and with adaptations allowed but under the same conditions).

To understand the use of these workshop materials, a brief outline of the international course is useful. It contains eight modules, grouped into four sessions: (a) general concepts, (b) curriculum development, (c) assessment and entrustment decisions, and (d) faculty development and faculty support through peer consultation.

Readiness assurance test questions

A series of multiple-choice best-answer questions about EPAs and related concepts is provided. They have been used in the international course many times and always evoke group discussions to elaborate the preferred best answers, often with the exchange of arguments about distractors of the of the multiple choice questions. Note that the purpose of these (voluntary) questions is primarily to evoke such discussions among workshop participants, rather than to evaluate or assess individual participants. Readiness assurance questions are to be completed before workshop attendance.

The items can be downloaded as Appendix with Chapter 25 which contain readiness assurance questions for general concepts (16), curriculum development (10) and assessment/entrustment (10).

Workshop exercise 'EPAs 101'

This 30-minute exercise, in small groups (of four to six), asks participants to provide, one by one, a definition or explanation of a concept from the list below; other participants may then supplement the offered definition or explanation. As a reference, the glossary in this chapter may be used to back up and extend this exercise.

1. Can you provide a one-sentence definition of 'EPA'?
2. What is the purpose of CBME and why may EPAs add to that purpose?
3. Can you list at least five features of an EPA?
4. What is the difference between competencies and EPAs?
5. How do ad hoc and summative entrustment decisions differ?
6. Which are commonly used levels of supervision?
7. What is a STAR?
8. Why may entrustment extend the 'does' level of Miller's pyramid?

Workshop exercise 'The faculty meeting discussion'

This 30-minute exercise, in small groups (of four to six), splits each small group into two cohorts (cohort A: two to three play critical faculty members; cohort B: two to three play EPA implementation committee members). Three examples of critical faculty questions require a response from the committee.

- 'Competency-based education is a fad. The clinician cannot be reduced to competencies and subcompetencies. Assessing knowledge and skills is difficult enough and I fear that moving to competencies and EPAs will create graduates with an even smaller knowledge base'
- 'You have defined competency-based education without a fixed duration. How will we ever accommodate that?'
- 'Our specialty has made a list of diseases trainees should learn about. Can't we just relabel them as EPAs?'

The workshop time may be split into two units of 15 minutes each. After 15 minutes, the cohorts switch roles.

Workshop exercise: 'Create an EPA framework with a nominal group technique'

A domain for EPA development that is intuitive for most participants, independent of specialty and profession, is 'parenting,' that is, the everyday task of raising a baby. This 20-minute workshop exercise, in small groups (of four to six), uses an adapted nominal group technique (NGT). NGT has four phases:

1. Everyone lists, in silence, as many relevant items (tasks) as possible for parenting, in about five minutes
2. Going around the table (or screen) one by one, each participant adds a single item to the group list, without interference from other participants, until the round-robin procedure yields no more items to add

3. Participants work together to clean and clarify the list by lumping and splitting items on the list
4. Participants prioritize items on the list by voting

Workshop exercise: 'Elaborate an EPA'

This is a 20-minute exercise for small groups (of four to six). The group identifies one EPA title and then elaborates the EPA using a template that is derived from AMEE Guide 140.[a] The template can be downloaded as Appendix with Chapter 25.

The exercise can be combined with the workshop exercise 'Create an EPA framework with a nominal group technique,' in which case, after the NGT procedure, one of the high-priority suggested EPAs is selected to be elaborated. The combined exercise is described in a worksheet that can be downloaded as Appendix with Chapter 25.

Workshop exercise 'Curriculum development with EPAs'

Curriculum development with EPAs is an important topic for faculty development and curricula are usually developed over a long period of time, ranging from months to years. A brief workshop can therefore only scratch the surface of what it means to develop an educational program.

This 45-minute exercise focuses on a discussion in a small group (of four to six) about education (teaching and assessment) that should prepare trainees for readiness to execute an EPA with indirect or no supervision. The exercise uses five sample EPAs, all available in elaborated format:

- Obtaining informed consent
- Oral and written reporting to document a clinical encounter
- Patient handover
- Virtual patient consultation
- Health promotion and preventive care

The exercise provides a worksheet with a blank table organized into three columns (preclinical education, clinical education, postgraduate education) and four rows: targeted level of supervision for each stage, content, education methods, and assessment methods. The 12 cells can be filled with curricular suggestions for one EPA; each parallel small group may cover a different EPA from the list of five. A worksheet, including the elaborated EPAs, can be downloaded as Appendix with Chapter 25.

Workshop exercise 'Entrustment-based discussion'

The EBD is a 10- to 20-minute conversation with a focus on risk assessment when anticipating an entrustment decision, either directly after an EPA has been performed or before an upcoming activity. The conversation checks the trainee's full understanding of the activity with its associated risks and assesses the trainee's readiness to act in unfamiliar situations with 'what would you do if…' questions.

The exercise was created for a broad audience and therefore uses everyday examples of entrustment in the private setting (i.e., asking a neighbor's child to babysit for your child and asking a

[a] ten Cate O, Taylor D. The recommended description of an entrustable professional activity, AMEE guide 140. *Med Teach*. 2021;43(10):1106–1114.

neighbor's teenager with a restricted driver's license to pick up your mother from the airport). The exercise can be downloaded as Appendix with Chapter 25.

Workshop exercise 'Clinical competency committee meeting'

Clinical competency committees are charged with evaluating trainees to make summative decisions about readiness and permission to execute EPAs with only distant supervision. In this 20-minute small group exercise, committee members (five or six) are played by participants. The five or six roles (less than half a page each) are distributed in advance and each role is only read by the participant assuming the role. All participants review the same summary of one trainee's portfolio. This resident opts for a 'level 4' summative entrustment decision with a STAR to start practicing unsupervised. The committee members review the portfolio and their own experiences and must come to a decision, in a 15-minute discussion led by one participant whose role is that of committee chair. The exercise can be downloaded as Appendix with Chapter 25 and includes a general worksheet as well as six dedicated roles.

Workshop exercise 'Faculty development for specific target groups'

This 30-minute exercise is meant to elaborate the different needs, goals, practices, and required resources for faculty development, training, and instruction for various stakeholder groups (leaders, frontline clinical teachers, trainees, clinical competency committee members, champions). Divided into small groups (of four to six), each group handles one target group, and, if there is enough time, a second one. The exercise can be downloaded as Appendix with Chapter 25.

Workshop exercise 'Troika peer consultation'[b]

This 45-minute exercise requires every participant to have prepared a personal pressing question for consultation. The question should be related to EPAs, entrustment decision making, or competency-based education. The whole group is divided into small groups of three and enacts the consultation in three rounds. In every round, one participant is the 'client,' poses a pressing question, and receives peer consultation in a structured format. The exercise instructions can be downloaded as Appendix with Chapter 25.

The EQual Rubric tool to evaluate the fit-for-purpose validity of entrustable professional activities

This EQual rubric tool,[c] created in Microsoft Excel, provides EPA development teams with a resource to evaluate the quality of the construction of individual EPAs. The application of the tool is described in detail in Chapter 11. This downloadable resource includes 14 quality questions about the EPA, each scored on a five-point scale, with anchor values explained. It calculates the overall score and scores for each section of the rubric, and highlights when comments were provided by those using the tool. The tool can also be adapted for use with survey software,

---

[b] This exercise was derived from the Liberating Structures website https://www.liberatingstructures.com/8-troika-consulting/.

[c] Taylor DR, Park YS, Egan R, et al. EQual, a novel rubric to evaluate entrustable professional activities for quality and structure. *Acad Med*. 2017 Nov;92:11:S110–117.

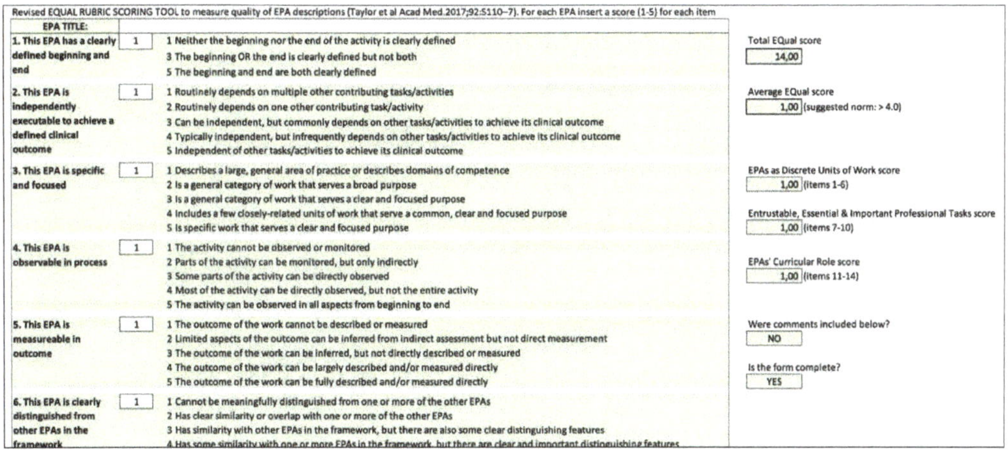

Revised EQUAL RUBRIC SCORING TOOL to measure quality of EPA descriptions (Taylor et al Acad Med.2017;92:S110–7). For each EPA insert a score (1-5) for each item

EPA TITLE:

1. This EPA has a clearly defined beginning and end — 1
1 Neither the beginning nor the end of the activity is clearly defined
3 The beginning OR the end is clearly defined but not both
5 The beginning and end are both clearly defined

2. This EPA is independently executable to achieve a defined clinical outcome — 1
1 Routinely depends on multiple other contributing tasks/activities
2 Routinely depends on one other contributing task/activity
3 Can be independent, but commonly depends on other tasks/activities to achieve its clinical outcome
4 Typically independent, but infrequently depends on other tasks/activities to achieve its clinical outcome
5 Independent of other tasks/activities to achieve its clinical outcome

3. This EPA is specific and focused — 1
1 Describes a large, general area of practice or describes domains of competence
2 Is a general category of work that serves a broad purpose
3 Is a general category of work that serves a clear and focused purpose
4 Includes a few closely-related units of work that serve a common, clear and focused purpose
5 Is specific work that serves a clear and focused purpose

4. This EPA is observable in process — 1
1 The activity cannot be observed or monitored
2 Parts of the activity can be monitored, but only indirectly
3 Some parts of the activity can be directly observed
4 Most of the activity can be directly observed, but not the entire activity
5 The activity can be observed in all aspects from beginning to end

5. This EPA is measureable in outcome — 1
1 The outcome of the work cannot be described or measured
2 Limited aspects of the outcome can be inferred from indirect assessment but not direct measurement
3 The outcome of the work can be inferred, but not directly described or measured
4 The outcome of the work can be largely described and/or measured directly
5 The outcome of the work can be fully described and/or measured directly

6. This EPA is clearly distinguished from other EPAs in the framework — 1
1 Cannot be meaningfully distinguished from one or more of the other EPAs
2 Has clear similarity or overlap with one or more of the other EPAs
3 Has similarity with other EPAs in the framework, but there are also some clear distinguishing features
4 Has some similarity with one or more EPAs in the framework, but there are clear and important distinguishing features

Total EQual score: 14,00
Average EQual score: 1,00 (suggested norm: > 4.0)
EPAs as Discrete Units of Work score: 1,00 (items 1-6)
Entrustable, Essential & Important Professional Tasks score: 1,00 (items 7-10)
EPAs' Curricular Role score: 1,00 (items 11-14)
Were comments included below? NO
Is the form complete? YES

Figure 25.1: EQual Rubric Excel tool—fragment.

which may provide additional options for data analysis. The tool can be opened with the password 'EQual.' Figure 25.1 shows a fragment of the tool. Click here to download the tool.

References

1. Englander R, Flynn T, Call S, et al. Toward defining the foundation of the MD degree: core entrustable professional activities for entering residency. *Acad Med.* 2016;91(10):1352–1358. DOI: https://doi.org/10.1097/ACM.0000000000001204
2. Englander R, Cameron T, Ballard AJ, Dodge J, Bull J, Aschenbrener CA. Toward a common taxonomy of competency domains for the health professions and competencies for physicians. *Acad Med.* 2013;88(8):1088–1094. DOI: https://doi.org/10.1097/ACM.0b013e31829a3b2b
3. Sherbino J, Frank JR, Flynn L, Snell L. 'Intrinsic roles' rather than 'armour': renaming the 'non-medical expert roles' of the CanMEDS framework to match their intent. *Adv Health Sci Educ Theory Pract.* 2011;16(5):695–697. DOI: https://doi.org/10.1007/s10459-011-9318-z
4. Dreyfus SE. The five-stage model of adult skill acquisition. *Bull Sci Technol Soc.* 2004;24(3): 177–181. DOI: https://doi.org/10.1177/0270467604264992
5. ten Cate O, Hoff RG. From case-based to entrustment-based discussions. *Clin Teach.* 2017;14(6):385–389. DOI: https://doi.org/10.1111/tct.12710
6. ten Cate O, Jarrett JB. Would I trust or will I trust? The gap between entrustment determinations and entrustment decisions for trainees in pharmacy and other health professions. *Pharmacy (Basel).* 2023;11(3). DOI: https://doi.org/10.3390/pharmacy11030107
7. ten Cate O. When I say … entrustability. *Med Educ.* 2020;54(2):103–104. DOI: https://doi.org/10.1111/medu.14005
8. ten Cate O, Schwartz A, Chen HC. Assessing trainees and making entrustment decisions: on the nature and use of entrustment-supervision scales. *Acad Med.* 2020;95(11):1662–1669. DOI: https://doi.org/10.1097/ACM.0000000000003427
9. ten Cate O, Hart D, Ankel F, et al. Entrustment decision making in clinical training. *Acad Med.* 2016;91(2):191–198. DOI: https://doi.org/10.1097/ACM.0000000000001044
10. Hennus MP, van Dam M, Gauthier S, Taylor DR, ten Cate O. The logic behind entrustable professional activity frameworks: a scoping review of the literature. *Med Educ.* 2022;56(9): 881–891. DOI: https://doi.org/10.1111/medu.14806

11. Montgomery KB, Mellinger JD, McLeod MC, et al. Decision-making confidence of clinical competency committees for entrustable professional activities. *JAMA Surg.* May 8, 2024. DOI: https://doi.org/10.1001/jamasurg.2024.0809
12. ten Cate O, Chen HC, Hoff RG, Peters H, Bok H, van der Schaaf M. Curriculum development for the workplace using entrustable professional activities (EPAs): AMEE guide no. 99. *Med Teach.* 2015;37(11):983–1002. DOI: https://doi.org/10.3109/0142159X.2015.1060308
13. Schumacher DJ, Michelson C, Winn AS, Turner DA, Martini A, Kinnear B. A realist synthesis of prospective entrustment decision making by entrustment or clinical competency committees. *Med Educ.* December 13, 2023. DOI: https://doi.org/10.1111/medu.15296
14. ten Cate O, Chen HC. The ingredients of a rich entrustment decision. *Med Teach.* 2020;42(12):1413–1420. DOI: https://doi.org/10.1080/0142159X.2020.1817348
15. Goldhamer MEJ, Pusic MV, Nadel ES, Co JPT, Weinstein DF. Promotion in place: a model for competency-based, time-variable graduate medical education. *Acad Med.* 2024;99(5): 518–523. DOI: https://doi.org/10.1097/ACM.0000000000005652
16. ten Cate O, Scheele F. Competency-based postgraduate training: can we bridge the gap between theory and clinical practice? *Acad Med.* 2007;82(6):542–547. DOI: https://doi.org/10.1097/ACM.0b013e31805559c7
17. ten Cate O. Supervision and entrustment in clinical training: protecting patients, protecting trainees. WebM&M Case Studies. https://psnet.ahrq.gov/webmm/case/461. November 9, 2018:1.
18. Pool I, Hofstra S, van der Horst M, ten Cate O. Transdisciplinary entrustable professional activities. *Med Teach.* 2023;45(9):1019–1024. DOI: https://doi.org/10.1080/0142159X.2023.2170778

Index

Page numbers in *italic* or **bold** refer to a figure or table respectively. Page numbers in ***bold italic*** refer to boxed material (case studies and examples).

The abbreviation EPA is used in places for 'entrustable professional activities'.

F

G

H

I

J

K

L

M

N

O

P

Q

R

S

www.ingramcontent.com/pod-product-compliance
Lightning Source LLC
LaVergne TN
LVHW070907210926
848482LV00017B/1014
* 9 7 8 1 9 1 4 4 8 1 6 0 4 *